AF615708

VOCATIONAL REHABILITATION for Persons with Traumatic Brain Injury

Edited by

Paul Wehman, PhD
Professor of Rehabilitation Medicine
and Special Education

Jeffrey S. Kreutzer, PhD
Associate Professor
Departments of Rehabilitation Medicine
and Neurological Surgery

Medical College of Virginia
Richmond, Virginia

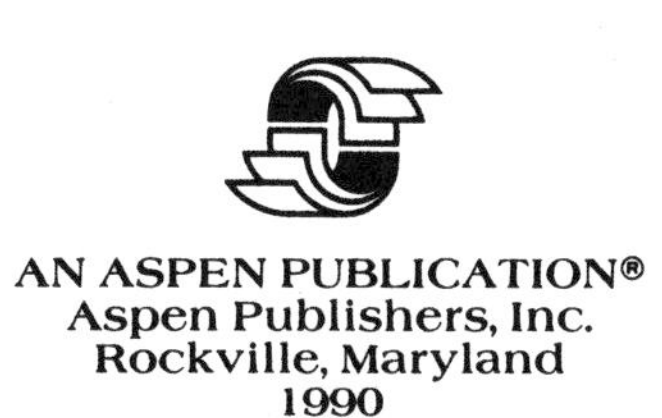

AN ASPEN PUBLICATION®
Aspen Publishers, Inc.
Rockville, Maryland
1990

Library of Congress Cataloging-in-Publication Data

Vocational rehabilitation for persons with traumatic brain injury / edited by
Paul Wehman, Jeffrey S. Kreutzer.
p. cm.
"An Aspen Publication."
Includes bibliographical references.
ISBN: 0-8342-0135-6
1. Brain damage—Patients—Rehabilitation. 2. Occupational Therapy.
I. Wehman, Paul. II. Kreutzer, Jeffrey S., 1953-
[DNLM: 1. Brain Injuries—Rehabilitation. 2. Rehabilitation, Vocational.
WL 354 V872]
RC387.5.V63 1990
362.4—dc20
DNLM/DLC
for Library of Congress
89-18529
CIP

Editorial Services: Ruth Bloom

Library of Congress Catalog Card Number: 89-18529
ISBN: 0-8342-0135-6

Printed in the United States of America

1 2 3 4 5

Table of Contents

Contributors

Patricia L. Bennett, MEd
Assistant Director
Maryland Rehabilitation Center
Baltimore, Maryland

Al Condeluci, PhD
Program Director
United Cerebral Palsy Association of Pittsburgh
Pittsburgh, Pennsylvania

Joel F. Diambra, MEd
Behavioral Intervention Program Coordinator
Virginia Commonwealth University
Richmond, Virginia

Leonard Diller, PhD
Professor, Clinical Rehabilitation Medicine
Research and Training Center on Head Trauma and Stroke
New York City Medical Center
New York, New York

David A. Ellerd, MS
Director, Re-Entry Vocational Services
California Association of Rehabilitation Professionals
Torrance, California

Evelyn F. Esposito
Virginia Head Injury Foundation
Richmond, Virginia

Frederick W. Esposito
President
First Financial Services of Virginia
Richmond, Virginia

Robyn Linn Fry
Employment Specialist
Department of Rehabilitation Medicine
Medical College of Virginia
Richmond, Virginia

Patricia Goodall, EdS
Training Associate and Training Consultant
Rehabilitation Research and Training Center
Virginia Commonwealth University
Richmond, Virginia

Christine H. Groah, MEd
Intake Coordinator
Department of Rehabilitation Medicine
Medical College of Virginia
Richmond, Virginia

Elizabeth V. Horn, MIA
Executive Director
Virginia Head Injury Foundation
Richmond, Virginia

Trudie Hughes, MEd
TBI Lead Employment Specialist
Rehabilitation Research and Training Center
Richmond, Virginia

Susan G. Killam, MEd
Lead Employment Specialist
Rehabilitation Research and Training Center
Richmond, Virginia

Jeffrey S. Kreutzer, PhD
Associate Professor
Departments of Rehabilitation Medicine and Neurological Surgery
Medical College of Virginia
Richmond, Virginia

Bruce E. Leininger, MS
Predoctoral Fellow in Clinical Neuropsychology
Department of Rehabilitation Medicine
Medical College of Virginia
Richmond, Virginia

Kali Mallik, MS, MTech
President
Baltimore County Economic Development and Rehabilitation Alliance, Inc.
Baltimore, Maryland

Pamela D. Sherron, MEd
Program Manager for Supported Employment
Department of Rehabilitation Medicine
Medical College of Virginia
Richmond, Virginia

Mary C. Stapleton, MA
Staff Psychologist, Project Coordinator
Maryland Rehabilitation Center
Maryland State Department of Education
Pathways Project
Baltimore, Maryland

Linda C. Veldheer, MEd, DPA
Director of Developmental Disabilities
Virginia Department of Mental Health, Mental Retardation and Substance Abuse Services
Developmental Disabilities Office
Richmond, Virginia

R. Timm Vogelsberg, PhD
Associate Professor, Department of Psychological Studies in Education, College of Education
Temple University
Philadelphia, Pennsylvania

Paul Wehman, PhD
Professor of Rehabilitation Medicine and Special Education
Medical College of Virginia
Richmond, Virginia

Michael West, MEd
Research Analyst
Rehabilitation Research and Training Center
Virginia Commonwealth University
Richmond, Virginia

William W. Woolcock, PhD
Assistant Professor
Department of Teacher Education
University of Arkansas at Little Rock
Little Rock, Arkansas

Nathan D. Zasler, MD
Assistant Professor and Director, Brain Injury Rehabilitation Services
Department of Rehabilitation Medicine
Medical College of Virginia
Richmond, Virginia

Foreword

There are now more than 700 hundred programs in the United States which offer services to individuals who have suffered the effects of traumatic brain injury. Ten years ago there were less than 70, and 20 years ago there were only a handful of such programs. During this period the professionals in the field of rehabilitation and the public-at-large have become aware of a major public health problem brought about in part by the presence of high speed roads and the automobile. It has been estimated that the rehabilitation of individuals with traumatic brain injury is now a $1 billion-a-year industry. Aside from the increased public need, it used to be thought that (a) individuals with traumatic brain injury could not be helped very much by rehabilitation and that return to the community was mostly a matter of spontaneous recovery or (b) individuals with traumatic brain injury were no different from any other group of individuals and that no special considerations were needed with regard to their rehabilitation. Since it was also thought that traumatic brain injury was an event that generally occurred in war time and America was at peace, no serious attention had to be paid to this population. However, the awareness of the growing incidence of the problem along with advances in management of the problem led to a paradigm shift.

Thomas Kuhn[1] used the term "paradigm shift" to describe periods in the history of a scientific field when a radical shift, a revolution with major changes in ideas and methods, takes place. *Vocational Rehabilitation for Persons with Traumatic Brain Injury* expresses a paradigm shift in clinical thinking about traumatic brain injury and rehabilitation. It captures the notion that individuals with severe traumatic brain injury can be returned to successful employment. This notion was not considered in a serious way 20 years ago and until the present was still widely questioned in scholarly studies. This book makes the case for successful vocational rehabilitation outcomes by combining a careful search of existing knowledge in several allied fields, identifying the most salient factors to be considered, organizing the information in a cogent way and providing case materials and guidelines for patterns of actions. These guidelines are specific enough to be helpful but not overly detailed in a cookbook fashion to lull the reader into a false mechanical approach to a complex problem.

The approach brings together insights generated by two different lines of research and clinical practice that have emerged in recent years. One approach is based on the idea that the presence of traumatic brain damage, which causes changes in behavior and personality, does not necessarily mean that nothing can be done to help the individual improve his abilities attitudes. It moves the field of neuropsychology away from a focus on diagnostic issues around brain behavior relationships to a closer examination of how the person actually performs and what can be done to alter that performance—a rehabilitation issue. The second thrust is to move the field of vocational rehabilitation beyond its former level of development. Vocational rehabilitation for individuals with disabilities had moved from aptitude testing to job sampling techniques of assessment after World War II. Simulating an actual work situation to sample behaviors was better than using tests that on the surface had little resemblance to what individuals were required to do on the job. "Supportive employment," a method that departs even further from the psychometric tradition of comparing an individual's performance with that of a normative group, is concerned with establishing a person/job fit by providing as much assistance as possible in the work situation to both the client and the employer, and then removing the support as needed. If the aim of rehabilitation is to reduce the burden of disability or handicap, supportive employment follows this aim. It provides the levels of assistance needed to ultimately reduce the burden of dependency—for the person, for the family, for the employer, and for the tax payer. Just as levels of assistance is the guiding idea behind facilitating independence in activities of daily living for the person undergoing retraining in motoric impairments, supportive employment provides assistance in a vocational setting. This opens up a new way of thinking about the techniques and the possibilities for a population group in great need.

Vocational Rehabilitation for Persons with Traumatic Brain Injury goes even further. It points out that successful rehabilitation may often require work with the community and the integration of a variety of support services, e.g., transportation and housing which may be needed to maintain the individual in the community.

At a time in our national life when there may be increasing concern that social programs do not work, the developments in this field are very exciting and are captured very well in this stimulating volume.

Leonard Diller, PhD
Chief, Behavioral Science
Rusk Institute of Rehabilitation Medicine
Director, Research and Training Center—Head
Trauma and Stroke
Professor, Clinical Rehabilitation Medicine
New York University Medical Center
New York, New York

NOTE

1. Thomas Kuhn, "The Structures of Scientific Revolutions," *Foundations of the Unity of Science*, 2nd ed., vol. 2, no. 2 (Chicago: University of Chicago Press, 1970).

Preface

Fifteen years ago few persons would have thought that a vocational rehabilitation text about persons who experienced a severe head injury would be relevant. During this era very few people survived serious motor vehicle accidents. Yet in the past decade, striking medical advances have allowed this new field to develop.

The purpose of this book is to describe job placement techniques and vocational rehabilitation for persons who have survived traumatic brain injury. We have gathered a number of the leading workers in this field and prevailed upon them to write a chapter. What has resulted is a remarkably practical collection of clinical, personal, and research experiences in supported employment, job placement, and vocational service delivery. Work reentry programs are no longer unique; *excellent* work reentry programs are, however. In this book we present several examples of excellent work reentry programs.

We believe that the material presented will be extremely helpful to understanding how to provide vocational services to persons with traumatic brain injury. Four chapters specifically address supported employment implementation with a full cadre of case studies. These chapters provide program information on how to develop supported employment programs. Several other chapters cover information related to supportive aspects of vocational rehabilitation programs such as prognostic indices, critical medical information, work generalization, and community support services. In addition, two chapters address work from the perspectives of parents and of an advocate with the Virginia Head Injury Foundation.

This book is for rehabilitation counselors, rehabilitation nurses, occupational and physical therapists, vocational evaluators and employment specialists, special educators as well as university students who are in training. A number of case studies and sample program forms illustrate *how* to implement vocational programs, which would be of tremendous use to the direct service provider and counselor.

Paul Wehman
Jeffrey S. Kreutzer

Acknowledgments

We hope that this book will be read and used by professionals in the brain injury field and family members as well who wish to educate themselves. We believe this to be one of the first books that directly addresses vocational outcome, and we hope that it will help advance the vocational rehabilitation knowledge base for those who have traumatic brain injuries. We are extremely grateful to the survivors, families of the survivors, and direct service staff with whom we work daily. We also owe a debt of gratitude to J. Paul Thomas, PhD, and Richard Melia, PhD, the project officers from the National Institute on Disability and Rehabilitation Research. Funds from the National Institute have partially supported this work. The support these project officers have shown us in our work has been gratifying.

In addition to these individuals, we are most grateful to Guy Clifton, MD, Henry Stonnington, MD, Cheryl Burns, Jenny Harris, Bruce Leininger, Paul Sale, John Kregel, and David Banks. These colleagues have helped shape our thinking and research. Finally, a special thank you to Tricia Baker, Jan Smith, Brenda Robinson, and Jeanne Dalton, whose editorial work was invaluable.

Chapter 1

Return to Work: Critical Issues in Employment

Paul Wehman and Patricia Goodall

Within the past decade, a major emphasis has been placed on the rehabilitation and treatment of persons who have experienced traumatic brain injuries. The reason is that more people than ever are surviving moderate and severe traumatic injuries sustained in motor vehicle and other accidents as a result of advances in neurosurgery, emergency evacuation procedures, rehabilitation techniques, and psychopharmacology. Unfortunately, most of these people are sufficiently compromised to require specialized vocational services if they are to return to the workforce.

Consider the case of John. Recently discharged from the United States Navy and ready to enter graduate school for an advanced degree in engineering, John is hit at a crosswalk by a drunk driver. Suffering massive injuries to his head and chest, John is taken to the nearest hospital trauma center. Within days, he medically stabilizes but stays unconscious for several months. Slowly, John wakes up and over months begins to physically recover. Cognitively and emotionally, however, he has significant problems. He has memory difficulties, his planning and organizing skills are limited, and he becomes angry and frustrated for no apparent reason. What is his prognosis for reentering the workforce and developing a career?

Severely head injured persons have been shown to have poor return to work employment rates (Brooks, McKinlay, Symington, Beattie, & Campsie, 1987; McMordle, Barker, & Paolo, 1989; Oddy, Coughlan, Tyerman, & Jenkins, 1985). But research information is too limited at this point to discern the work reentry prognosis for all moderately and severely head injured clients. Much more needs to be learned in this realm.

The purpose of this book is to improve vocational outcome for persons with traumatic brain injuries by exploring different rehabilitation approaches. The chapters that follow express the best information currently available on providing meaningful job placement, intervention, and training at the workplace.

CURRENT MODELS AND APPROACHES

Several approaches are being used to facilitate vocational placement and work reentry for persons with traumatic head injury. Prigatano (1986) and Ben-Yishay and his colleagues (1987) have described a combination of cognitive training, day rehabilitation, and occupational trials, although neither program emphasizes behavior modification or intensive support activities at the job site. Their work has shown the way in helping professionals in the field.

Wesolowski et al. (1988) make these comments on the Ben-Yishay and Prigatano programs.

> Ben-Yishay (1985; 1987) reported that 84 percent of his clients were *rated* employable following occupational trials, and three years postdischarge 50 percent to 60 percent were reported to be successfully employed. Prigatano (1986) reported that 65 percent of the clients completing his program were employed at discharge, and 50 percent had maintained successful employment 12 months postdischarge. These two programs had rigid entrance criteria and only accepted clients who had no behavior problems and were able to live independently. (p. 319)

Wesolowski, Burke, and Guth (1988) themselves describe a model of intense behavior modification and structured programming in a controlled residential environment. In their study, conducted at the New Mexico Center in New Hampshire, outcome data were analyzed from 44 brain injured clients discharged from the center. Their mean length of coma was approximately 20 days. Results revealed that 1 year later, 50 percent of their clients maintained successful employment.

The strength of this approach lies in its comprehensive treatment of all aspects of an individual's life. The weakness lies in the client's discharge back to communities that cannot or will not provide this programming intensity and support. A similar approach was a highly structural, applied behavior analysis by Wesolowski et al. (1988).

Finally, Wehman, Kreutzer, Wood, Morton, et al. (1988) articulate a comprehensive individual placement model of supported employment; that is, a professionally trained employment specialist or job coach accompanies the head injured client to a job as long as special assistance is required. This model of supported employment has so far met with similar to slightly higher success rates than the other models. Approximately 70 percent of the clients placed have been retained (Wehman, Kreutzer, Stonnington, et al., 1988), although a number of others have required re-placement. There were no entrance criteria to the program other than (1) evidence of severe head injury, (2) willingness to work, and (3) willingness to seek treatment if alcohol or drug use was a problem. More than 90 percent of the clients did not live independently; the average coma length was 67 days and 92 percent resulted from motor vehicle accidents. Most postinjury jobs were in the $4 to $7 an hour range and all were in competitive employment. Almost all of these clients consistently required intervention throughout supported placement.

The following general conclusions can be drawn about post-traumatic brain injury vocational programs.

1. Several models are being tried and tested to evaluate work reentry success.
2. Few are prospective in nature; that is, few of them provide long-term follow-along after the 1- or 2-year postdischarge evaluation.
3. Different programs use varied patient entrance criteria, which makes comparing the programs difficult.
4. The programs show varying levels of employment outcome.

IMPLEMENTING COMMUNITY-BASED EMPLOYMENT PROGRAMS

It is well known that persons with traumatic brain injuries have a myriad of complex problems, some that are acute and others that are ongoing or chronic. The major problems experienced in placement and retention have been unrealistic vocational aspirations of clients, substance abuse problems, and psychiatric or interpersonal difficulties (Eames, 1988).

An effective work reentry program must consider these multidimensional problems throughout the job development and job placement process. Exhibit 1-1 indicates 21 critical employment compatibility issues that should be analyzed prior to or *concurrent with* placement. These issues are described below and are presented only as guidelines for program planning, not as hard and fast rules.

Preinjury Vocational Competence and Motivation

A person's preinjury vocational competence, specific work history, and interest in advancement are important for a complete evaluation by vocational staff and provide the clinical data necessary in steering appropriate job development. Three questions must be asked.

Exhibit 1-1 Traumatic Brain Injured Employment Compatibility Analysis

	Yes	No
I. Preinjury Vocational Competence and Motivation		
1. The client showed a stable work history for at least 12 months prior to injury.	___	___
2. The client showed an interest in work advancement.	___	___
3. The client has specific vocational skills.	___	___
II. Postinjury Vocational Competence and Motivation		
4. The client has shown a stable work history for at least 12 months since injury.	___	___
5. The client consistently indicates a desire and willingness to work.	___	___
6. The client has specific job/vocational preferences.	___	___
III. Physical and Medical Status		
7. The client has no physical problems other than the brain injury.	___	___
8. The client has been medically evaluated within the past 6 to 12 months.	___	___
9. The client takes medication as prescribed by a physician.	___	___
IV. Psychiatric or Maladaptive Behavior		
10. The client has no history of *persistent* psychiatric problems or maladaptive behavior.	___	___
11. The client has no history of *persistent* socially inappropriate behavior in a variety of settings.	___	___
12. The client has no history of *consistent* physical or verbally abusive behavior.	___	___
V. Substance Use/Abuse		
13. The client has no history of substance use or abuse that caused social problems.	___	___
14. The client currently abstains from alcohol.	___	___
15. The client currently abstains from the use of illicit drugs.	___	___
VI. Family or Marital Stability		
16. The client's family is supportive of his/her employment.	___	___
17. The client and/or the family has received counseling/support services for adjustment to consequences of the injury.	___	___
VII. Vocational Goals and Expectations		
18. The client consistently indicates the type of job and pay he/she likes and dislikes.	___	___
19. The client has realistic expectations of the type of work in which he/she can reasonably be expected to succeed at this time.	___	___
VIII. Job Match (see Consumer Screening Form, Exhibit 1-2)		
20. An appropriate job has been matched to the client's abilities and desires.	___	___
21. Transportation is available.	___	___

1. Did the client show a stable work history for at least 12 months prior to the injury?
2. Did the client show an interest in work advancement?
3. Did the client have specific vocational skills?

Accurate answers to these questions give the vocational staff information on the type of worker an individual was in the past, the quality of work habits, and the industry in which to focus job development efforts, at least initially.

A number of persons with traumatic brain injury who need services may *not* have had a good preinjury work record. This type of history can complicate further the job development and job placement process.

Postinjury Vocational Competence and Motivation

In a study (Wehman, Kreutzer, West, et al., 1989) it was noted that 42 traumatic brain injury survivors worked only 13 percent of the total months that they could have following their hospital release. This was contrasted with almost 75 percent of the total months worked when the same group of survivors was in the preinjury status.

The 12-month period after hospital release is a time when people with traumatic brain injuries are fraught with discouragement, frustration, anger, and indecision about work. However, it is during this critical time that the tone and direction of the client's work reentry program are set.

Prigatano (1988) has suggested that long-term postacute (more than 12 months postinjury) survivors might be more ready for placement after working out frustrations and unrealistic expectations. Others have suggested that immediate vocational intervention after hospital release is most beneficial (Stonnington, 1986). No clear data exist to help guide clinicians in this regard.

Some observations indicate that postinjury vocational competence may be more affected by the amount of motivation and competence a person has or can develop rather than by length of time since injury. Ellerd (personal communication, January, 1989) has indicated that many of the traumatic brain injury placements being made in a Sacramento program require two, three, and even four jobs before stability is established. This is discussed further in Chapter 6. Wehman, Kreutzer, West, et al., (1989) also supports the need for re-placements.

In evaluating progress, vocational staff must ask the following questions:

1. Has the client shown any stable work history (12 months or more) since injury?

2. Does the client consistently indicate a desire and willingness to work?
3. Does the client consistently indicate the same or similar job preferences?

The latter question is vital because many survivors are highly inconsistent in stating what jobs they will or will not accept. This makes it difficult for the job developer to select an acceptable job.

Physical and Medical Status

Whether caused by motor vehicle accidents, firearms, assaults, falls, or pedestrian accidents, persons with moderate and severe traumatic head injuries often require extensive hospitalization due to coma or other conditions. The injured persons then may require weeks and months of intense physical and cognitive rehabilitation. Even then, many individuals continue to experience physical, social, and cognitive problems that interfere with gaining and maintaining employment (Brooks et al., 1987). In the supported work approach to job placement, clients are not excluded on the basis of cognitive or physical disability (Wehman, Kreutzer, Wood, et al., 1989).

To assure the safety of an individual being placed and to assist in the job matching process, it is necessary to obtain detailed information on a client's physical and medical status. Each individual referred for supported employment should undergo a physical and medical evaluation within the 12 months before placement begins. The evaluation by a physician should approve and release the individual for employment and indicate physical strengths and problems (e.g., seizures or diabetes). The physician should list medication prescribed for the client, including dose and frequency.

This information should be used to increase the likelihood for success on the job. For example, a digital watch could be set to remind a worker to take seizure medication throughout the day. Forgetting to take the medication could result in seizures on the job, which could lead to termination by the employer.

Psychiatric or Maladaptive Behavior

Major barriers to achieving stable employment and job retention for individuals with traumatic brain injury are emotional or interpersonal difficulties (Hendryx, 1989; Wehman, Kreutzer, Stonnington, et al., 1988).

During job development, information from client records, family members, and other professionals should be examined to discern if the individual has a history of psychiatric or emotional difficulties, severe and persistent maladaptive behaviors, or physically or verbally abusive behavior.

If severe depression or aggressive outbursts can be controlled and stabilized with therapy and/or medication, the individual likely would remain a candidate for supported employment. At the work site during supported employment, a professional employment specialist helps the client to adjust socially and manages inappropriate behavior using behavioral techniques (Wehman & Kregel, 1985).

Severe and persistent behavior that is dangerous or grossly inappropriate will adversely affect job placement and job retention, causing further frustration and loss of self-esteem for the client. The best recourse for the employment specialist at this point is to refer the client to a neuropsychologist or psychiatrist for services.

Substance Use/Abuse

Research studies show a relationship between alcohol use and traumatic brain injury (Goodall, 1989). Although most such studies focus on alcohol or other drug use at the time of injury or preinjury, a recent Medical College of Virginia survey found approximately 23 percent of individuals surveyed with traumatic brain injury were problem drinkers at a mean recovery period of 18 months postinjury (Kreutzer, 1988).

Postinjury substance abuse may be as serious a problem as the brain injury itself (Substance Abuse Task Force, National Head Injury Foundation, 1988). Beyond the physical dangers, such abuse can affect adversely an individual's employment and may be the reason for loss of employment (Eames, 1988; Wehman, Kreutzer, Wood, et al., 1988).

Some professionals believe drug and alcohol abstinence should be a requirement for persons referred for supported employment services who exhibit substance abuse problems. (Kreutzer & Goodall, 1989). One supported employment program lists an "absence of evidence indicative of substance abuse" as one of its criteria for accepting a candidate for placement (Wehman, Kreutzer, Wood, et al., 1989).

Supported employment programs can screen for evidence of substance use via a questionnaire and/or structured interview (Wehman, Kreutzer, Stonnington, et al., 1988). A *history* of alcohol or other drug use, particularly at the time of the injury, should be carefully noted. If the client and the family indicate that the client does not use alcohol or other drugs, then it can be assumed that no problem currently exists. However, assessment for substance abuse should occur throughout an individual's employment, especially if there were signs of use or abuse either preinjury or at the time of injury.

Any evidence of *current* substance abuse must be addressed before job placement. A substance abuse problem is not alleviated by employment; in fact, employment may provide additional income with which to purchase alcohol or illicit drugs.

In either case, assessing an individual's substance-abuse behavior should be done by a trained substance abuse or addiction specialist. Each job placement program also should have a substance use/abuse policy for individuals referred for services. Ignoring a problem this serious and widespread among persons with traumatic brain injury is to ignore a critical issue involved in successfully implementing community-based employment programs.

Family or Marital Stability

Family systems theory posits that when something happens to anyone within a system, all members within that system are affected (Minuchin, 1974). If a family member experiences a traumatic brain injury, the entire family is affected and altered by the consequences of the injury, which include physical, emotional, and behavioral changes in the individual (Livingston & Brooks, 1988). Lezak (1978) found that role changes that inevitably take place when an adult becomes dependent can be emotionally distressing for all concerned, particularly for spouses.

It is generally accepted that the family of an individual with a disability is important in the successful implementation of supported employment services (Moon, Goodall, Barcus, & Brooke, 1986; Wehman & Kregel, 1985). Rosenthal and Young (1988) stated that "a failure to understand family dynamics following head injury . . . is likely to limit the potential success of any rehabilitation program."

Some families may be overprotective or nonsupportive; others may be dysfunctional and in need of family counseling or therapy. It is common for relationships to dissolve following an injury; during the initial weeks or months of employment, the result can be problems on the job or possibly job separation.

In light of the changes that occur within the family and the family's importance in rehabilitation efforts, family members must be included as a vital part of the supported employment team. The employment specialist's role includes providing the family with information about supported employment services and assessing the family's feelings about employment for the injured family member.

Vocational Goals and Expectations

Most quality vocational programs for special populations concentrate on an individual's interests and preferences (Fraser, 1988), given that people work most effectively in jobs they like. This assumption is perhaps more relevant for persons with traumatic brain injury because they often feel a need to gain control over at least some aspects of their life.

In determining vocational goals and expectations for an individual referred for supported employment services, the following should be considered during the assessment process:

- What type of work is the client interested in doing?
- What type of work has the client done preinjury? Postinjury?
- What are the family's work expectations for the client?
- What are the client's existing skills?
- What is the client's ability to learn new skills?

If these issues are not considered before job development, clients may repeatedly turn down potential job interviews, sabotage job placements, or, worse yet, land in jobs in which they are unhappy.

On the other hand, many individuals hold unrealistic vocational expectations because the brain injury itself may cause diminished self-sight and lowered ability to solve problems and perceive situations correctly. Families may contribute to the denial by predicting a complete recovery in which the individual will return to preinjury employment (Corthell & Tooman, 1985; Kreutzer, Wehman, Morton, & Stonnington, 1988).

Intervention through education or counseling may be necessary if the desires and work expectations of the client and family conflict with the professional opinions of the supported employment staff.

Job Match

Matching specific characteristics of a client and a given job is critical to a successful job match. In the supported employment approach, an employment specialist engages in client-specific job development. A job match is the culmination of the employment specialist's thorough analysis of job requirements and client abilities. Based on existing skills and the potential to learn certain tasks, the client is matched to a suitable job (Kreutzer et al., 1988; Wehman & Kregel, 1985; Wehman, Kreutzer, West, et al., 1989 [in press]).

Moon et al. (1986) describe the job-matching process as locating, then analyzing a potential job. If the employment specialist feels the client can perform or learn the job duties involved and will be comfortable in that job environment, a job interview is arranged. The employment specialist also considers issues of transportation, family support, physical/medical status, and social and behavioral skills. Exhibit 1-2, Consumer Screening Form, lists the specific aspects of a work environment that should be assessed.

Exhibit 1-2 Consumer Screening Form

CONSUMER:

Name: ______________________

Social Security #: ______________________

Date of screening (month/day/year): ______________________

Type of screening: Initial ________ Ongoing/Employed ________ Ongoing/Unemployed ________

Total number of hours per week presently working: ________ months per year: ________

STAFF MEMBER COMPLETING FORM:

Name: ______________________

I.D. Code: ______________________

General Directions: PLEASE DO NOT LEAVE ANY ITEM UNANSWERED

Indicate the most appropriate response for each item based on observations of the consumer and interviews with individuals who know the consumer (i.e., family members, adult service providers, school personnel, employers).

1. Availability: (Circle yes or no for each item)	Will Work Weekends	Will Work Evenings	Will Work Part-Time	Will Work Full-Time
	Yes / No	Yes / No	Yes / No	Yes / No

Specifics/Comments:

2. Transportation: (Circle yes or no for each item)	Transportation Available	Specialized Travel Services Accessible	Lives on Bus Route	Family Will Transport	Provides Own Transportation (Bike, Car, Walks, Etc.)
	Yes / No	Yes / No	Yes / No	Yes / No	Yes / No

Specifics/Comments:

3. Strength: Lifting and Carrying	Poor (< 10 lbs.)	Fair (10–30 lbs.)	Average (30–40 lbs.)	Strong (> 40 lbs.)
	________	________	________	________

Specifics/Comments:

4. Endurance: (without break)	Works < 2 hours	Works 2–3 hours	Works 3–4 hours	Works > 4 hours
	________	________	________	________

Specifics/Comments:

5. Orienting:	Small Area Only	One Room	Several Rooms	Building-Wide	Building and Grounds
	______	______	______	______	______
Specifics/Comments:					

6. Physical Mobility:	Sit/Stand in One Area	Fair Ambulation	Stairs/Minor Obstacles	Full Physical Abilities
	______	______	______	______
Specifics/Comments:				
7. Independent Work Rate: (no prompts)	Slow Pace	Steady/ Average Pace	Above Average/ Sometimes Fast Pace	Continual Fast Pace
	______	______	______	______
Specifics/Comments:				
8. Appearance:	Unkempt Poor Hygiene	Unkempt/ Clean	Neat/Clean but Clothing Unmatched	Neat/Clean and Clothing Matched
	______	______	______	______
Specifics/Comments:				
9. Communication:	Uses Sounds/ Gestures	Uses Key Words/Signs	Speaks Unclearly	Speaks Clearly, Intelligibly to Strangers
	______	______	______	______
Specifics/Comments:				
10. Appropriate Social Interactions:	Rarely Interacts Appropriately	Polite, Responds Appropriately	Initiates Social Interactions Infrequently	Initiates Social Interactions Frequently
	______	______	______	______
Specifics/Comments:				

continues

Exhibit 1-2 continued

11. Unusual Behaviors:	Many Unusual Behaviors ________		Few Unusual Behaviors ________	No Unusual Behaviors ________
Specifics/Comments:				
12. Attention to Task/ Perserverance:	Frequent Prompts Required ________	Intermittent Prompts/High Supervision Required ________	Intermittent Prompts/Low Supervision Required ________	Infrequent Prompts/Low Supervision Required ________
Specifics/Comments:				
13. Independent Sequencing of Job Duties:	Cannot Perform Tasks in Sequence ________	Performs 2–3 Tasks in Sequence ________	Performs 4–6 Tasks in Sequence ________	Performs 7 or More Tasks in Sequence ________
Specifics/Comments:				
14. Initiative/ Motivation:	Always Seeks Work ________	Sometimes Volunteers ________	Waits for Directions ________	Avoids Next Task ________
Specifics/Comments:				
15. Adapting to Change:	Adapts to Change ________	Adapts to Change with Some Difficulty ________	Adapts to Change with Great Difficulty ________	Rigid Routine Required ________
Specifics/Comments:				
16. Reinforcement Needs:	Frequently Required ________	Intermittent (daily) Sufficient ________	Infrequent (weekly) Sufficient ________	Paycheck Sufficient ________
Specifics/Comments:				

17. Family Support:	Very Supportive of Work	Supportive of Work with Reservations	Indifferent About Work	Negative About Work
Specifics/Comments:				
18. Consumer's Financial Situation:	Financial Ramifications No Obstacles	Requires Job with Benefits	Reduction of Financial Aid Is a Concern	Unwilling To Give Up Financial Aid
Specifics/Comments:				
19. Discrimination Skills:	Cannot Distinguish Among Work Supplies	Distinguishes Among Work Supplies with an External Cue	Distinguishes Among Work Supplies	
Specifics/Comments:				
20. Time Awareness:	Unaware of Time and Clock Function	Identifies Breaks and Lunch	Can Tell Time to the Hour	Can Tell Time in Hours and Minutes
Specifics/Comments:				
21. Functional Reading:	None	Sight Words/ Symbols	Simple Reading	Fluent Reading
Specifics/Comments:				
22. Functional Math:	None	Simple Counting	Simple Addition/ Subtraction	Computational Skills
Specifics/Comments:				

continues

Exhibit 1-2 continued

23. Independent Street Crossing:

None	Crosses Two-Lane Street with Light	Crosses Two-Lane Street without Light	Crosses Four-Lane Street with Light	Crosses Four-Lane Street without Light
______	______	______	______	______

Specifics/Comments:

24. Handling Criticism/Stress:

Resistive/ Argumentative	Withdraws into Silence	Accepts Criticism/ Does Not Change Behavior	Accepts Criticism/ Changes Behavior
______	______	______	______

Specifics/Comments:

25. Acts/Speaks Aggressively:

Hourly	Daily	Weekly	Monthly	Never
______	______	______	______	______

Specifics/Comments:

26. Travel Skills: (Circle yes or no for each item)

Requires Bus Training	Uses Bus Independently/ No Transfer	Uses Bus Independently/ Makes Transfer	Able To Make Own Travel Arrangements
Yes / No	Yes / No	Yes / No	Yes / No

Specifics/Comments:

27. Benefits Consumer Needs (Circle yes or no for each choice):

Yes / No	0 = None	Yes / No	4 = Dental Benefits
Yes / No	1 = Sick Leave	Yes / No	5 = Employee Discounts
Yes / No	2 = Medical/Health Benefits	Yes / No	6 = Free or Reduced Meals
Yes / No	3 = Paid Vacation/Annual Leave	Yes / No	7 = Other (Specify): ______

28. Check all that consumer has performed:

___ Buffing	___ Bussing Tables	___ Sweeping	___ Using Dishwasher	___ Keeping Busy
___ Vacuuming	___ Food Preparation	___ Assembly	___ Mopping (Indust.)	___ Clerical Work
___ Food Line Supply	___ Pot Scrubbing	___ Dusting	___ Restroom Cleaning	___ Trash Disposal
___ Washing Equipment	___ Stocking	___ Food Serving	___ Other___________	

Medications: ______________________ Medical Complications/Conditions: ______________________

Source: Form developed by the Rehabilitation Research and Training Center, Virginia Commonwealth University, in cooperation with the Virginia Departments of Mental Health and Mental Retardation and Rehabilitative Services.

SUMMARY

This chapter has introduced several key issues that impinge upon return to work for persons with traumatic brain injury. Many of these issues are described in far greater depth in the chapters that follow. This book is designed to be a useful guide to vocational services providers and other practitioners involved in work reentry programs. Strong emphasis has been placed on practical problem guidelines.

REFERENCES

Ben-Yishay, Y., Silver, S.M., Piasetsky, E., & Rattock, J. (1987). Relationship between employability and vocational outcome after intensive holistic cognitive rehabilitation. *The Journal of Head Trauma Rehabilitation, 2*(1), 35–48.

Brooks, N., McKinlay, W., Symington, C., Beattie, A., & Campsie, L. (1987). Return to work within the first seven years after head injury. *Brain Injury, 1*, 5–19.

Corthell, D.W., & Tooman, M. (Eds.). (1985). *Rehabilitation of TBI (traumatic brain injury)*. Menomonie, WI: Research and Training Center, University of Wisconsin–Stout.

Eames, P. (1988). Behavior disorders after severe head injury: Their natural causes and strategies for management. *The Journal of Head Trauma Rehabilitation, 3*(3), 1–6.

Ellerd, D.A., personal communication with author, January, 1989.

Fraser, R. (1988, November). Work reentry for persons with traumatic brain injury. Cognitive Rehabilitation Conference, Richmond, VA.

Goodall, P. (Ed). (1989). *Return to work following traumatic brain injury*, Special issue newsletter, *5*(1). Richmond, VA: Rehabilitation Research and Training Centers on Supported Employment and Traumatic Brain Injury, Virginia Commonwealth University.

Hendryx, P.M. (1989). Psychosocial changes perceived by closed-head-injured adults and their families. *Archives of Physical Medicine and Rehabilitation, 70*, 526–530.

Kreutzer, J.S. (1988, September). *Alcohol, drugs, and crime: Before and after injury*. Paper presented at the Second Annual Meeting, Cognitive Rehabilitation: Community Reintegration through Scientifically Based Practice, Richmond, VA.

Kreutzer, J.S., & Goodall, P. (1989, June). *Incidence, assessment, and treatment of substance abuse*. Workshop conducted at the Postgraduate Course on Rehabilitation of the Brain Injured Adult and Child, Williamsburg, VA.

Kreutzer, J., Wehman, P., Morton, M.V., & Stonnington, H.H. (1988). Supported employment and compensatory strategies for enhancing vocational outcome following traumatic brain injury. *Brain Injury, 2*(3), 205–223.

Lezak, M.D. (1978). Living with the characterologically altered brain injured patient. *Journal of Clinical Psychiatry, 39*, 592–598.

Livingston, M.G., & Brooks, D.N. (1988). The burden on families of the brain injured: A review. *The Journal of Head Trauma Rehabilitation 3*(4), 6–15.

McMordle, W., Barker, S.L., & Paolo, T. (1989). Return to work after head injury. *Brain Injury* (in press).

Minuchin, S. (1974). *Families and Family Therapy*. New York: Basic Books.

Moon, M.S., Goodall, P., Barcus, J.M., & Brooke, V. (1986). *The supported work model of competitive employment for citizens with severe disabilities: A guide for job trainers* (rev. ed.). Richmond, VA: Rehabilitation Research and Training Center.

Oddy, M., Coughlan, T., Tyerman, A., & Jenkins, D. (1985). Social adjustment after closed head injury: A further follow-up seven years after injury. *Journal of Neurology, Neurosurgery, and Psychiatry, 48*, 564–568.

Prigatano, G.P., Fordyce, D.J., Zeiner, H.K., Roueche, J.R., Pepping, M., & Wood, B.C. (1986). *Neuropsychological Rehabilitation after Brain Injury*. Baltimore: Johns Hopkins University Press.

Prigatano, G. (1988). Rehabilitation interventions after traumatic brain injury. *Brain Injury, 4*(2), 30–37.

Rosenthal, M., & Young, T. (1988). Effective family intervention after traumatic brain injury: Theory and practice. *The Journal of Head Trauma Rehabilitation, 3*(4), 42–50.

Stonnington, H.H. (1986). Traumatic brain injury rehabilitation. *American Rehabilitation, 12*(4), 4–7.

Substance Abuse Task Force. (1988). *White paper*. Southborough, MA: National Head Injury Foundation.

Wehman, P., & Kregel, J. (1985). A supported work approach to competitive employment of individuals with moderate and severe handicaps. *The Journal of the Association for Persons with Severe Handicaps, 10*(1), 3–11.

Wehman, P., Kreutzer, J.S., Stonnington, H.H., Wood, W., Sherron, P., Diambra, J., Fry, R., & Groah, C. (1988). Supported employment for persons with traumatic brain injury: A preliminary report. *The Journal of Head Trauma Rehabilitation, 3*(4), 82–94.

Wehman, P., Kreutzer, J., West, M., Sherron, P., Diambra J., Fry, R., Groah, C., Sale, P., & Killam, S. (1989, December). Employment outcomes of persons following traumatic brain injury: Preinjury, postinjury, and supported employment. *Brain Injury, 3*(4), 397–412.

Wehman, P., Kreutzer, J., Wood, W., Morton, M.V., & Sherron, P. (1988). Supported work model for persons with traumatic brain injury: Toward job placement and retention. *Rehabilitation Counseling Bulletin, 31*(4), 298–312.

Wehman, P., Kreutzer, J., Wood, W., Stonnington, H., Diambra, J., Morton, M.V. (1989). Helping traumatically brain injured patients return to work with supported employment: Three case studies. *Archives of Physical Medicine and Rehabilitation, 70*, 109–113.

Wesolowski, M., Burke, W., & Guth, M.L. (1988). Comprehensive head injury rehabilitation: An outcome evaluation. *Brain Injury, 2*, 313–322.

Chapter 2

Literature and Public Policy Review

Linda C. Veldheer

Until recently, rehabilitation of brain injury meant remediating as many medical and physical problems as possible in a hospital or inpatient facility, then discharging the individual with limited or no continued services or follow-up (Hayden & Hart, 1986).

Today, the study of traumatic head injury rehabilitation is in the developmental stages. In the 1980s, many new theories, models, and strategies were presented at conferences, in professional journals, and in texts.

Descriptive literature is available on treatment and rehabilitation approaches intended to benefit persons with traumatic head injury, but there is little empirical research. Goldstein and Ruthven (1983, p. 92) emphasize that the present state of knowledge is limited with regard to what is and is not possible for brain injured persons and what are the best approaches to their rehabilitation.

A variety of treatment and rehabilitation approaches in various settings involve a number of professionals and disciplines (Goldstein & Ruthven, 1983, chap. 2). Such treatment has become a specialty for a number of medical, allied health, and academic disciplines (Hawley, 1984).

The approaches are based on one or more philosophical orientations and borrow heavily from models of treatment originally intended for persons with physical or sensory problems, mental retardation, or psychiatric disorders. The most important contributions come from the fields of physical, cognitive, psychosocial, and vocational rehabilitation.

Very limited empirical evidence shows any benefit from these borrowed approaches to people with brain injury. The literature indicates that even a simple multidisciplinary approach, where various professionals apply their specialty, is not adequate (Hayden & Hart, 1986). Rather, an integrated multimodal and interdisciplinary approach seems to be emerging as the most beneficial for persons with traumatic head injury. This approach requires communication and overlap among professional disciplines to jointly determine expectations and implement strategies. Unfortunately, such collaboration is difficult to achieve in any service setting.

Several general reference texts published in recent years focus on comprehensive rehabilitation of persons with head injury. They cover broad issues of treatment approaches, assessment, community integration, family education, and advocacy. Notable books include those by Brooks (1984); Goldstein and Ruthven (1983); Jennett and Teasdale (1981); Prigatano, Fordyce, Zeiner, Roueche, Pepping, and Wood (1986); Rosenthal, Griffith, Bond, and Miller (1983); Yvlisaker (1985); and Ylvisaker and Gobble (1987).

REHABILITATION: ACUTE TO POSTACUTE PERIODS

Most literature on traumatic head injury describes a hypothetical natural course of recovery for brain damage (Bond, 1979).

Three periods of recovery are described. Medical treatment and clinical interventions dominate the acute medical period, which extends from injury until resolution of post-traumatic amnesia, or about 3 to 6 months postinjury.

A specialized trauma center or acute care hospital is the usual setting for inpatient treatment during this acute medical period. The caliber and success of acute medical treatment will affect short- and long-term outcome (Bowers & Marshall, 1982; Habermann, 1982; Roberts, 1979).

A great deal of variation currently exists in the courses of treatment and rehabilitation received by persons with traumatic brain injury. In fact, the fate of a patient depends on many factors, including the availability of emergency trauma services and care at this early time after injury.

During this period, the dominant disciplines are neurology, neurosurgery, psychopharmacology, and critical care nursing. The focus is on saving the patient's life and ameliorating the amount and effects of brain damage and accompanying medical conditions.

Some survivors who remain in coma, in persistent vegetative states, or with severe brain damage and chronic medical conditions may eventually be transferred to a skilled nursing home or other long-term care facility.

Continued medical management and physical rehabilitation are the major focus during the acute rehabilitation period lasting about 6 to 12 months after injury. During this period, most persons with brain injury will remain in an acute care hospital or enter a specialized inpatient rehabilitation hospital or facility. Some persons also may receive outpatient services in such settings. A multidisciplinary approach may involve neuropsychiatry, neuropsychology, psychopharmacology, physical medicine/physiatry/rehabilitation medicine, general medicine, physical therapy, occupational therapy, speech therapy, and social work. The predominant focus is maximum restoration of physical and sensory functions. Progressive programs also attempt to remediate cognitive functioning and promote psychosocial adjustment (Cope & Hall, 1982; Imes, 1985; Zahara & Cuvo, 1984).

For some persons with mild to moderate head injuries, this phase may culminate in a return to normal functioning and resumption of preinjury life activities. However, for most persons with severe injuries a return to normal functioning is not feasible (Oddy & Humphrey, 1980; Thomsen, 1984).

Generally, the ability of persons with traumatic head injury to access good acute rehabilitation will depend on personal or public financial resources available for expensive therapeutic programs and the ability of such programs to deal effectively with clients who have multiple disabilities due to brain damage. Many persons with head injury do not receive adequate acute rehabilitation services.

It is during the *chronic (postacute) rehabilitation period* (more than 12 months after injury) that persons with traumatic head injury apparently reach a state of plateaued improvement and stabilized functional status. Community reentry is considered to be a dynamic process that evolves over the postinjury course of the survivor's life (Traphaghan, 1988). Any functional improvements during the chronic phase seem to result only from intensive and comprehensive rehabilitation efforts (Griffith, 1983). These efforts must involve a variety of rehabilitation approaches to address the multiple functional disabilities and other problems resulting from the injury.

Continued rehabilitation efforts in some form are likely to be made in a variety of service settings for an indefinite period. The specific direction of formal and informal rehabilitation activities will vary among individuals, depending on many factors such as functional status and needs, private and public financial resources available to the person, programs and services available and appropriate in the community, and the initiative and persistence of the person or family to seek and obtain assistance.

Some persons with traumatic brain injury become clients of service systems designed for persons with mental retardation, psychiatric disorders, or physical impairments. In general, these programs are unable to provide appropriate and comprehensive rehabilitation services to persons with head injury.

A rehabilitation hospital or other specialized rehabilitation facility also may provide some long-term rehabilitative services to head injured persons, usually on an outpatient basis. However, these services or other community-based programs specialized to deal with traumatic brain injury often are not available or affordable. Due to limited program options and financial support, many people with head injury remain in a condition of dependency, usually on family members. Very often, persons with traumatic head injury receive no long-term specialized rehabilitation (Jacobs, 1987).

IMPORTANCE OF ONGOING ASSESSMENT

What distinguishes the rehabilitation needs of persons with traumatic brain injury from other client groups is the diversity in potential types and levels of multiple impairments, and resulting disabilities that vary from one individual to the next. Assessment, therefore, is the key during both acute and chronic rehabilitation.

Professional literature from a variety of disciplines addresses general issues of assessment and evaluation of persons with traumatic head injury (Eson, Yen, & Bourke, 1978; Jennett & Bond, 1975; Kay & Silver, 1988). Much of the available literature focuses on assessment of specific areas of functioning, such as physical/sensory (Harvey & Jellinek, 1981; Nelson, 1983; Smith, 1983; Wahlstrom, 1983), intellectual/cognitive (Holland, 1980; Kear-Colwell & Heller, 1980; Lezak, 1983; Lynch, 1983), and emotional/behavioral (Cronholm, 1972; Lynch, 1984; Prigatano, Pepping, & Klonoff, 1986; Weismann, 1975). Several authors address special issues of assessment relevant to vocational evaluation of persons with head injury (Twelfth Institute on Rehabilitation Issues, 1985; Musante, 1983; Wachter, Fawber, & Scott, 1987; Weiss, 1980).

A consensus is that assessment and evaluation of persons with traumatic head injury is complex and multifaceted. The most prominent theme is the need for continuing assessments and reassessments over time, in different environments, and under varying conditions (Torkelson, 1985).

Because of the potential combinations of problems and limitations that persons with traumatic brain injury may experience, because of individual variations in recovery or improved functioning, and because the use of standardized assessment instruments with the head injured population is still in its infancy, an eclectic approach to evaluation is necessary. This involves careful and pragmatic use and adaptation of a variety of formal and informal assessment instruments and evaluation methods (Miller, 1983).

All professionals and disciplines contributing to a comprehensive approach to assist persons with head injury should be involved in assessment.

THE PHYSICAL DISABILITY MODEL

A predominant focus of rehabilitation literature is the physical disability model and physical rehabilitation. This interdisciplinary approach involves medical treatment and therapeutic interventions to restore an individual to normal or improved motor functioning, mobility, vision, speech, hearing, and physical stamina. It involves such specialties as neurology, physical medicine/physiatry/rehabilitation medicine, physical therapy, speech therapy, occupational therapy, and physical conditioning (Twelfth Institute on Rehabilitation Issues, 1985).

Various physical/sensory impairments are a primary focus in the acute rehabilitation period, but may continue to need attention during the chronic rehabilitation period (Najenson, Grosswasser, Mendelson, & Hackett, 1980; Panikoff, 1983). For many individuals with moderate or severe head injury, the recovery of functional motor abilities (gross-motor, fine-motor, and motor-speech skills) may take a prolonged period and can be assisted by both physical and cognitive therapeutic efforts.

A substantial amount of literature on applying traditional physical rehabilitation techniques to persons with traumatic brain injury has been reviewed and summarized by Bray, Carlson, Humphrey, Mastrilli, and Valko (1987); Nelson (1983); and Rinehart (1983). The various therapeutic strategies focus on remediating whatever physical and/or sensory impairments are present and compensating for abilities not yet recovered or permanently lost. There is much emphasis on achieving maximum independence in personal care and activities of daily living. Many persons with brain injury will require compensatory devices, such as mobility aids (e.g., wheelchairs, limb braces, crutches, and canes), communication aids (e.g., hearing aids, sign language, communication boards, and electronic message devices), and environmental control devices (e.g., adapted personal care and household equipment, adapted driving equipment, and adapted appliances and tools). The individual also will require training in the use of such compensatory devices. This training is often complicated by the impaired cognitive functioning and learning ability experienced and the attitudinal factors of persons with head injuries.

There is significant evidence from both empirical research and clinical experience that suggests the interrelationships among the various physical/sensory, intellectual/cognitive, and emotional/behavior impairments in a person with traumatic brain injury will exaggerate all the functional deficits and interfere with physical rehabilitation (Bray et al., 1987; Prigatano, 1987). Therefore, physical rehabilitation approaches should be carefully integrated with a larger program of rehabilitation services that addresses the cognitive and psychosocial correlates that are present. The rising field of cognitive rehabilitation, based on several neuropsychological models, has become the popular keystone for efforts to improve the functioning of persons with traumatic head injury (Imes, 1985).

WHERE THE SERVICES ARE

The most significant resource for persons with traumatic head injury is the state-federal Vocational Rehabilitation Program. This federally funded, state-administered program provides a wide range of services to help persons with disabilities to obtain or return to employment (Office of Special Education and Rehabilitative Services, 1988). This program originated with the National Vocational Rehabilitation Act of 1920, which created a system of state vocational rehabilitation agencies. The Act was revised and adopted as the Vocational Rehabilitation Act in 1954. It was completely rewritten in 1973 (Public Law 93–113) to place more focus on clients with severe handicaps. In 1978 (Public Law 95–602), provisions were added to create comprehensive independent living services for persons with severe handicaps and research activities were expanded by creating the National Institute on Disability and Rehabilitation Research. In 1986, Public Law 99–506 was passed to strengthen emphasis on clients with severe handicaps and make formal provisions for supported employment services. All programs designated under the amended Rehabilitation Act are administered by the Office of Special Education and Rehabilitative Services (OSERS) within the U.S. Department of Education.

Although the long-term and broad service needs of persons with severe disabilities have been acknowledged with recent amendments to the Vocational Rehabilitation Act, the federal/state services continue to focus on short-term vocational evaluation, specific vocational training, and employment placement (Whitehead & Marrone, 1986). Thus, the popular concept of rehabilitation is time limited and strictly vocational. However, many persons with severe disabilities may require comprehensive and long-term services to address deficits across all domains of life activities.

There are many problems with attempting to improve and expand traditional vocational rehabilitation services to respond to the many needs of persons with severe and multiple disabilities, such as may result from traumatic head injury. Paramount is the expenditure of finite resources on clients who need expensive, specialized, long-term services (that are primarily nonvocational) but who are high-risk for successful vocational rehabilitation (Twelfth Institute on Rehabilitation Issues, 1985, chap. VII). In addition to insufficient funding for nontraditional rehabilitation approaches—such as independent living services and supported employment services—there is also a lack of trained personnel for such services. While an expanded role for vocational rehabilitation is slowly evolving, there is not yet strong public demand and support for it. However, there is increasing advocacy among individuals with severe disabilities who seek a more meaningful life and among rehabilitation professionals and other advocates to respond more appropriately and equitably to the needs of persons with severe handicaps.

Relevant Federal Programs

The Administration on Developmental Disabilities in the U.S. Department of Health and Human Services funds and directs a number of programs for persons who become severely disabled by traumatic head injury before age 22.

The Administration assists states to develop comprehensive, coordinated, and state-of-the-art services and assistance for persons with substantial disabilities that begin in childhood and continue throughout life (Elder, Conley, & Noble, 1986). Each state receives a Basic State Grant to establish a State Planning Council to function as a systems advocate in planning and coordinating services, to promote policy development, and to demonstrate innovative approaches to service delivery. Each state also receives funds to operate a Protection and Advocacy System to secure the civil rights of persons with developmental disabilities.

The Administration on Developmental Disabilities also funds university-affiliated programs that provide interdisciplinary training to personnel who will provide services to persons with developmental disabilities and their families.

The Rehabilitation Service Continuum

While some services for persons with traumatic brain injury have developed rapidly since 1980, these have been predominately in the areas of acute medical care and acute rehabilitation. These are much more extensively available and funded than services for long-term rehabilitation. *The National Directory of Head Injury Rehabilitation Services*, issued by the National Head Injury Foundation (1988), gives this breakdown for services available in the United States:

TYPE OF PROGRAM	NUMBER OF PROGRAMS
Coma Treatment	102
Acute Inpatient Rehabilitation	179
Extended Inpatient Rehabilitation	120
Outpatient Rehabilitation	158
Lifelong Care	50
Transitional Living	103
Independent Living	58
Behavioral Treatment	53
Respite/Recreation	36

The coma treatment programs are provided in acute care hospitals or acute rehabilitation facilities. Lifelong care programs are provided in nursing care facilities or other special residential facilities. Independent living programs consist of services and supports provided in the community. Transitional living programs may be either facility-based or community-based.

Independent living, behavioral treatment, and respite/recreation programs are among long-term rehabilitation services needed by persons with brain injury. These least-developed services are not available everywhere. In fact, many of the programs currently available are concentrated in a few states and communities.

Part of the explanation for the slow development of long-term rehabilitation service for persons disabled by traumatic brain injury is the relative newness of this disability constituency and the fact their long-term service needs become apparent with the years following the traumatic event. Where they have appeared are at a number of large, private facilities that created acute treatment and transitional services early in the 1980s and expanded their operations into development of long-term supported living programs for persons with head injury. Others have appeared as components of preexisting programs for other disability groups. Unfortunately, they remain the least-developed and least-funded component of services needed by persons with traumatic brain injury.

The major reason for limited evolution of community-based or institutional long-term care is the current status of funding. There are few funding mechanisms available for persons with head injury except private funding options such as workers' compensation, liability settlements, the occasional long-term care insurance coverage, and personal and family financial resources. Even these options are frequently limited or become exhausted in supporting a variety of programs and services for an indefinite period.

For the most part, the long-term programs that have been developed are established in states where public funding mechanisms are more readily available for long-term care services. This may mean that funding available for elderly citizens is also available for younger disabled persons for community-based services or that Medicaid funds are available for both nursing home programs and community-based programs for persons with head injury.

Although many states have allocated some federal, state, and local funding for specific services for persons with head injury, usually for vocational services through the state's vocational rehabilitation agency, only a few states have attempted a broader approach to address long-term comprehensive rehabilitation needs:

- In Connecticut, three agencies provide services to the traumatically brain injured population. The Department of Human Resources has funding available for behavioral treatment services. The Department of Rehabilitative Services is involved in vocational training through job coaching and other services. The Department of Income Maintenance provides funding for head injured persons when eligibility requirements are met. A "hardship release" Medicaid rate, established in 1984, allows for a higher reimbursement rate for the level of care needed by persons with catastrophic head injury. This has served as an incentive for the development of private services within the state. At the present time, no agency coordinates all services for head injured persons in Connecticut (Connecticut Department of Health Services, January 1984).

- In 1983, the Governor of Wisconsin directed the Department of Developmental Disabilities to serve the traumatically brain injured population through its County boards. In 1986, legislation provided a statutory inclusion of brain injury in the developmental disabilities definition, rather than the previous inclusion by interpretation. Services for the traumatic brain injured population have not developed, however, because funding to the County boards for all services for developmental disabilities has been cut. An interagency task force repeated many of the recommendations originally made to the Governor in 1983 on the need for services for persons with head injury (Wisconsin Department of Health and Social Services, April 1986).
- A Head Injury Advisory Council advises the Governor of Missouri on the current status of needs and services and acts as lead agency for the head injured population. The Council conducted a survey and needs assessment of the population and drafted a comprehensive 5-year plan for the development of services in Missouri. This plan has not been implemented because of lack of funding (Missouri Head Injury Advisory Council, July 1986).
- In 1985, Massachusetts developed the Statewide Head Injury Program, known as SHIP, that is administered through the Massachusetts Rehabilitation Commission. SHIP is mandated to provide: (1) case management services; (2) technical assistance and training; (3) program development; and (4) purchase of services as a provider of last resort. SHIP's case management services are available to all persons diagnosed with externally caused traumatic brain injury. The program provides technical assistance and training to other state agencies, to professionals, and to the general public through its staff and through consultants. SHIP has funds available to purchase services for clients who have no other means of receiving those services (Massachusetts Rehabilitation Commission, July 1986).
- Various agencies in Minnesota help to meet the service needs of head injured persons. The Department of Human Services and the Department of Vocational Rehabilitation serve persons with traumatic brain injury, although activities are not formally coordinated. Case management is offered through both agencies, but neither one has the capacity to serve all of the brain injured population. The Department of Human Services provides a personal care attendant program, which also staffs group home facilities for head injured persons. An extensive Medicaid program funds many community-based services needed by traumatically brain injured persons. The majority of the community-

based services in Minnesota have been developed in the Minneapolis-St. Paul area, where local funding has augmented state funds (Minnesota Brain Injury Committee, September 1987).

- California's state Medicaid system, Medical, reimburses persons with severe disabilities for a number of needed community-based and institutional services. This has been an incentive for the development of private services for persons with head injury. California also created a statewide information and referral system for neurologically impaired persons. Regional centers throughout the state provide information on services available in that region and funding sources available in California for these services. Regional centers also provide respite and other family support services (Friss, 1988).

These examples reflect the complex administrative and funding issues that confront states in mediating federal, state, and local roles and functions to effectively respond to the needs of a disability constituency that requires comprehensive, long-term services and support.

Advocacy: Critical Role in Rehabilitation

Development and subsequent efforts of advocacy organizations are instrumental in raising awareness of and mobilizing action for disability constituencies. Organized advocacy activity on behalf of persons with traumatic head injury has evolved rapidly during the current decade, mostly because of the leadership provided by the National Head Injury Foundation (NHIF) established in 1980. NHIF and its state and local units are nonprofit organizations composed of persons with head injury, family members, friends, professionals, service providers, and other persons (Horn, November 7, 1988). In 1989 there were 55 state associations and support groups and 375 local chapters or support groups in the NHIF advocacy network (NHIF Newsletter, Summer 1989).

The NHIF is concerned with all aspects of traumatic brain injury from prevention to comprehensive rehabilitation. Major goals include stimulating public and professional awareness of the problem of head injury, providing information and referral resources, developing a network of support groups for persons with head injury and for family members, and promoting the establishment of specialized rehabilitation programs and supportive living arrangements for head injured persons (National Head Injury Foundation, 1986). NHIF also advocates establishment of central registries for traumatic head injury in all states.

At both national and state levels the NHIF attempts to influence policy and direct and redirect funding that would benefit persons with head injuries and their families (Twelfth Institute on Rehabilitation Issues, 1985). This includes focusing on establishment of cooperative agreements among federally assisted programs at national and state levels that would make conventional services more accessible and responsive to persons with head injuries. There are also activities to promote the funding of specialized model programs, professional training, basic and applied research, and prevention efforts specific to head injury; maximize use of social security and Medicare/Medicaid benefits by persons with head injury; and draw attention to and address the problems and gaps in public/private insurance coverage (National Head Injury Foundation, February 1988).

NHIF has signed a cooperative agreement with the Office of Special Education and Rehabilitation, U.S. Department of Education, which outlines strategies for making several major programs under this critical government agency more accountable to the educational and vocational/independent living needs of persons with traumatic brain injury (Office of Special Education and Rehabilitative Services, 1985). This has resulted in the targeting and funding of several research studies, model service demonstration projects, and personnel training projects that pertain specifically to head injury by the Office of Special Programs (OSEP), the Rehabilitation Services Administration (RSA), and the National Institute of Disability Rehabilitation and Research (NIDRR).

The NHIF has itself received a multiyear grant from NIDRR to develop and conduct a national program for public education on traumatic brain injury (NHIF Newsletter, Spring 1988). Project *TAP* (traumatic head injury awareness and prevention) has focused its efforts on extending access to specialized information about head trauma through a variety of national and state activities as well as developing and disseminating resource materials. Several minigrants have been awarded to six states to extend the national program at the state and local levels.

At the federal level, the NHIF is lobbying for annual budget appropriations for federal programs relevant to persons with head injury (National Head Injury Foundation, April 1988) as well as special initiatives to increase available resources for this population, such as through Medicaid reform (National Head Injury Foundation, March 1988). State and local NHIF units are also involved in systems and legislative advocacy to improve service opportunities for persons with head injury.

Advocacy to influence public policy that will promote the productivity and independence of persons with traumatic head injury is in an early stage. Several states, including New York, Connecticut, Minnesota, Texas, Massachusetts, Virginia, Maine, and Wisconsin, have special task forces or permanent advisory bodies to study the problem of head injury and recommend improved service delivery to this population. While such activities have raised awareness, there has been limited progress in mobilizing appreciable resources to assist head injured persons with severe disabilities to attain optimal productivity and independence.

Among the significant results of the advocacy efforts of the NHIF and its state associations, local affiliates, and support groups was the establishment of a federal Interagency Head Injury Task Force.

In 1987, the U.S. Department of Health and Human Services directed the National Institute of Neurological and Communicative Disorders and Stroke (NINCDS) to organize the Task Force to study and address a wide range of issues related to traumatic brain injury. Members represent 12 diverse federal agencies, including all major programs designed to respond to the needs of persons with head injury.

Through the NHIF and its state associations, much has been achieved in a few years to promote public and professional interest in the problems and needs of persons with brain injury. However, NHIF recognizes that major barriers exist in current service delivery systems that prevent survivors of head trauma from receiving comprehensive, long-term rehabilitation (NHIF Newsletter, Fall 1988). These include failure to formally accept and classify traumatic brain injury as a discrete category of disability; overburdened agendas and budgets in existing federally assisted programs; lack of specialized programs and trained personnel to provide appropriate services to persons with head injury; and lack of funding to expand existing programs or to create new programs and services needed by this constituency. NHIF is rapidly becoming sophisticated in principles and techniques of systems and legislative advocacy. With its vision and level of activism, NHIF anticipates it can influence public policy and service delivery that will result in improved opportunities for persons disabled as a result of traumatic head injury.

For more on advocacy, see Chapter 16.

SUMMARY

This chapter has reviewed descriptive and empirical literature pertinent for a background understanding of traumatic head injury. Included was information related to existing government and advocacy programs that are available to persons with traumatic brain injuries and their families.

REFERENCES

Bond, M. (1979). The stages of recovery from severe head injury with special reference to late outcome. *International Rehabilitation Medicine, 1*, 155–159.

Bowers, S., & Marshall, L. (1982). Severe head injury: Current treatment and research. *Journal of Neurosurgical Nursing, 14*, 210–219.

Bray, L., Carlson, F., Humphrey, R., Mastrilli, J., & Valko, A. (1987). Physical rehabilitation. In M. Ylvisaker & E. Gobble (Eds.), *Community re-entry for head injured adults* (pp. 25–85). Boston: Little, Brown.

Brooks, D. (1984). *Closed head injury: Psychological, social, and family consequences.* New York: Oxford University Press.

Connecticut Department of Health Services. (1984, January). *Governor's task force on traumatic brain injury: Final report.* Hartford, CT: Author.

Cope, D., & Hall, K. (1982). Head injury rehabilitation: Benefit of early intervention. *Archives of Physical Medicine and Rehabilitation, 63*, 433–437.

Cronholm, B. (1972). Evaluation of mental disturbance after head injury. *Scandinavian Journal of Rehabilitation Medicine, 4*, 35–47.

Elder, J., Conley, R., & Noble, J. (1986). The service system. In W. Kernan, & J. Start (Eds.), *Pathways to employment for adults with developmental disabilities* (pp. 53–66). Baltimore, MD: Paul H. Brookes.

Eson, M., Yen, K., & Bourke, R. (1978). Assessment of recovery from serious head injury. *Journal of Neurology, Neurosurgery, and Psychiatry, 41*, 1036–1042.

Friss, L. (1988, Summer). *Resource center for families of brain-damaged adults.* San Francisco, CA: Family Survival Project.

Goldstein, G., & Ruthven, L. (1983). *Rehabilitation of the brain-damaged adult.* New York: Plenum Press.

Griffith, E. (1983). Types of disability. In M. Rosenthal, E. Griffith, M. Bond, & J. Miller (Eds.), *Rehabilitation of the head injured adult* (pp. 23-32). Philadelphia: F.A. Davis Co.

Habermann, B. (1982). Cognitive dysfunction and social rehabilitation in the severely head injured patient. *Journal of Neurosurgical Nursing, 14*, 220–224.

Harvey, R., & Jellinek, H. (1981). Functional performance assessment: A program approach. *Archives of Physical Medicine and Rehabilitation, 62*, 456–461.

Hawley, L. (1984). *A family guide to the rehabilitation of the severely head injured patient.* Austin, TX: Healthcare International.

Hayden, M., & Hart, T. (1986). Rehabilitation of cognitive and behavioral dysfunction in head injury. *Advanced Psychosomatic Medicine, 16*, 195–229.

Holland, A. (1980). *Communicative abilities in daily living.* Baltimore, MD: University Park Press.

Horn, E. (1988, November 7). Personal communication.

Imes, C. (1985). Cognitive rehabilitation of brain-damaged patients: An annotated bibliography. *Cognitive Rehabilitation, 3*(3), 8–19.

Interagency task force holds public hearing. (1988, Fall). *NHIF Newsletter*, pp. 1; 8; 12.

Jacobs, H. (1987). *The Los Angeles head injury survey: Procedures and initial findings.* Unpublished paper. UCLA Medical Center-Department of Psychiatry, University of California, Los Angeles.

Jennett, B., & Bond, M. (1975). Assessment of outcome after severe brain damage. *Lancet, 1*, 480–489.

Jennett, B., & Teasdale, G. (1981). *Management of head injuries.* Philadelphia: F.A. Davis.

Kay, T., & Silver, S. (1988). The contribution of the neuropsychological evaluation to the vocational rehabilitation of the head injured adult. *The Journal of Head Trauma Rehabilitation, 3*(1), 65–76.

Kear-Colwell, J., & Heller, M. (1980). The Wechsler Memory Scale and closed head injury. *Journal of Clinical Psychology, 36*, 782–787.

Lezak, M. (1983). *Neuropsychological assessment* (2nd ed.). New York: Oxford University Press.

Lynch, W. (1983). Neuropsychological assessment. In M. Rosenthal, E. Griffith, M. Bond & J. Miller (Eds.), *Rehabilitation of the head injured adult* (pp. 291-308). Philadelphia: F.A. Davis.

Lynch, W. (1984). *Behavioral assessment and rehabilitation of the traumatically brain-damaged.* New York: Plenum Press.

Massachusetts Rehabilitation Commission. (1986, July). *The status of people with brain injuries in Massachusetts: Epidemiological aspects and service needs.* Boston: Author.

Miller, J. (1983). Early evaluation and management. In M. Rosenthal, E. Griffith, M. Bond, & J. Miller (Eds.), *Rehabilitation of the head injured adult* (pp. 37–58). Philadelphia: F.A. Davis.

Minnesota Brain Injury Committee. (1987, September). *FY87 annual report and action plan: Statewide service delivery system.* Minneapolis, MN: Author.

Missouri Head Injury Advisory Council. (1986, July). *Proposed service delivery system for rehabilitation of Missourians with head injury.* St. Louis, MO: Author.

Musante, S. (1983). Issues relevant to the vocational evaluation of the traumatically head injured client. *Vocational Evaluation and Work Adjustment Bulletin, 16*, 45–49, 68.

Najenson, T., Grosswasser, Z., Mendelson, L., & Hackett, P. (1980). Rehabilitation outcome of brain damaged patients after severe head injury. *International Rehabilitation Medicine, 2*(1), 17–22.

National Head Injury Foundation. (1986, September). *Trauma: The silent epidemic.* Framingham, MA: Author.

National Head Injury Foundation. (1988). *National directory of head injury rehabilitation services, the 1988 edition.* Southborough, MA: Author.

National Head Injury Foundation. (1988, February). *Traumatic head injury: A review of gaps and problems in insurance coverage.* Framingham, MA: Author.

National Head Injury Foundation. (1988, March). *Testimony of the National Head Injury Foundation to the Senate Finance Subcommittee on Health relative to the Medicaid Home and Community Quality Services Act.* Southborough, MA: Author.

National Head Injury Foundation. (1988, April). *Testimony of the National Head Injury Foundation to the House Appropriations Subcommittee on Labor, Health and Human Services, Education relative to fiscal year 1989 appropriations for programs serving persons with head injury.* Southborough, MA: Author.

Nelson, A. (1983). Motor assessment. In M. Rosenthal, E. Griffith, M. Bond, & J. Miller (Eds.), *Rehabilitation of the head injured adult* (pp. 241–269). Philadelphia: F.A. Davis.

NHIF/NIDRR project TAP update. (1988, Spring) *NHIF Newsletter*, 5.

Oddy, M., & Humphrey, M. (1980). Social recovery in the year following severe head injury. *Journal of Neurology, Neurosurgery, and Psychiatry, 43*, 798–802.

Office of Special Education and Rehabilitative Services. (1985). *Report on issues relating to traumatic brain injury.* (Program Assistance Circular 85–14). Washington, D.C.: Rehabilitation Services Administration, U.S. Department of Education.

Office of Special Education and Rehabilitative Services. (1988). *Summary of existing legislation affecting persons with disabilities* (Publication No. E-88-22014). Washington, D.C.: Rehabilitation Services Administration, U.S. Department of Education.

Panikoff, L. (1983). Recovery trends of functional skills in the head injured adult. *American Journal of Occupational Therapy, 37*, 754–760.

Prigatano, G. (1987). Neuropsychological deficits, personality variables, and outcome. In M. Ylvisaker & E. Gobble (Eds.), *Community re-entry for head injured adults* (pp. 1–23). Boston: Little, Brown.

Prigatano, G., Fordyce, D., Zeiner, H., Roueche, J., Pepping, M., & Wood B. (1986). *Neuropsychological rehabilitation after brain injury.* Baltimore, MD: The Johns Hopkins University Press.

Prigatano, G., Pepping, M., & Klonoff, T. (1986). Cognitive, personality, and psychosocial factors in the neuropsychological assessment of brain-injured patients. In B. Uzzell, & Y. Gross (Eds.), *Clinical neuropsychology of intervention* (pp. 135–166). Boston: Martinuz Nihoff.

Public Law 93-113. (1973). *The rehabilitation act of 1973.* 29 USC 701.

Public Law 95-602. (1978). *The rehabilitation, comprehensive services and developmental disabilities amendments of 1978.* 29 USC 796.

Public Law 99-506. (1986). *The rehabilitation act amendments of 1986.* 29 USC 732.

Rinehart, M. (1983). Considerations for functional training in adults after head injury. *Physical Therapy, 63*, 1975–1982.

Roberts, J. (1979). Pathophysiology, diagnosis, and treatment of head trauma. *Topics in Emergency Medicine, 1*(1), 41–62.

Rosenthal, M. (1983). Behavioral sequelae. In M. Rosenthal, E. Griffith, M. Bond, & J. Miller (Eds.), *Rehabilitation of the head injured adult* (pp. 197–208). Philadelphia: F.A. Davis.

Senate hearing and interagency task force milestones for NHIF. (1988, Spring). *NHIF Newsletter*, pp. 1; 4.

Smith, R. (1983). Speech and language assessment. In M. Rosenthal, E. Griffith, M. Bond, & J. Miller (Eds.), *Rehabilitation of the head injured adult* (pp. 279–289). Philadelphia: F.A. Davis.

Support groups and NHIF state associations (1989, Summer). *NHIF Newsletter*, p. 9.

Thomsen, I. (1984). Late outcome of very severe blunt head trauma: A 10–15 year second follow-up. *Journal of Neurology, Neurosurgery, and Psychiatry, 47*, 260–268.

Torkelson, R. (1985). *Rehabilitation of persons with head injuries.* Washington, D.C.: D:ATA Institute.

Traphaghan, J. (1988). *Community re-entry.* Southborough, MA: National Head Injury Foundation.

Twelfth Institute on Rehabilitation Issues. (1985). *Rehabilitation of traumatic brain injury.* Menomomie, WI: Stout Vocational Rehabilitation Institute.

Wachter, J., Fawber, H., & Scott, M. (1987). Treatment aspects of vocational evaluation, and placement for traumatically brain injured adults. In M. Ylvisaker, & E. Gobble (Eds.), *Community re-entry for head injured adults* (pp. 259–299). Boston: Little, Brown.

Wahlstrom, P. (1983). Occupational therapy assessment. In M. Rosenthal, E. Griffith, M. Bond, & J. Miller (Eds.), *Rehabilitation of the head injured adult* (pp. 271–278). Philadelphia: F.A. Davis.

Weismann, M. (1975). The assessment of social adjustment. *Archives of General Psychiatry, 32*, 357–361.

Weiss, L. (1980). Vocational evaluation: An individualized program. *Archives of Physical Medicine and Rehabilitation, 61*, 453–464.

Whitehead, C., & Marrone, J. (1986). Time limited evaluation and training. In W. Kiernan & J. Stark (Eds.), *Pathways to employment for adults with developmental disabilities* (pp. 163–176). Baltimore, MD: Paul H. Brookes.

Wisconsin Department of Health and Social Services. (1986, April) *Brain injury task force final report to the Secretary.* Madison, WI: Author.

Ylvisaker, M. (Ed.). (1985). *Head injury rehabilitation, children and adults.* San Diego, CA: College-Hill Press.

Ylvisaker, M., & Gobble, E. (Eds.). (1987). *Community re-entry for head injured adults.* Boston: Little, Brown.

Zahara, D., & Cuvo, A. (1984). Behavioral applications to the rehabilitation of traumatically head injured persons. *Clinical Psychology Review, 4*(4), 477–491.

Chapter 3

Managing Psychosocial Dysfunction

Jeffrey S. Kreutzer, Bruce E. Leininger,
Pamela D. Sherron, and Christine H. Groah

When Brooks, McKinlay, Symington, Beattie, and Campsie (1987) reviewed vocational outcome literature, they found return to work rates varying from 50 to 99 percent among persons with traumatic brain injury. Their own investigation provided data that suggested cause for greater pessimism. Of 98 severely injured persons interviewed 2 to 7 years postinjury, 86 percent were employed preinjury, whereas only 29 percent were employed postinjury. Regression analyses that examined postinjury personality characteristics revealed that emotionalism and difficulty controlling anger were closely associated with vocational failure. Brooks et al. concluded that physical disability was only minimally related to employability, whereas cognitive and behavioral disturbance and personality factors were significantly related to employability.

Ben-Yishay, Silver, Piasetsky, and Rattok (1987) reviewed the return to work literature and similarly concluded that vocational failure following traumatic brain injury was related to cognitive dysfunction, disinhibition, lack of initiative, poor interpersonal skills, and impaired self-awareness. They cited findings from a number of studies suggesting that vocational potential is related to learning, memory, and personality factors.

Lezak (1987) investigated the interrelationships among vocational, personality, cognitive, physical, and social disturbances after brain injury. When 42 postinjury patients were evaluated annually for periods lasting 3 to 5 years, most performed within normal limits on standard measures of intellectual function by 3 years postinjury. Nevertheless, problems in anger management, anxiety, depression, adynamia, social isolation, unemployment, and socially inappropriate behavior were commonly reported at 3 years postinjury. Statistical analyses revealed that personality and emotional disorders were more disabling than physical or cognitive impairments within this population.

This chapter provides practical information to rehabilitation professionals on five client psychosocial problems that represent major obstacles to vocational success: depression, aggressive behavior, family dysfunction, impaired self-awareness, and substance abuse. For each problem, factors are reviewed that can help determine whether a client is at risk for work separation because of the problem. This discussion of at-risk factors is intended to help vocational rehabilitation professionals address problems proactively. The greater the number of at-risk factors, the greater the likelihood the problem will negatively influence employability. Information is provided about how to recognize each problem on the basis of common symptoms. The greater the number of symptoms observed, the greater the seriousness of the problem and the greater the likelihood that professional intervention will be required. Finally, intervention approaches are recommended for enhancing employment success and a case vignette is presented within each section for illustrative purposes.

DEPRESSION

Depression is a natural consequence of the many losses as well as restrictions and limitations imposed on the individual with brain injury. Many persons are denied the opportunity to participate in formerly pleasurable activities, which include interpersonal relationships (loss of friends) as well as restrictions on driving, alcohol consumption, and other activities designed to ensure personal safety and maximize rehabilitation gains. Losses and restrictions also appear to be common for family members of head injury patients. For example, 74 percent of wives surveyed by Mauss-Clum and Ryan (1981) reported diminished social contacts. Kozloff (1987) and Lezak (1978) have also commented on the social isolation that typically follows traumatic brain injury. Social isolation in turn limits the availability of support systems that could buffer against depression.

Often, individuals with traumatic brain injury pass through a grieving process during which they gain insight into their losses, which then leads to depression. For example, during the initial postinjury period, clients suffer from a variety of severe linguistic, intellectual, and psychomotor deficits (Levin, Benton, & Grossman, 1982). Poor self-awareness is often observed and characterized by limited insight into the long-term negative consequences arising from injury. As cognitive skills improve, self-awareness develops and depression often results.

Mauss-Clum and Ryan (1981) conducted a survey of perceived changes in patients following brain injury. Fifty-seven percent of the 30 family members who responded to the survey reported that depression was a problem for their injured family member. An identical incidence of depression was reported by Brooks et al. (1986) in their 5-year follow-up investigation of severe head injury. Relatives of 42 patients were surveyed regarding perceptions of problems for the patient, and 57 percent of the relatives indicated that depression was a significant problem for the patient.

Mauss-Clum and Ryan (1981) also found a high incidence of depression in family members of patients with brain dysfunction. A total of 79 percent of wives surveyed and 45 percent of mothers surveyed reported depression. Because family members play an important role in providing long-term support for the client, depression in family members may interfere with their ability to provide needed emotional support to the client.

The frequent incidence of depression following traumatic brain injury is not surprising given the high rates of unemployment within this population. Winegarden, Simonetti, and Nykodyn (1984) studied the effects of unemployment in the normal population and said that unemployment may be perceived as "living death." Investigating the potential effects of unemployment in persons without disability, Brenner (1976) estimated that a 1 percent increase in the national unemployment rate would result in a 4.1 percent national increase in suicides and a 3.4 percent increase in first-time admissions to psychiatric hospitals.

One might expect depression to diminish following vocational placement. However, clinical experience suggests that symptoms of depression may initially increase after placement. The new work environment is likely to be stressful, test the client's limits, and contribute to fears of failure and inadequacy. Symptoms of depression are most likely to subside if coworkers and supervisors provide a supportive environment and client mistakes are accepted as a normal part of learning the job. Ultimately, each phase of job mastery contributes to self-esteem and self-confidence, which improves job performance and life satisfaction.

At-Risk Factors

Examination of medical records and client and family interviews using the following checklist can suggest whether a client is at risk for serious depression:

__ preinjury or postinjury treatment for depression

__ preinjury or postinjury suicide attempts or threats; clients who have a specific plan are at greater risk than those who do not have a specific plan; those who have previously attempted suicide are at greater risk than those who have only threatened to commit suicide

__ psychological or psychiatric evaluation indicating significant depression; results of examination may appear in psychological or psychiatric treatment records

__ lack of social and family support systems; family members who are antagonistic toward the client

__ environmental stressors, including financial difficulties; long-term failure to gain or maintain employment; severe physical or cognitive disability especially with acute self-awareness; loss of significant other(s) due to death, medical illness, or desire for separation; recent displacement or threat of displacement from residence

Symptoms of Depression

Careful observation and regular discussions with the client, family, coworkers, and employers will help identify symptoms of serious depression as shown on this checklist:

__ poor physical appearance or hygiene

__ frequent self-criticism and expressions of worthlessness and hopelessness

__ expressed lack of interest in sexual, recreational, social, or employment activities

__ excessive sleep or sleep disturbance evident by frequent wakening, nightmares, difficulty falling asleep, or early morning wakening; sleep disturbance may contribute to work tardiness

__ flat or blunted affect characterized by little or no change in emotional expression and lack of correspondence between verbalizations and facial expression

__ tearfulness

__ negative or pessimistic attitude

__ weight gain or loss of (±) 10 pounds or more over a brief period of time

__ threats of intent to harm self reported by client or others especially if a specific plan is expressed; the greater the frequency of threats, the greater the risk for self-harm and patients with ready access to means of self-harm (e.g., firearms, poison, potentially harmful medications) are at greater risk

__ attempts to harm self possibly indicated by unusual or frequent accidents of a suspicious nature and blatant disregard of obvious warnings

Considerations for Treatment

Analysis of the client's social and family situation will help the rehabilitation professional understand sources of stress that contribute to depression. For example, family members may exacerbate a client's depression by being critical and establishing overly optimistic goals for the client. Family and friends who focus on the client's efforts and positive behaviors can facilitate development of a positive self-image. Substance abuse and guilt associated with use of alcohol or illicit drugs also may contribute to depression.

Many clients are confused and overwhelmed by the losses and alterations in lifestyle brought about by head injury. They and family members may view the injury as punishment for prior sins. These clients should be helped to understand that grieving is a normal adjustment process to an abnormal event, and that the injury occurred as a result of bad luck, not deserved punishment. Pastoral counseling may benefit those who believe they have been punished for past transgressions.

Components of depression, such as hopelessness, can affect the client's work productivity, collegial relationships, and supervisor ratings. Hopelessness may be manifested as inappropriate dress, poor hygiene and grooming, or low motivation. Clients must learn that poor appearance negatively impacts interpersonal relationships and work evaluations. Praise should be provided for appropriate appearance. Patients with severe memory deficits or impaired self-awareness will benefit from using a checklist that specifies the personal hygiene tasks (e.g., shower, comb hair, brush teeth, etc.) that need to be completed before work. In some cases, family members or significant others may be required to help the client prepare for work.

Work responsibilities should begin with a few simple tasks to assist clients who express hopelessness or other indices of depression. Clients should be permitted to master tasks at a comfortable rate because overwhelming the client will lead to greater pessimism and depression. Individuals who are overly sensitive to efforts to help them feel comfortable may express anger at being patronized if they view tasks as overly simple. Comments about perceived patronizing should be responded to with expressions of honest intent to help the employee feel more comfortable with his or her performance. Clients should be encouraged to produce at maximum levels while attending to work quality. New job responsibilities should be added only as criteria for success are met on previously introduced tasks. Praise for effort rather than quality of work may be most appropriate for clients who are sensitive to failure and have difficulty meeting production standards.

Sleep disturbance is another characteristic of depression that may affect productivity. Employment specialists can often help clients with sleep problems by providing these few simple suggestions:

1. Clients should develop a log to record hours spent not sleeping. The log will help establish an accurate description of sleep and wake cycles. Clients should establish regular routines for sleeping and waking to avoid excessive sleep.
2. Clients should limit napping during the day. Napping is occasionally a result of boredom and can contribute to difficulty sleeping at normal bedtime. Job coaches can phone unemployed clients during work hours to limit their "sleeping in" or excessive napping.
3. Clients should not eat or do physical exercise immediately before bedtime because this heightens arousal.
4. Clients should do relaxation exercises to reduce sleep initiation difficulties.
5. Clients can read or do chores before bedtime to facilitate falling asleep.
6. Clients should not force themselves to sleep as this strategy paradoxically results in heightened alertness and ensuing frustration. After unsuccessfully trying to fall asleep for 20 to 30 minutes, clients should get out of bed and not return until sleep seems imminent.

Clients sometimes become preoccupied with feelings of personal failure, grief, and worthlessness. In these cases, employment specialists are encouraged to perform active listening, provide encouragement, focus on positive attributes and accomplishments, and assist clients with their problem-solving skills. Clients may be perseverate, which interferes with efficient problem solving. Perseveration adds to social isolation by discouraging mutually beneficial friendships. Redirecting the content of conversation can help reduce perseverate thinking. The employment specialist also may need to discuss with clients rules concerning appropriate topics for discussion in the workplace to avoid negative impact on coworkers and customers. Expressions of pessimism and other complaints should be limited to specific people and scheduled times. Every effort should be made to reinforce positive client statements. However, excessive attention for negative statements can inadvertently be reinforcing. A structured social skills program often will help the client improve conversational skills.

A client's expression of suicidal ideation or intent is often frightening to employment specialists and family members. Expressions of suicidal intent should be taken seriously in every case. It is more prudent to pay mistakenly too much attention to a suicide threat than too little attention. In every case, contact a mental health professional for specific recommendations. This professional can determine the client's potential for self-harm and coordinate appropriate treatment referral. The employment specialist should inform clients that their suicide threats are acknowledged as serious and illustrate how badly they must be feeling. Concern for the client's well-being should be communicated along with the promise that every effort will be made to prevent self-injury. Ideally, a contract should be established in which the client agrees not to inflict self-harm before conversing with a professional brought to the scene. Family members and friends can help prevent suicide attempts by communicating their concern for the client. Suicide threats and gestures usually suggest that hospitalization and psychoactive medications will be required. In nearly every state, evidence of serious intentions to hurt oneself constitutes grounds for involuntary psychiatric hospitalization.

Psychotherapeutic approaches to the treatment of depression, such as cognitive-behavior therapy and family therapy, often emphasize perspective. Traumatic brain injury clients frequently are self-preoccupied and direct all energy into becoming the same person they were preinjury. This feat rarely if ever occurs considering the findings from long-term head injury outcome studies. Those who focus on returning to the past self will only be frustrated and disappointed. Clients should be encouraged to adopt a perspective that focuses on their improvements relative to their status immediately postinjury. Discussion should focus on the potential benefits achieved through persistence and participation in rehabilitation. Altering a client's perspective is usually difficult but the benefits of doing so are certain.

Psychotherapy is provided in individual, marital, family, and group formats. Clinicians help identify maladaptive behaviors and inappropriate communication systems. Adaptive behaviors, clear communication patterns, and mutually supportive behaviors are reinforced. Marital and family therapy are often effective because family members may either contribute to depression or themselves require psychological support. Group therapy is often beneficial because clients are sometimes more willing to accept advice from peers than from professional therapists. Groups also allow clients to benefit from the successes and failures reported by others in similar situations.

Psychotherapy can be especially beneficial to the client who can respond to direction and verbalize the sources of depression. Depression may be relieved by increasing the client's participation in pleasurable activities and decreasing time spent in unpleasant activities. Clinicians should focus on affecting changes in behavior that will produce corresponding changes in mood. Psychotherapy provides clients with a more objective source of support, which is especially helpful when relationships with family, friends, and colleagues have been strained or lost. A psychotherapist also can provide respite to the family members who typically provide the main source of emotional support for clients.

Mental health professionals can provide a variety of treatments for symptoms of depression. Treatment begins with a thorough assessment of prior treatment records, mental status examination, behavior observations, client interview, and interview with family members. A number of standardized assessment instruments have proven clinically useful. For example, the Depression scale of the Minnesota Multiphasic Personality Inventory (MMPI) provides valuable information about depressive symptoms such as pessimism, appetite and sleep disturbance, and poor self-esteem (Dahlstrom, Welsh, & Dahlstrom, 1972; Graham, 1987). Particular MMPI scale configurations also suggest whether a person is at risk for suicide. The Beck Depression Scale (Beck, 1967; Beck, Ward, Mendelson, Mock, & Erbaugh, 1961) has also proven to be a valuable tool in evaluating depression severity.

Psychiatrists have medical training and are specially skilled in prescribing and monitoring the effect of medications intended to benefit emotional status. Medications are often useful for persons who are severely depressed. Clients with poor memory, minimal verbal skills, and inability to verbalize the source of their depression may especially benefit from pharmacological management. Medications can alleviate feelings of hopelessness, sleep disturbance, restricted affect, and adynamia (diminished drive and energy). Rehabilitation professionals should be aware of any medications taken by their clients and be sensitive to potential side affects. Failure to take medications as prescribed can adversely affect work productivity. Optimal dosages may vary with activity levels, productivity, diet, and work schedules. Many medications have side affects that may contribute to fatigability and cognitive impairments. The employment specialist should work closely with the psychiatrist by providing feedback to attain the maximum overall benefit from medications.

Finally, structured activity, exercise, proper nutrition, and recreational programs contain various benefits for depressed clients. Many persons with brain injury are inactive. Weight gain is common and contributes to poor self-esteem. Participation in group physical activities will increase activity levels and result in weight loss. Group activities also enable opportunities for developing friendships and support systems. Activity offers a form of escape from the self-preoccupation that may result from social isolation and inactivity. It also may be helpful for clients to consult nutritionists or physicians to improve their diets. Proper nutrition and maintaining weight within health guidelines will enhance productivity.

Case Presentation

K.N. is a 32-year-old male injured while riding his motorcycle 7 months before referral for supported employment services. He sustained a severe head injury and was in a coma for 4 days. He attended college for 18 months, but left when offered a job with a vending company. K.N. was employed with this firm for 7 years, felt unfulfilled in his work, and was considering other employment immediately before injury. The client's head injury resulted primarily in cognitive impairments, including problems with learning, memory, and executive functions.

K.N. began to experience mood swings soon after returning to his preinjury job. His mood vacillated between inappropriate optimism and self-assurance to self-criticism and feelings of worthlessness. K.N. complained of difficulty sleeping, fatigability, and poor concentration. Also, K.N.'s appetite decreased and he began to lose weight. The client expressed negativity toward his job and marriage, and he was often tearful when discussing these topics. K.N. was referred to a psychologist for treatment when the mood swings first appeared. The client attended appointments initially but discontinued his sessions during a period when he felt inappropriately optimistic about his situation. Despite his resistance, the employment specialist encouraged continued involvement in therapy, Alanon meetings, a support group, and YMCA activities.

One weekend, K.N.'s wife went out of town to visit her family. Soon after she left, K.N. contacted the employment specialist and said he was contemplating suicide and had several guns that could be used to take his life. The employment specialist attempted to reduce K.N.'s feelings of desperation by expressing concern for his well-being. Furthermore, she suggested that he not spend the weekend alone but instead use the available time to visit friends. She also extracted a promise that he would call again if he felt imminently suicidal. The employment specialist then conferred with K.N.'s therapist regarding the recent changes in the patient's status. A day later and upon his therapist's recommendation, K.N. entered an inpatient psychiatric unit for more intensive therapy. Daily psychotherapy sessions were initiated and K.N. was started on antidepressant medication.

AGGRESSIVE BEHAVIOR

Aggressive behavior occurs in many forms, may be expressed actively or passively, verbally or physically, and may or may not be directly expressed toward the source of the aggressor's frustration. Although all aggression is not the result of frustration, clinicians generally agree that frustration contributes to aggressive behavior. Environmental contingencies, including anticipated punishment or retaliation, also affect the probability that an individual will behave aggressively.

Passive forms of aggression aggravate others and prevent them from attaining their goals. In a sense, the aggressor knowingly fails to cooperate with instructions. The passive aggressive employee who is angry at his employer may deliberately slow his production rate. Active forms of aggression also prevent victims from accomplishing their goals. For instance, an angry employee puts kerosene into a gasoline powered lawn mower, which ruins the engine and prevents completion of the job. Passive forms occur more commonly than active forms of aggression probably because the latter are more likely to result in punishment, retaliation, or other negative contingencies.

Aggressive behavior ranks next to suicidal threats as the second most serious obstacle to long-term employment. Employers may tolerate low productivity levels, poor work quality, inappropriate sexual comments, or tardiness for a while. But a physically aggressive act can result in immediate termination, arrest, and even incarceration, and intentional destruction of property represents an intolerable expense. Hundreds of hours invested in job development, placement, and training can be wasted as a consequence of a single impulsive act. Furthermore, aggression can disrupt the entire workplace and reduce the productivity of many workers. Tension levels throughout the work environment will increase with each aggressive act. Aggression may invite retaliation and draw other workers into conflict. In addition, the aggressive employee with traumatic brain injury is often feared and occasionally ridiculed by other employees. The quality of collegial relationships is negatively impacted by aggressive behavior in virtually all instances.

Aggressive behavior also occurs outside the workplace. Mauss-Clum and Ryan's (1981) survey of family members provided important information about the incidence and characteristics of aggressive behavior in persons with traumatic brain dysfunction. A total of 53 percent of the patients were considered irritable, 50 percent had temper outbursts, and 47 percent had decreased self-control. Approximately one fourth of wives reported they had been verbally abused and threatened with physical violence; of mothers, one third reported being verbally abused and nearly one fifth were threatened with physical violence. Lezak (1978) also reported a high incidence of aggression following brain injury and indicated that aggressive behaviors were a significant contributor to family distress. Case histories of 15 death row inmates revealed that each had sustained at least one traumatic brain injury before committing violent crimes against others (Lewis, Pincus, Feldman, Jackson, & Bard, 1986).

Researchers in Europe have provided cross-cultural corroboration of the high incidence of aggressive behavior after traumatic brain injury. Oddy, Coughlan, Tyerman, & Jenkins (1985) monitored the behavior of 34 patients with severe head injuries. At follow-up 7 years postinjury, 31 percent of the relatives of these patients reported that the patient frequently lost his or her temper. Brooks et al. (1986) reported on a sample of 42 patients 5 years following severe brain injury. Relatives described 64 percent of patients as irritable and possessing a bad temper. The investigators compared their 5-year outcome data with information obtained at 1 year postinjury. The percentage of patients described as irritable or having a bad temper did not change. However, threats of violence actually increased with time, from 15 percent of the sample at 1 year to 54 percent at 5 years. Furthermore, 20 percent of the relatives had been assaulted on one or more occasions, and 31 percent of the patients had been in trouble with the law one or more times following injury.

Doherty, Kreutzer, and Harris (1989) contrasted preinjury and postinjury criminal behavior in 135 head injury patients. Family members, primarily wives and parents, provided historical information about injured family members. Of the head-injured sample, 16 percent were arrested preinjury and 10 percent were convicted. Postinjury, 6 percent were arrested and 4 percent were convicted. The criminal offenses most commonly committed were driving under the influence of alcohol, public drunkenness, assault, and drug possession. Other offenses reported included breaking and entering, reckless driving, and disorderly conduct. One patient was arrested for assault on ten different occasions following his injury.

To summarize, aggression occurs in various forms and may be intended to directly harm victims or interfere with goal attainment. Aggressive behavior unfortunately appears to be a common sequel of traumatic brain injury. Aggression may be partly a consequence of frustrations resulting from disability or diminished self-control arising from injury to frontal brain centers. Several studies also suggest that a high proportion of persons with brain injury displayed antisocial behavior before injury. For some, postinjury aggressiveness may simply reflect a continuation or exacerbation of preinjury behavioral tendencies.

At-Risk Factors

The client's potential for aggressive behavior can be estimated based on evidence of the factors on the following checklist:

__ preinjury or postinjury arrest, conviction, or aggressive behavior

__ inability to describe reasons why society provides negative consequences for aggressive acts; often reflects immature moral development or developmental regression arising from severe cognitive impairment

__ aggressive role models in the environment, especially when they are friends, family, or coworkers

__ heightened anxiety levels combined with oversensitivity and impulsiveness

__ failure or inability to anticipate the reactions of others; especially common in egocentric individuals who fail to demonstrate empathy

__ belief on the part of family members, friends, coworkers, or supervisors that aggressive behaviors are inevitable or excusable because of the client's head injury

__ frequent frustration arising from disability and failure to reach goals; common for persons having poor self-awareness and overly high expectations

Symptoms of Aggressive Behavior

Rehabilitation professionals are encouraged to use this checklist and consider the following behaviors as forms of aggression:

__ expressed intent to harm someone; the likelihood of aggressive behavior is more serious when the individual expresses a specific plan of action and the threat is expressed directly to the victim (expressing a threat to an intended victim enhances the potential for escalating conflict)

__ noncompliance as indicated by failure to perform assigned tasks or follow instructions; be aware that individuals who appear noncompliant may simply not understand instructions or expectations because of brain dysfunction

__ negativism or oppositional behavior characterized by expressed unwillingness to follow instructions or deliberately carrying out assigned tasks in a manner that differs from stated instructions; noncompliance is a form of *passive* aggression whereas negativism is an *active* form of aggression

__ throwing or breaking objects or defacing property

__ verbal or physical abuse directed at others, such as insults, obscene gestures, yelling, screaming, pushing, or hitting

Considerations for Treatment

No well-established self-report measures of aggressiveness exist for use with the traumatic brain injury population. However, the empirically derived Psychopathic Deviate scale from the Minnesota Multiphasic Personality Inventory provides information about past antisocial behavior and aggressive potential (Dahlstrom et al., 1972; Graham, 1987). Persons who achieve a high score on this scale are typically rebellious toward authority figures, impulsive, antagonistic, hostile, resentful, and excessive users of drugs and alcohol. Persons who also score high on the Paranoia scale may be overly sensitive and particularly prone to act aggressively.

The best predictor of future behavior is past behavior. Historical information about clients can be gathered from academic, employment, medical, legal, and military records as well as family members, friends, and clients themselves. Be aware, however, that clients generally underreport their aggressive actions. Some clients may even fail to report past transgressions in the hope of creating a favorable impression or beginning anew.

Employment specialists should monitor the client's aggressive behavior and its natural consequences in work, home, and social settings. Eliminating aggressive behavior is especially difficult when inappropriate actions are tolerated in some settings but not others. Family members and friends should identify aggressive behavior as it occurs, voice the unacceptibility of the physical act or verbalization, recommend alternate means of venting frustration, reinforce assertive behaviors, and provide consistent negative consequences for aggressive actions.

Some clients and family members may believe that clients have limited, if any, control over aggressive tendencies. They must be educated about the causes and consequences of aggressive behavior. Family members who want to protect the client by not providing negative feedback must acknowledge that the world penalizes aggressive actions and withholding feedback will ultimately hamper the client's long-term adjustment. The client and family must learn to recognize that aggressive behavior is the client's *choice* of action, which is inappropriate and can be eliminated if desired.

Appreciation for the natural consequences of aggressive actions should be established and appropriately reinforced without lengthy discussion into why aggressive behaviors are unacceptable. Employment specialists should avoid positively reinforcing clients by giving them special attention after aggressive actions. If breaking or throwing objects is frequent, it may be helpful to remove dangerous, highly breakable, or expensive objects from the client's immediate environment. Rehabilitation professionals should make every effort to observe the full sequence of events leading to aggressive behavior and intervene early to prevent an aggressive act from occurring. For example, clients display heightened anxiety by pacing, preoccupation, or verbalizations. Encouragement to relax or temporarily withdrawing the employee from the scene may prevent the aggressive act. Some clients will feel more in control of their aggressive behavior when their ideas are integrated into contracts that identify aggressive behaviors and agreed upon consequences. Additional reinforcement programs should be implemented to reward assertive behaviors.

Clients should be informed that expressed intent to harm another individual will not be taken lightly. Nevertheless, honesty in expressing feelings to the rehabilitation professional should be encouraged and praised. Otherwise, clients may simply fail to verbalize intentions and act without warning. Clients should be encouraged to vent negative feelings to friends or family members rather than the object of their anger. Employment specialists may also find it helpful during the work day to schedule several brief sessions with clients for venting and considering alternatives to aggression.

One alternative is an assertive approach to improving a client's relationship with the intended victim. Assertiveness training involves exploring the perceived consequences of alternative actions. Consideration of short- and long-term consequences of specific assertive and aggressive behaviors will usually reduce the likelihood of aggression. The employment specialist should point out the natural consequences of aggressive behavior when clients are unable to do so themselves. Self-monitoring of appropriate assertive and inappropriate aggressive responses may be helpful in improving self-control.

Although the long-term consequences of aggressive behavior are certainly negative, they sometimes are gratifying initially. Aggressive behaviors elicit attention from others, which is especially reinforcing for clients who perceive little control over their environments. Employment specialists are encouraged to caution coworkers and supervisors about inadvertently reinforcing aggressive behaviors.

Psychotherapy is often helpful for the aggressive individual with brain injury. Therapy sessions provide a safe, objective environment for aggressive clients to voice frustrations and vent anger. Psychotherapy entails assertiveness training, problem solving into goals and consequences of behavior, and relaxation training to reduce tension. Family therapy is indicated when family members exacerbate already high tension levels, model aggressive acts, or excuse aggressive behavior. Pharmacological management or an exercise program that allows the client to discharge tension may also be beneficial. As with persons who threaten suicide, individuals who are clearly dangerous to others may be involuntarily committed to psychiatric facilities.

Case Presentation

E.H. is a 31-year-old male who sustained a severe head injury in a motorcycle accident approximately 15 years ago. He was in coma for 3 months following his injury and has since had difficulty controlling his temper. Family members reported E.H.'s temper had caused him to lose numerous jobs.

E.H. was arrested for assault, trespassing, and disorderly conduct within the first 10 years following his accident. Family members said he was often impatient, impulsive, and prone to make inappropriate comments and behave oddly. They added that he was lonely, often misunderstood by others, and had difficulty maintaining friendships. E.H. had received treatment for his aggressiveness through psychologists and psychiatrists at various times since his injury.

E.H. was referred to the supported employment program 13 years following his head injury, when he was living independently. He reportedly consumed alcohol three to four times a week, drinking three alcoholic beverages most of the time but occasionally consuming six or more drinks at one sitting. E.H. claimed that drinking made him more likable and at ease around others and less likely to act aggressively toward or alienate others. Interestingly, at the time of his motorcycle accident, E.H. had a blood alcohol level of .25 g/dl. (over twice the .10 g/dl. legal limit in many states).

E.H.'s neuropsychological evaluation revealed only minimal cognitive and motor impairments at 13 years postinjury. However, the evaluator had considered discontinuing the testing session prematurely because of the client's difficulty controlling frustration. On several occasions, E.H. banged on the testing table, shouted, and verbally abused the examiner. The client's agitation was expressed with such intensity that the evaluator concluded that others in the workplace would most certainly feel uncomfortable around him. E.H.'s greatest disability was clearly his inability to control his anger and aggressive behavior.

E.H. was placed as a warehouse person at a local automotive parts retailer after extensive job development and consideration of his behavioral dysfunction. His job duties included stocking warehouse merchandise and retrieving merchandise for customer orders. E.H. displayed initiative and independent work from his first day on the job. However, he had difficulty accepting the established method of stocking merchandise. Furthermore, he disliked being praised for good work performance and would often reply, "Don't patronize me." E.H. was upset by the fact that the employment specialist had to inspect his work. In time, the employment specialist began to examine E.H.'s work only when the client was not present.

One day, E.H. told a coworker to lower her voice because he had "exceptionally acute hearing" and her talking was bothering him. E.H.'s abruptness and intensity took the coworker by surprise and she later communicated her hurt feelings to the employment specialist. When confronted about what happened, E.H. responded, "That's how people treat me." In another incident, the employment specialist suggested an easier way of changing the price on a price gun. E.H. yelled and stormed off, returning to the task a minute later but refusing to respond to the employment specialist's directions for the rest of the shift. E.H. was unable to meet productivity standards and his employment specialist helped him by sharing his responsibilities. On day 19 of employment, E.H. suddenly grabbed boxes out of the job coach's hands and shouted, "Go home!"

Problems in temper management and aggression were still present 1 month following placement. For instance, E.H. threatened to hit a coworker who offered help in completing a difficult task. On another occasion, E.H. complained about a scratch on his arm but raised his fist when the employment specialist attempted to examine him. The employment specialist questioned the client as to what might happen if he ever hit a coworker, but E.H. never responded. Potential consequences were subsequently outlined by the employment specialist.

At almost 2 months into the job, the store supervisor, E.H., and the employment specialist discussed areas that needed improvement. The supervisor encouraged E.H. to improve his morale, learn to work as a team member, and be more reserved in his interactions with coworkers. E.H. asked for immediate feedback following inappropriate behavior so he could respond accordingly and he asked that his supervisors not offer verbal praise for good job performance. E.H. also commented that he did not appreciate being called "Iceman" whenever the supervisor wanted him to "cool down."

The store supervisor also contacted the employment specialist during the third and sixth months of E.H.'s employment. The reason for the first call was that E.H. had kissed a female store manager. A contract was subsequently implemented that required E.H. to contact a selected chain of supervisors in resolving work disagreements. Furthermore, he agreed to end all contact with the female manager.

Several store managers also expressed concern over E.H.'s arrogance, overreaction to comments, repeated requests for money and transportation, requests for sympathy, object throwing, body odor, and explicit preference for retrieving only lightweight customer orders. E.H.'s behavior had improved little if any by 6 months. The client claimed the management's report was a pack of lies but conceded that he had occasionally kicked boxes of merchandise. The employment specialist introduced a behavioral monitoring system in which E.H. recorded instances of raised voice, raised voice and threatening comment, tenseness and shakiness, physical threats to coworkers, and physical aggression. E.H. also began to see a psychiatrist who placed him on medication to reduce his episodic dyscontrol syndrome and aggressive behavior. Unfortunately, these interventions had limited impact, and E.H. was terminated at 1 year on the job after initiating a brawl with a coworker.

DYSFUNCTIONAL FAMILY SYSTEMS

Our clients are not the only victims of traumatic brain injury. Family members often suffer as much as, and in many cases more than, clients do. The emotional, behavioral, and cognitive consequences of the injury; the drastic shift in roles and responsibilities; and the severely limited community and rehabilitation resources all place a tremendous burden on family members. At the same time, Jacobs (1988) and Kozloff (1987) have evidence that social networks diminish in size following injury, leaving the primary burden of long-term care to family members. This means that rehabilitation professionals can best achieve goals for the client only with full family cooperation.

Several investigators have provided evidence of the negative impact of traumatic brain injury on the mental health of family members. Mauss-Clum and Ryan (1981) studied the reactions of family members after a loved one sustained head injury. The majority of mothers in the sample reported feelings of frustration, irritability, and annoyance. Wives, who were more adversely affected, reported feelings of irritability, depression, anger, and insecurity. Prayer, involvement in work, talking with friends, and attending support group meetings served as primary coping mechanisms. To some extent, family members also relied on denial, vacations, tranquilizers, and alcohol.

Livingston, Brooks, and Bond (1985) interviewed more than 40 family members in the home setting at 3, 6, and 12 months post-trauma. Statistical analyses revealed consistently high anxiety levels throughout the first year as measured by the Leeds Anxiety Scale (Snaith, Bridge, & Hamilton, 1976). The authors concluded that nearly 40 percent of the relatives examined suffered from psychiatric disorders within the first year postinjury and that relatives' well-being is directly linked to patient status.

McKinlay, Brooks, Bond, Martinage, and Marshall (1981) interviewed primary caretakers for 55 patients in the first year postinjury. The investigators focused on the mental status of relatives and *levels of burden*. Objective burden was defined as the number of physical, intellectual, and emotional problems sustained by the patient and reported by family members. Information on subjective burden was provided by caretakers via responses to questions about stress levels. Analyses revealed no significant relationships between language or physical impairment and subjective burden. However, there was a significant relationship between the number of emotional and behavioral changes reported by family members and their own perceptions of subjective burden. Greater levels of burden were associated with higher incidences of emotional and behavioral aberrations. The authors concluded that emotional stress in family members was primarily related to personality and behavioral changes, and less related to physical disability.

At-Risk Factors

Clinicians are encouraged to collect thorough historical and descriptive information about clients and their relationships with family members. The factors in the checklist below can help identify families who may have difficulty providing adequate support and may represent obstacles to successful employment:

__ preinjury or postinjury family problems, including substance abuse, divorce, or criminal behavior

__ preinjury or postinjury family psychiatric problems, especially if inpatient treatment was required

__ ignorance or denial on the part of family members regarding effects and implications of injury; in some cases family members may not wish to actively solve problems in the belief that the client's complete recovery will occur in time

__ distrust of professionals indicated by a history of noncompliance with treatment recommendations or doctor shopping

__ absence of respite opportunities

__ disruption of normal family roles, especially in cases where one member must assume additional role(s) held by the client preinjury

__ presence of stressors, including forced unemployment, medical illness, displacement or threat of displacement from residence, acute medical problems that directly affect client or family members, and recent death of family member

Symptoms of Dysfunctional Family System

Clinicians are encouraged to observe family interactions for the following symptoms that may indicate family dysfunction:

__ frequent expression of expectations for patient that are inconsistent with ability

__ overprotectiveness as characterized by either displaying excessive concern or treating the client as totally incompetent

__ expressed unwillingness to assist patient

__ current or past psychiatric/psychological treatment of family members

__ verbal or physical abuse among family members

__ social isolation, especially in situations where support systems are available (e.g., Head Injury Foundation and other support groups)

__ absence of displays of affection, physical distance maintained by family members, and criticism of one another by family members

__ unkempt house or poor hygiene demonstrated by family members

__ unwillingness of family members to consider their contribution to client's problems or unwillingness to assist in problem solving

General Considerations for Treatment

Employment specialists are encouraged to develop an impression of the family's emotional health before offering placement services. Observations gathered during home interviews will usually provide helpful clues. Family expectations about placement services and family estimates of client work capacity should be reviewed and appraised for accuracy. The employment specialist then can estimate whether family members will facilitate the client's return to the workforce, and decide whether family education or family therapy is needed.

Family structure and support can be formally appraised through the use of standardized assessment instruments available only recently. The Family Assessment Device (Epstein, Bishop, & Levin, 1978) is a 60-item questionnaire that contains seven subscales. Scale scores, which provide information about the adequacy of affective responsiveness, communication, problem-solving ability, family roles, and rules for behavior, can be used to rank intervention priorities and select appropriate treatments. The seventh subscale, the General Functioning Scale, provides an overall index of family health. Other measures include the Family Environment Scale (Moos & Moos, 1974) and the Family Adaptability and Cohesion Scales (Olson, Portner, & Lavee, 1985). Bishop and Miller (1988) provide additional information on quantitative means of family assessment.

Ideal family support systems possess a number of characteristics relevant to a vocational rehabilitation program. Family members should possess realistic expectations for clients and help them pursue reasonable goals. Clients, families, and employment specialists should share similar perceptions of clients' strengths, limitations, expectations for placement, and potential productivity. Overly optimistic and unreasonable expectations will doom clients to failure and result in lowered self-esteem, anxiety, and depression. Overprotectiveness and minimal goal-setting will not enable clients to fully use residual strengths and may result in lifelong dependence, feelings of inadequacy, and resentment. Employment specialists should work with family members to develop reasonable expectations and regularly discuss the nature and effectiveness of employment interventions.

Families should also have open and honest communication. Assertive communication is more constructive than sarcasm or hesitancy to share thoughts. Facial expressions and body language should be congruent with verbal messages. Poor communication skills developed and maintained over long periods can require lengthy intervention before significant changes appear. Establishing common family goals, pointing out obstacles, and developing strategies for problem solving can improve family communication.

Good interpersonal communication among rehabilitation professionals, clients, and families is essential to effective rehabilitation systems, especially during job development and immediately following placement. Employment specialists can develop positive relationships with family members by sharing information about community resources, focusing on positive client points, speaking in practical terms, and avoiding jargon. The use of jargon will not only create interpersonal distance between employment specialists and families but also may cause families to feel ignorant and overwhelmed.

Rosenthal and Young (1988) described six types of family interventions that may be useful following traumatic brain injury. *Family education* focuses on providing family members with general information about traumatic brain injury and specific information about the patient. *Family counseling* focuses on the family unit and is intended to help overcome feelings of loss and helplessness. *Marital and sexual counseling* focuses on the marital unit and on restructuring marital roles and redeveloping a healthy sexual relationship. *Family support groups* furnish emotional support and education. Family members and clients are encouraged to participate in groups primarily composed of other families having a loved one with brain injury. Sharing similar experiences and solutions to problems is cost effective. *Family networking* is a process of developing the extended family system to share the burden of care for clients and provide mutual support. *Family advocacy* entails working with families to help them take full advantage of existing community resources, modify existing resources to better meet the needs of persons with head injury, and develop new, needed resources.

The employment specialist is encouraged to learn about community support and rehabilitation programs and share this information with clients and families. Licensed professionals, such as psychologists, counselors, and social workers, are best qualified to provide marital counseling, family counseling, and family networking services. Family support groups are offered through community support agencies, such as the local Head Injury Foundation. Qualified nonprofessionals, including the employment specialist, may be involved in the development, implementation, and leadership of family groups.

Employment specialists are encouraged to network with experienced mental health professionals in the community to facilitate rapid and effective responses to referrals. Rapid intervention is especially critical in crises. Although employment specialists can provide some basic family support services, professionals can help in deciding when professional help is required. If individual family members have preexisting mental health problems that are exacerbated by stresses related to the client's brain injury, referral for long-term psychotherapy or psychopharmacologic intervention may be required for those family members.

The client is part of a rehabilitation system and a family system and should not be viewed as an independent entity. Family members can pose unquestionably serious obstacles to gaining and maintaining employment.

Conversely, meeting family needs and building support systems can help assure successful placement and long-term employment.

Case Presentation

C.F. is a 29-year-old male high school graduate who sustained a severe head injury in a diving competition 17 years ago. A second traumatic experience occurred 1 year later, when C.F.'s father, a pilot, died in a midair collision. After completing high school, C.F. worked many jobs but only for short periods. He reportedly has difficulty concentrating on work and displays limited interest in maintaining employment. C.F. lived with his widowed mother until age 26, when he moved into a supervised apartment dwelling for psychiatric patients. He was forced to leave his apartment within the first month after he repeatedly violated the apartment's alcohol and drug use policies. C.F.'s mother immediately rescued him and took him back into her residence. Unable to live with his mother's restrictions, C.F. moved into a mobile home that he purchased with money from his head injury settlement.

C.F.'s neuropsychological evaluation revealed mild-to-moderate deficits in learning, memory, concentration, processing, executive functions, and bilateral dexterity. However, C.F.'s most significant problem was motivation. His employment history was marked by a tendency to give up when faced with difficult or unappealing work. Furthermore, he had overly optimistic expectations for an appropriate salary.

C.F.'s first placement within the supported employment program was at a home for physically handicapped children. His job duties primarily consisted of preparing and serving meals for the residents. Beginning with the first day of employment, C.F.'s mother telephoned him every morning and woke him or arrived at his home and fixed breakfast. The employment specialist was initially unaware of this. However, during the second week of employment, C.F. arrived at work an hour late and complained no one had wakened him. The employment specialist learned that C.F.'s mother had been out of town that day. An alarm clock was subsequently purchased and C.F. was shown how to use it. A checklist also was developed to ensure C.F. would take everything he needed for the job each day. (i.e., keys, uniform, lunch, etc.). The employment specialist had several discussions with C.F. and his mother over the next weeks and stressed that it was essential that C.F. become more independent. Nevertheless, the client's mother continued to call or stop by every morning despite repeated confrontations.

Over the next few weeks, C.F. repeatedly claimed to lose his way while driving the 15 miles to his job. Travel training was subsequently provided. The employment specialist initially rode along with the client, then followed behind him as he drove to work each day. Finally, C.F. drove independently but met the employment specialist at certain points along the way. Written instructions were mounted on the dash along with a number to call if he became lost. Quite unexpectedly, C.F.'s mother drove behind the client on the first day he was supposed to journey to his job unassisted. The mother abruptly pulled off the road upon seeing the employment specialist's car ahead in the distance. C.F. arrived at the job site upset and informed the employment specialist that his mother had followed him. The mother denied she had deliberately followed her son, claiming she had been on her way to the post office. Once again, the employment specialist encouraged the mother not to interfere with her son's program.

Three months later, the client's mother drove C.F. to work one day. The client claimed he had not driven his car because he was having it repainted. However, C.F.'s mother was still providing transportation for her son 2 weeks later. The client then said he had been arrested for driving under the influence of alcohol while parked at a friend's house and seated in the passenger seat of his car. After the employment specialist attempted to confirm C.F.'s story with the state police, the client finally admitted he had been arrested for marijuana possession, and his mother had taken his car from him. The employment specialist contacted the client's mother, who then admitted having told C.F. to lie about the reasons for not driving to work because she felt her son would be terminated from the program. C.F. conceded he had been afraid to tell the employment specialist the truth about his situation because he knew his mother would be angry with him. The employment specialist subsequently arranged substance abuse counseling for C.F. and monitored his adherence to the treatment program through weekly meetings.

IMPAIRED SELF-AWARENESS

Ben-Yishay et al. (1987) have identified poor self-awareness as a frequent contributor to employment problems following traumatic brain injury. Poor self-awareness, or inaccurate self-perception, may be manifested in a variety of forms and influenced by a number of factors.

Head injury often results in drastic changes in personality and personal abilities (Lezak, 1978; Thomsen, 1984). Following injury, many patients are transformed physically, intellectually, emotionally. These alterations are primarily negative and consequently difficult for patients and family members to accept. For example, Mauss-Clum and Ryan (1981) interviewed wives of patients with acquired brain dysfunction and found that 32 percent reported, "I am married to a stranger;" 42 percent reported, "I'm married but don't have a husband." These startling revelations highlight how dramatic personality and emotional changes can be after head injury.

Traumatic brain injury is very different from most illnesses that patients and their families have encountered. A broken arm, for example, is not only overtly evident, but also heals in a short time. Recovery from most illnesses is rapid and complete because of medical science. However, the nervous system is unique and nerve cells cannot regenerate like other types of cells in the body. Consequently, the common expectations of complete and rapid recovery after head injury are rarely realized.

The challenge of rediscovering oneself following injury is further complicated by variability in the recovery process. Improvements occur in neurological status, functional abilities, emotional control, and intellectual skills at differing rates (Mandelberg & Brooks, 1975; Thomsen, 1984); they actually may deteriorate in some, particularly older, individuals. Accurate self-awareness requires a complex interaction of many brain centers that may be compromised months and even years postinjury. Family members and friends may be hesitant to provide clients with accurate feedback about negative changes to protect the patient's self-esteem. Parents often become overprotective after injury and treat the individual more like a child than an adult (Mauss-Clum & Ryan, 1981; Gardner, 1973). Given these many obstacles, there is little wonder why restoring accurate self-awareness represents such a difficult hurdle.

Some clinicians have found that disabled persons, regardless of whether they suffer from brain injury, pass through a series of stages soon after injury. Schontz (1975) suggested that the early stages of injury are characterized by shock and confusion, when disabled individuals have difficulty viewing their problems as long- rather than short-term. In the second stage, in which the individual encounters repeated frustrations because of limitations and restrictions arising from the disability, the possibility of long-term or permanent disability is seriously considered for the first time. This stage is often characterized by grieving and depression. Ideally, the final stage in adjusting to injury is characterized by acknowledgment. The individual accepts disability as a long-term impairment, plans accordingly, and participates more fully in rehabilitation. Lezak (1986) suggested that families of persons with traumatic brain injury pass through similar stages characterized by denial, depression, and acknowledgment.

Poor self-awareness is also a consequence of physiological damage to the brain. Neuronal damage following injury is typically diffuse and affects most brain regions. The ability to accurately perceive oneself is a complex skill dependent on integrating the individual's perception of performance quality and feedback from others. Memory impairment is among the most common and debilitating effects of injury, and many persons simply forget what they have learned about the impact of their injury. Furthermore, memory impairment limits the extent to which a person can benefit from experience and accurately recall feedback provided by others. Lezak's classic article (Lezak, 1978), which outlined characterological changes after brain injury, identified poor self-awareness as among the most disabling consequences of brain injury.

At-Risk Factors

The following checklist can help identify persons who are especially at risk for problems related to poor self-awareness:

__ less than 12 months since injury
__ severe level of injury, especially characterized by reasoning or memory impairment
__ expression by significant others of goals that exceed or grossly underestimate the client's abilities
__ inability to anticipate consequences of behavior
__ unwillingness to accept valid feedback from others as potentially valuable
__ inability to accurately describe personal changes resulting from injury

Symptoms of Poor Self-Awareness

The following checklist of symptoms can help rehabilitation professionals identify both obvious and subtle signs of poor self-awareness:

__ unrealistic expectations regarding vocational alternatives
__ self-rating of job performance inconsistent with that provided by employment specialists or employers
__ frequent failures, especially in academic or vocational situations
__ numerous errors on vocational and daily living tasks without apparent signs of error recognition (e.g., facial grimace suggesting frustration)
__ denial or disagreement when provided with feedback, particularly when similar feedback is provided by various individuals

General Considerations for Treatment

With few exceptions, most individuals with traumatic brain injury gradually develop improved self-awareness through experience and accurate feedback from others in a supportive environment. A thorough and regular evaluation by rehabilitation professionals is often the cornerstone to developing reasonable goals for clients and educating them and their families to establish reasonable expectations. The clinician who performs an evaluation also assumes the responsibility of providing feedback to the patient, family, and rehabilitation team in practical and understandable terms.

The importance of involving families in providing accurate feedback to clients cannot be underestimated. Information concerning the immediate and long-term effects of injury is highly valued by family members (Mauss-Clum & Ryan, 1981) and can usually be easily communicated to them. Distribution of appropriate literature pertaining to head trauma and encouraging networking with other affected families is recommended. In most cases, families should be encouraged gently not to reflexively become overprotective, limiting the client's ability to progress and learn from experience. During the earliest phase postinjury, family members often have difficulty acknowledging the patient's impairments and the long-term consequences of injury (Romano, 1974). Clinicians must work closely with family members to help them develop accurate perceptions of the patient's strengths and limitations.

The accuracy of client self-awareness can be improved by providing regular feedback about the adequacy of performance levels. Every effort should be made to focus on positive behavior, particularly because negative behavior can inadvertently become the focus of attention and thereby be reinforced. Clients are more likely to be responsive and develop a more positive attitude when presented with positive, rather than negative, feedback. Encouraging clients to become involved in peer support groups can also be beneficial. Feedback provided by others with traumatic brain injury, when accurate, is often more easy to accept than feedback provided by parents, spouses, or therapists. Repeated videotaping of actual work and simulated activities allows clients to view their behavior from the outside and can have a potent impact on self-awareness.

Rehabilitation professionals may wish to visit the workplace and encourage coworkers or supervisors to provide feedback to clients. Consistent feedback provided by several individuals is more likely to be effective than inconsistent feedback by one or two individuals. When the client's performance is poor, it may be helpful to reinforce effort rather than quality of performance.

Several important factors regarding client self-awareness should be kept in mind. Persons with traumatic brain injury face numerous frustrations and failures following injury. They are likely to be especially sensitive to negative feedback, so every attempt should be made to delineate positive behavior. Furthermore, denial, a psychological function, often serves an appropriate protective role. Professionals are encouraged to view denial as an indication of the patient's emotional strength. Direct confrontation in the face of denial is likely to be met with defensiveness and dislike rather than improvements in behavior. Frequent indications of denial by clients may signal that clinicians should lower goals and expectations that will enable a series of successes that will bolster self-esteem.

Case Presentation

S.S. is an 18-year-old male who sustained a severe head injury after falling from a tree at age eight. Since his accident, S.S. has received extensive treatment for problems involving depression, poor judgment, and interpersonal difficulties. He has been arrested three times over the past 3 years for removing food from grocery stores without paying. He is often impulsive and frequently treats others inappropriately without considering the impact of his actions. He also disregards the validity of feedback provided by others about perceived problems with his temperament, thinking, behavior, and even physical status (i.e., residual left hemiparesis [weakness in left half of the body affecting the arm and leg]).

S.S. denies he has any residual disability from his fall, although he admits having suffered two broken arms. He has been unable to maintain employment chiefly because of interpersonal and behavioral difficulties. When initially referred for supported employment services, S.S. insisted his vocational choices were limited to car repair and chemical engineering. S.S.'s family has come to tolerate numerous undesirable behaviors as a result of feeling defeated in their efforts to change their son's behavior. S.S.'s neuropsychological evaluation revealed primarily impairments in concentration, memory, reasoning, judgment, and work organization.

S.S. was placed in a sales associate position for a shoe store. His employment was already in serious jeopardy after only 3 days on the job because he demonstrated an apparently unquenchable interest in his female coworkers. He complimented them excessively and repeatedly asked for dates. Much to the embarrassment of his female coworkers, S.S. reported to male coworkers specific sexual activities that had occurred on dates. Furthermore, as time passed, S.S. emphasized socializing with coworkers over completing job duties.

S.S. became angry and defensive when his supervisor pointed out that he was not adequately completing his work. The client also repeatedly asked for favors not granted to other coworkers, such as additional breaks. S.S. also falsified his timecard to extend his break time. He was threatened with job termination immediately after being blatantly discourteous to a customer while standing next to his store manager. Interestingly, S.S. rated his job performance as good to excellent even after repeatedly being told that his job was on the line.

The employment specialist initially addressed S.S.'s inappropriate behaviors by arranging weekly meetings among the program manager, the employment specialist, and the client and updating the young man's parents and psychiatrist on his progress. These interventions were only minimally successful. The client was subsequently required to participate in weekly counseling sessions to develop a behavior intervention plan incorporating S.S.'s input and to review the successes and failures associated with use of the plan. S.S.'s employment specialist also began to provide immediate feedback when the client was acting inappropriately. In addition, she often cued him to "stop and think" about how he would approach store customers.

These interventions were only marginally successful and it became clear that S.S.'s interactions with customers would need to be continually supervised. Consequently, S.S.'s job responsibilities were changed so that his primary duties involved unloading product shipments and stocking warehouse merchandise. The client remained in this new position for 9 months before leaving his job to pursue a college education despite serious reservations voiced by his parents and the employment specialist.

SUBSTANCE ABUSE

Motor vehicle accidents are a primary cause of traumatic brain injury and alcohol is a frequent contributor to motor vehicle, as well as pedestrian, recreational, and aviation, accidents. Rimel, Giordani, Barth, and Jane (1982) completed a prospective study of 199 patients admitted for hospitalization with a diagnosis of moderate head injury. The primary mechanisms of injury were vehicular accidents (66 percent), falls (19 percent), and assaults (13 percent). Analysis of admission blood alcohol levels revealed that 73 percent of the patients had consumed alcohol prior to being injured. Twenty-seven percent had a blood alcohol level between .10 and .20 g/dl., and 26 percent of the sample had a blood alcohol level greater than twice the legal limit for intoxication ($>$ .20 g/dl.). Approximately one third of the patients had histories of alcohol abuse. In 102 patients admitted for hospitalization following traumatic brain injury, Sparadeo and Gill (1989) found that patients admitted with blood alcohol levels above .10 g/dl. required longer hospitalization, demonstrated greater behavioral disturbance, and displayed more cognitive impairment when discharged.

Substance abuse includes both alcohol and drug use. Despite the potentially adverse effects on long-term outcome, there has been little empirical research to indicate the actual incidence of preinjury and postinjury substance abuse. Following a survey of substance abuse policies in rehabilitation programs, Rohe and DePompolo (1985) chastised clinicians for ignoring substance abuse issues. These authors suggested that substance abuse problems can be resolved partly by establishing clear policies prohibiting use of alcohol and drugs by patients and educating staff and patients on the effects and potential dangers of substance abuse.

There are many reasons why abstinence is the best policy for persons with traumatic brain injury. First, the effects of alcohol and illicit drugs contribute to greater impairment of already impaired cognitive and psychomotor skills. Second, alcohol and drugs have the potential to interact dangerously with drugs prescribed by physicians. Third, these substances increase the likelihood of seizures; patients with traumatic brain injury are already at greater risk for seizures in comparison to the normal population. Fourth, while optimal nutritional status is essential for optimal recovery, patients who consume alcohol are less likely to ingest a nutritious diet, replacing calories normally available from healthy foods with calories derived from alcohol. Fifth, persons with traumatic brain injury are more sensitive to the effects of alcohol and drugs (Oddy et al., 1985), which places them at increased risk for a second injury. Finally, many patients are at risk for dependence given that alcohol and drugs provide only temporary relief from the many stresses that typically follow injury.

At-Risk Factors

The following checklist can help identify persons who are especially at risk for developing substance abuse problems:

__ preinjury or postinjury abuse or dependence
__ ignorance regarding potential dangers of substance abuse
__ unwillingness to acknowledge dangers of substance abuse
__ family members or close friends with substance abuse problems
__ social system characterized by substance use and abuse
__ history of arrest or conviction for alcohol-related crimes preinjury or postinjury
__ inconsistent views among family and staff about dangers associated with substance use
__ intoxication (blood alcohol level > .10 g/dl.) at time of injury
__ spontaneous and frequent discussion of alcohol and drug-related issues
__ age less than 25 years
__ irregular job history that may be characterized by frequent job changes or attribution of responsibility for job problems to supervisors; concerns expressed by prior supervisors may include excessive tardiness and absenteeism or failure to meet production rates
__ independent clients who have minimal physical disabilities; they are at greater risk than those who are less independent and more physically disabled

Symptoms of Substance Abuse

The following checklist will help rehabilitation professionals identify common symptoms of substance abuse:

__ anger and other forms of defensiveness in response to questions about substance use

__ late development of seizure disorder

__ excessive denial in response to questions about substance use

__ diminished work performance manifested by tardiness, irritability, low productivity, and excessive absenteeism

__ social and recreational situations that frequently include drinking

__ addictive behavior patterns as indicated by responses to standardized drinking assessment questionnaires such as the Michigan Alcoholism Screening Test and the Quantity Frequency Variability Index

General Considerations for Treatment

Given the high incidence of preinjury substance abuse and the potentially serious dangers endemic to the traumatic brain injury population, good clinical practice requires ongoing assessment of alcohol and illicit drug use throughout the rehabilitation process. To achieve a more accurate picture of alcohol and drug use, information should be obtained ideally from several sources including the patient, family members, friends, and employer. Usage patterns can be established via clinical interview or through the use of standardized assessment instruments, such as the Michigan Alcoholism Screening Test (MAST) and the Quantity Frequency Variability Index.

The 25-item diagnostic MAST questionnaire asks questions about behaviors associated with alcoholism. The MAST has demonstrated criterion-related and test-retest validity (e.g., Selzer, Gomberg, & Nordhoff, 1979; Zung & Charalampous, 1975) and is available in an abbreviated version (Zung, 1970). For the abbreviated version, responses are assigned a numeric value, weighted as prescribed by Zung (1970), and added to derive a total score. Both MAST versions assign drinkers to either of two categories: adjustive drinker or problem drinker.

The Quantity Frequency Variability Index (Cahalan & Cisin, 1968) obtains information about drinking frequency and the amount of alcohol consumed at each sitting. Information about preinjury and postinjury alcohol use can be obtained by appropriately altering the questionnaire format. This index classifies persons as abstinent, infrequent, light, moderate, or heavy drinkers.

Clinicians should gather information about preinjury alcohol and illicit substance use. Examination of medical records may reveal that the patient has been treated for alcohol-related illnesses; psychiatric or psychological treatment records may indicate the patient was previously treated for substance abuse problems. Arrest records may reveal a history of arrest for driving under the influence of alcohol or drugs. When permitted, discussion with previous employers also may provide important information concerning work productivity and absenteeism. Furthermore, most hospitals obtain blood alcohol levels in persons admitted for head injury. Admission blood alcohol levels beyond the legal definition for intoxication suggest the existence of a preinjury substance abuse problem.

Assessment for substance abuse should be ongoing throughout the rehabilitation process. Seriously injured patients often have little opportunity to drink because their mobility is restricted and they are closely supervised. The likelihood of substance abuse increases as clients achieve greater levels of independence and their financial status improves. Alcohol restriction is likely to be viewed by the patient as another one of the many limitations imposed by the injury. The abstinent patient is likely to feel isolated and restricted in social gatherings while in the presence of friends and family who drink.

Clinicians should be sensitive to the issues arising from abstinence and convey empathy toward clients in this regard. The likelihood of abstinence can be enhanced using several methods. Beyond educating clients and families about the potential dangers of substance abuse, rehabilitation professionals, including physicians, should communicate consistent instructions regarding abstinence and reinforce patients for compliance. Family and support staff should encourage patients to participate in social and recreational activities that do not involve the use of alcohol. Contracts with patients help to establish clear expectations, guidelines, and behavioral contingencies.

Even though few treatment programs exist specifically for helping disabled individuals with substance abuse problems, professionals are encouraged to network with community substance abuse treatment agencies to provide services for those in need. The experienced rehabilitation professional can educate substance abuse counselors regarding outcome and the special problems of persons with traumatic brain injury. The substance abuse counselor can provide intensive treatment and educate the rehabilitation professional about treatment mechanisms and related psychological issues. Given the frequently expensive costs of rehabilitation and the serious dangers of substance abuse, no one can afford to be ignorant of the dangers of alcohol and illicit drug use.

Case Presentation

D.N. is a 29-year-old male who sustained a severe head injury in a serious automobile accident. His car skidded off the road and hit a tree during a heavy thunderstorm. Following injury, D.N. was in coma for more than 2 months, with full hospitalization in excess of 4 months. Due to his injury, he walks with a leg brace and cane, shows static nerve palsy in the right leg, has right hand ataxia, and has visual impairment in the left eye. He was referred for supported employment services 4 years following his injury.

A neuropsychological evaluation revealed that D.N. performed in the Low Average to Borderline Impaired range on measures of arithmetic computation, spelling, remote memory/fund of information, visuomotor learning, common sense reasoning, judgment of safety, and visuoperceptual skills. Significant deficits were found on measures of auditory and visuomotor learning, right hand motor speed/dexterity, and hypothesis testing.

Information on the client's alcohol and illicit drug use patterns was provided by the client and his brother. Answers to the Quantity Frequency Variability Index indicated that preinjury, D.N. had one or more alcoholic drinks three or more times per day. Furthermore, when D.N. drank, he had six or more drinks more than half the time. Evidently, he was a heavy drinker preinjury, placing him at increased risk for postinjury abuse problems. The client's mother was reportedly an alcoholic.

Since his injury, Quantity Frequency Variability Index information obtained from the client's brother indicated that he drank one or more alcoholic drinks three or four times a week. When D.N. did drink, he had six or more drinks more than half the time. His brother felt his perception of the client's drinking patterns was accurate.

D.N. had been popular and active in high school, playing on the school's baseball and basketball teams. Before his injury, he had worked as a maintenance assistant, a spray painter, and an animal care attendant. He had also performed clerical work during a 3-year enlistment in the U.S. Army. Following extensive job development and discussions with his employment specialist, D.N. was hired and placed in a full-time microfilm clerk position at a large electronics retailer.

Within the first month of employment, the employment specialist received a call from D.N., who stated he was not going to work. D.N. had fallen off his porch and bruised his ribs. Upon further inquiry, it was revealed that D.N. was drinking when he fell. D.N. informed the employment specialist that he was celebrating notification of being promoted from temporary to permanent work classification. The client's drinking increased as he became more settled in his job and had accumulated savings. He had lived with his brother and several of his brother's friends who encouraged abstinence; however, his employment income allowed him to move into his own apartment where he lived unsupervised.

Four months after securing his own residence, D.N. was stopped by the police, questioned, and arrested for driving under the influence of alcohol. He was required to spend several days in the city jail. Unfortunately, D.N. had been scheduled to work during those days. His brother called the employment specialist to ensure that D.N.'s employer would be informed that he would not be coming into work for several days.

Later, the employment specialist met with the psychologist who had initially provided counseling to D.N. Both the employment specialist and the psychologist felt that more intensive intervention was necessary. Concern was expressed regarding the client's ability to maintain his job. Further investigation revealed that there were erratic changes in D.N.'s work production rate. Also, coworkers reported erratic changes in D.N.'s attitude toward work as well as his personal life. The employment specialist noticed that D.N. often reported being tired and his diet consisted almost entirely of snack foods and coffee. D.N. had been losing weight and concern was expressed about his nutritional status. The patient's brother also reported that D.N. and his mother were regularly going out for drinks.

The employment specialist and psychologist agreed that intervention was needed or D.N. might soon lose his job. Meetings were held with D.N. and his brother to provide them with information on the dangers of alcohol consumption and importance of good nutrition for good health. Expressions of concern by rehabilitation professionals and the patient's brother as well as the serious implications of pending charges contributed to the client's willingness to abstain from alcohol. More frequent contacts with the client were initiated to reinforce and monitor compliance.

On a final note, D.N. went to court to stand trial for charges related to driving under the influence of alcohol. Blood alcohol test results were made available and revealed a blood alcohol level only two-thirds the legal limit. The case was dismissed. D.N. later settled into his job, his productivity rate and moods became more stable, and he received several raises.

SUMMARY

The problem of returning persons with traumatic brain injury to community living and gainful employment represents a series of complex challenges because most clients have more than one problem. The number, complexity, and interaction of problems contribute to the difficulty in maintaining long-term employment.

This chapter does not pretend to cover all the difficulties experienced by persons with head injury. We intended only to discuss a subset of problems that should be considered priorities. The reader also must keep in mind that rehabilitation is a long-term process that necessarily involves many failures intermixed with successes. Those who attempt to quickly solve all the client's problems will no doubt be disappointed. An important immediate goal of rehabilitation is to help move the client forward. Several steps backward will usually be taken in this process. Furthermore, no program can guarantee success. Repeated attempts at success hopefully will result in overall improvement. It should be borne in mind that overly optimistic goals can negatively impact the rehabilitation professional in addition to the client.

The likelihood of successful community integration is undoubtably enhanced by a team approach. Team members may include psychologists, social workers, speech pathologists, employment specialists, substance abuse counselors, recreational therapists, educators, employers, occupational therapists, and family members, among others. The supported employment model (e.g., Wehman et al., 1988) is based on the concepts of long-term follow-along and proactive intervention, which professionals and employment specialists must adhere to for successful community integration. The role of team members and their contributions change over time as old problems are solved and new problems appear. Ironically, employment and independence often create a new set of problems.

Model systems of head injury care have appeared recently and continue to be perfected (Thomas, 1988). They begin with state of the art neurosurgical intervention and, following postacute rehabilitation, clients may be enrolled in day rehabilitation or transitional living programs. The final stages of long-term rehabilitation ultimately include finding and maintaining employment. Traumatic brain injury rehabilitation professionals are encouraged to network with other professionals who provide services to individuals with similar disabilities. Through a process of mutual education, rehabilitation services intended for other populations may be adapted for persons with traumatic brain injury. Furthermore, professionals are encouraged to remain abreast of newly developed treatment techniques by regularly reading professional journals, such as those listed in the references.

REFERENCES

Beck, A.T. (1967). *Depression: Clinical, experimental, and theoretical aspects.* New York: Harper & Row.

Beck, A.T., Ward, C., Mendelson, M., Mock, J., & Erbaugh, J. (1961). An inventory for measuring depression. *Archives of General Psychiatry, 4,* 561–571.

Ben-Yishay, Y., Silver, S.M., Piasetsky, E., & Rattok, J. (1987). Relationship between employability and vocational outcome after intensive holistic cognitive rehabilitation. *The Journal of Head Trauma Rehabilitation, 2,* 35–48.

Bishop, D., & Miller, I. (1988). Traumatic brain injury: Empirical assessment techniques. *The Journal of Head Trauma Rehabilitation, 3*(4), 16–30.

Brenner, H. (1976). *Estimating the social costs of economic policy: Implications for mental health, physical health, and criminal aggression* (Report prepared for the Joint Economic Committee of the United States Congress). Washington, DC: United States Government Printing Office.

Brooks, N., Campsie, L., Symington, C., Beattie, A., & McKinlay, W. (1986). The five year outcome of severe blunt head injury: A relative's view. *Journal of Neurology, Neurosurgery, and Psychiatry, 49*, 764–770.

Brooks, N., McKinlay, W., Symington, C., Beattie, A., & Campsie, L. (1987). Return to work within the first seven years of severe head injury. *Brain Injury, 1*(1), 5–19.

Cahalan, D., & Cisin, I. (1968). American drinking practices: Summary of findings from a national probability sample: Extent of drinking by population subgroups. *Quarterly Journal of Studies on Alcohol, 29*, 130–151.

Dahlstrom, W.G., Welsh, G.S., & Dahlstrom, L.E. (1972). *An MMPI handbook* (Vol. 1). Minneapolis: University of Minnesota Press.

Doherty, K., Kreutzer, J., & Harris, J. (1989, June). *Incidence and characteristics of antisocial behavior pre- and post-brain injury*. Paper presented at the 13th Annual Postgraduate Course on the Rehabilitation of the Brain Injured Adult and Child, Williamsburg, VA.

Epstein, N., Bishop, D., & Levin, S. (1978). The McMaster model of family functioning. *Journal of Marriage and Family Counseling, 4*, 19–31.

Gardner, R.A. (1973). *The family book about minimal brain dysfunction*. New York: Jason Aronson.

Graham, J.R. (1987). *The MMPI: A practical guide* (2nd ed.). New York: Oxford University Press.

Jacobs, H.E. (1988). The Los Angeles Head Injury Survey: Procedures and initial findings. *Archives of Physical Medicine and Rehabilitation, 69*, 425–431.

Kozloff, R. (1987). Networks of social support and the outcome from severe head injury. *The Journal of Head Trauma Rehabilitation, 2*(3), 14–23.

Levin, H.S., Benton, A.L., & Grossman, R.G. (1982). *Neurobehavioral consequences of closed head injury*. New York: Oxford University Press.

Lewis, D., Pincus, J., Feldman, M., Jackson, L., & Bard, B. (1986). Psychiatric, neurological, and psychoeducational characteristics of 15 death row inmates in the United States. *American Journal of Psychiatry, 143*(7), 838–845.

Lezak, M.D. (1978). Living with the characterologically altered brain-injured patient. *Journal of Clinical Psychiatry, 39*, 592–598.

Lezak, M.D. (1986). Psychological implications of traumatic brain damage for the patient's family. *Rehabilitation Psychology, 31*, 241–250.

Lezak, M. (1987). Relationships between personality disorders, social disorders, social disturbances, and physical disability following traumatic brain injury. *The Journal of Head Trauma Rehabilitation, 2*(1), 57–69.

Livingston, M.G., Brooks, D.N., & Bond, M.R. (1985). Patient outcome in the year following severe head injury and relatives' psychiatric and social functioning. *Journal of Neurology, Neurosurgery, and Psychiatry, 48*, 876–881.

Mandelberg, I., & Brooks, D. (1975). Cognitive recovery after severe head injury: 1. Serial testing on the Wechsler Adult Intelligence Scale. *Journal of Neurology, Neurosurgery, and Psychiatry, 38*, 1121–1126.

Mauss-Clum, N., & Ryan, M. (1981). Brain injury and the family. *Journal of Neurosurgical Nursing, 13*(4), 165–169.

McKinlay, W., Brooks, D., Bond, M., Martinage, D., & Marshall, M. (1981). The short term outcome of severe blunt head injury as reported by relatives of the injured persons. *Journal of Neurology, Neurosurgery, and Psychiatry, 44*, 527–533.

Moos, R., & Moos, B. (1974). *Family Environment Scale: Manual*. Palo Alto, CA: Consulting Psychologists Press.

Oddy, M., Coughlan, T., Tyerman, A., & Jenkins, D. (1985). Social adjustment after closed head injury: A further follow-up seven years after injury. *Journal of Neurology, Neurosurgery, and Psychiatry, 48*, 564–568.

Olson, D., Portner, J., & Lavee, Y. (1985). *FACES:III*. Family Social Science, University of Minnesota, Minneapolis, MN.

Rimel, R., Giordani, B., Barth, J., & Jane, J. (1982). Moderate head injury: Completing the clinical spectrum of brain trauma. *Neurosurgery, 11*(3), 344–351.

Rohe, D., & DePompolo, R. (1985). Substance abuse policies in rehabilitation medicine departments. *Archives of Physical Medicine and Rehabilitation, 66*, 701–703.

Romano, M.D. (1974). Family response to traumatic brain injury. *Scandinavian Journal of Rehabilitation Medicine, 6*, 1–4.

Rosenthal, M., & Young, T. (1988). Effective family intervention after traumatic brain injury: Theory and practice. *The Journal of Head Trauma Rehabilitation, 3*(4), 42–50.

Schontz, F.F. (1975). *The psychological aspects of physical illness and disability*. New York: Macmillan.

Selzer, M., Gomberg, E., & Nordhoff, J. (1979). Men's and women's responses to Michigan Alcoholism Screening Test. *Journal of Studies on Alcohol, 40*, 502–504.

Snaith, R., Bridge, G., & Hamilton, M. (1976). The Leeds Scales for the self assessment of anxiety and depression. *British Journal of Psychiatry, 128*, 156–165.

Sparadeo, F.R., & Gill, D. (1989). Effects of prior alcohol use on head injury recovery. *The Journal of Head Trauma Rehabilitation, 4*(1), 75–82.

Thomas, J.P. (1988). The evolution of model systems of care in traumatic brain injury. *The Journal of Head Trauma Rehabilitation, 3*(4), 1–5.

Thomsen, I.V. (1984). Late outcome of severe blunt head trauma: a 10–15 year follow-up. *Journal of Neurology, Neurosurgery, and Psychiatry, 47*, 260–268.

Wehman, P., Kreutzer, J., Stonnington, H., Wood, W., Sherron, P., Diambra, J., Fry, R., & Groah, C. (1988). Supported employment for persons with traumatic brain injury: A preliminary report. *The Journal of Head Trauma Rehabilitation, 3*(4), 82–94.

Winegarden, D., Simonetti, J., & Nykodyn, N. (1984). Unemployment: "The living death?" *Journal of Employment Counseling, 21*, 149–155.

Zung, B., & Charalampous, K. (1975). Item analysis of the Michigan Alcoholism Screening Test. *Journal of Studies on Alcohol, 36*, 127–132.

Zung, B. (1970). Psychometric properties of the MAST and two briefer versions. *Journal of Studies on Alcohol, 40*, 845–850.

Chapter 4

The Role of the Physiatrist

Nathan D. Zasler

The Physiatrist (Fiz-ē-at'-rist), or specialist in Physical Medicine and Rehabilitation, is a physician concerned with the functional restoration of persons who are physically and/or cognitively challenged. The physiatrist's approach is holistic, relying heavily on a strong knowledge base in both the basic and clinical sciences. In the classic model of rehabilitative team care, the physiatrist serves as the team leader to optimize consolidation of the group's effort and maximize functional restoration of the brain injured person. Maximum interaction and problem solving are the goals of all team members, including physiatrist, nurse, physical therapist, occupational therapist, speech-language pathologist, recreational therapist, cognitive therapist, neuropsychologist, dietitian, pharmacist, social worker, case manager, and chaplain.

The care of traumatically brain injured persons by a physiatrist seems only natural in terms of the types of deficits these individuals incur and their resultant functional impairments, sometimes lifelong. A skilled brain injury rehabilitationist must have a good command of the latest developments in internal medicine, neurology, orthopedics, neurosurgery, psychiatry, and rehabilitation medicine. This broad base of scientific and clinical knowledge puts the physiatrist in a good position to direct the postacute and chronic care of the traumatically brain injured person. The complexity of the diagnostic and therapeutic interventions employed by the physiatrist will vary with the severity of the brain injury and the resultant neurological and functional deficits.

A well-structured rehabilitation program for traumatic brain injury must consider all aspects of care, including the composition and quality of staff, diversity of the program (i.e., acute, postacute, community reintegration, etc.), and the patient population it wishes to serve (i.e., severity of injury and compensation status). If we do not address *all* issues related to the traumatic brain injury, then we have failed to approach the problem from a holistic standpoint and thereby have failed to maximize the potential outcome. This ultimately results in greater burdens on the brain injured person, the family, and society. The best way to meet this challenge is through early and intensive intervention, preferably using a specialized brain injury rehabilitation unit under the direction of a physiatrist skilled in this area of rehabilitation.

Given that the incidence of traumatic brain injury has reached epidemic proportions in the United States—200 head injuries per 100,000 population per year (Krauss, Black, and Hessol, 1984) with an estimated 500,000 annual hospital admissions for head injury, of which 50,000 are left with significant long-term disability—it seems only logical that every effort should be made to provide an appropriate system of care encompassing all phases of treatment, both neurosurgical and rehabilitative, for every brain injury survivor.

MECHANISMS OF TRAUMATIC BRAIN INJURY

Before one can understand the consequences of traumatic brain injury on vocational pursuits, one must have a basic understanding of traumatic brain injury itself. Traumatic brain injury can be penetrating (open) or nonpenetrating (closed). Open brain injury typically occurs secondary to gunshot wounds. The resultant functional impairments being generally related to the area of the brain most severely affected. Closed brain injury occurs when there are acceleration and deceleration forces applied to the head, particularly when these are rotational. The three major categories of brain injury that can result from such trauma, specifically, focal cortical contusion, diffuse axonal (nerve) injury (DAI), and hypoxic ischemic injury, are related to the temporal sequence of sequelae, the mechanism of injury, and the clinical presentation (Adams, 1984). Injury can be classified as primary, occurring at the moment of injury, or secondary, occurring at some point post-injury. Primary brain injury occurs secondary to focal or localized brain damage (i.e., cortical contusions) and DAI. The areas of the brain most susceptible to focal injury are the frontal and temporal tips. This is felt to be due to the manner in which they come into contact with the surface of skull, thereby predisposing them to contusional injury. DAI occurs secondary to centripetal shearing forces that occur as the brain is accelerated/decelerated. The areas of the brain most likely to be damaged secondary to DAI are the corpus callosum and mesencephalon (Adams, Graham, Scott, Parker, & Doyle, 1980; Auerbach, 1986). In general, areas of transition between gray and white matter tend to be predisposed to DAI.

Brain stem structures are not immune to damage in traumatic brain injury; DAI and focal contusions can readily occur in this area (especially with rotational forces). Important causes of secondary brain injury that must be addressed as early as possible to minimize further cerebral damage include intracranial hematomas, brain edema, intracranial pressure elevations, hypoxia, and hydrocephalus.

PROGNOSIS AND FUNCTIONAL ASSESSMENT

The initial severity of brain injury can suggest long-term functional outcome. However, it is still impossible to predict outcome accurately enough to allocate resources for acute neurosurgical care and subsequent rehabilitative efforts. In general, the initial severity of injury is judged by the Glasgow Coma Scale (GCS) score (Teasdale & Jennett, 1974), which is also predictive of functional outcome. The scale uses three clinical parameters to measure initial severity of injury: eye opening, best verbal response, and best motor response. The individual scores are summed and can total from 3 to 15 points. A score of 3 to 8 indicates severe injury, 9 to 12 indicates moderate injury, and 13 to 15 implies minor injury. The duration of coma as well as post-traumatic amnesia (PTA) are theoretically tied to the extent/severity of brain injury, specifically to the magnitude of diffuse axonal injury. These factors and numerous others, including the patient's age, brain-stem findings, brain scans, evoked potential responses, and mechanism of injury, all influence outcome (Becker, Miller, & Greenberg, 1982).

Most neurosurgeons examining functional outcome in traumatic brain injury have used the Glasgow Outcome Scale (GOS). The GOS is composed of five categories: death, persistent vegetative state, severe disability, moderate disability, and good recovery (Jennett & Bond, 1975). The GOS has been shown to have poor sensitivity to functionally significant changes and to have suboptimal inter-rater reliability, thereby decreasing its validity (Maas, Braakman, Schouten, Minderhoud, & Van Zomeren, 1983). Functional scales developed to address the GOS shortcomings include the Disability Rating Scale (Rappaport, Hall, Hopkins, Belleza, & Cope, 1984) and Patient Evaluation Conference System (PECS) (Harvey & Jellinek, 1981). The result is there are no reliable tools available that allow the rehabilitationist to accurately predict which patient may or may not be capable of returning to work and, just as importantly, when a particular patient might be ready to return to work. At present, the prediction of vocational reintegration potential remains an educated clinical guess. A greater ability to predict the quality of vocational reintegration is the goal of continued research into and examination of parameters most highly correlated with successful vocational reintegration.

ONGOING INTERVENTION

Planning work reentry for the traumatic brain injured survivor really starts at the scene of the accident and never really stops until full vocational reintegration has occurred. If one considers all the potential morbidity factors associated with a traumatic brain injury and how these factors can potentially impair return to work, it is not at all unreasonable to advocate close monitoring and treatment from the day of the accident on. Early rehabilitative intervention has been proven without question to minimize morbidity and overall costs as well as maximize functional outcome (Cope & Hall, 1982). Yet even with early intervention, the sequelae of a traumatic brain injury can still be devastating and result in significant functional impairment, including the inability to return to gainful employment (Vogenthaler, 1987).

The skilled physiatrist can significantly decrease the functional/neurological morbidity and costs associated with traumatic brain injury, regardless of its severity, if ongoing care is provided to the injured person. Interventions can be directed to all areas of deficit, including medical, neurophysical, cognitive, and behavioral spheres. The relative permanency of many of the deficits incurred make it important to continue physiatric rehabilitative efforts even after the termination of acute inpatient rehabilitation. Unfortunately, many patients are lost to physiatric and general medical follow-up after discharge from acute brain injury rehabilitation programs. This is particularly true when there is not a structured continuum of care in place that secures adequate follow-up and/or when family support systems are lacking. All too often, a patient suffers medically, neurologically, psychosocially, and vocationally because of this breakdown in the provision of ongoing rehabilitative care.

POST-TRAUMATIC EPILEPSY

There are numerous neurological sequelae that can result from a traumatic brain injury and compromise work reentry. Probably the one with the greatest stigma attached to it is post-traumatic epilepsy (PTE). The patient who is diagnosed as having PTE often is considered unjustifiably an inappropriate candidate for work reentry. The incidence of PTE following traumatic brain injury is low (approximately 5 percent) and increases with the severity of the brain injury (Jennett, 1983). The pathogenesis of early and late seizures is thought to be quite different. Early seizures (during the first week postinjury) reflect acute pathophysiological changes such as edema, hypoxia, and increased intracranial pressure, whereas late seizures are theorized to be secondary to formation of scar tissue in the brain. PTE can take many forms, but most commonly is either of a partial nature or of a primary generalized/multifocal nature.

Risk factors for PTE include early seizures, depressed skull fractures, dural penetrations, presence of focal neurological findings, and intracranial hematomas (Jennett, 1975, 1983). A study questioning these risk factors indicated that the duration of coma was the strongest predictor of PTE and probably reflected the extent of gross brain injury secondary to DAI (Guidice & Berchou, 1987). Several authors have developed predictive formulas for PTE that allow the physician to calculate the overall risk for seizures at any particular time postinjury given the patient's risk factors (Feeney & Walker, 1979; Weiss, Salazar, Vance, Grafman, & Jabbari, 1986).

While most cases of PTE can be controlled with anticonvulsant medication, some rare cases are intractable to pharmacologic intervention. PTE has both cognitive and emotional consequences that can be totally unrelated to side effects of anticonvulsant medication, although this must always be taken into consideration (Bennett, 1987). Because anticonvulsants such as phenobarbital and phenytoin can suppress cognitive function (Reynolds, 1983; Trimble, 1987), it is critical for the physiatrist to have a working knowledge of these agents and their side effects. The drugs of choice for PTE are carbamazepine for partial seizures and valproic acid for primary generalized seizure disorders (Glenn, 1986; Pellock, 1989). Additional parameters for deciding on seizure medication include dosage schedules and cost.

Work restrictions also must be assessed relative to PTE risk. For example, the patient who incurred a brain injury secondary to a gunshot wound and has a PTE risk of 45 percent would best be advised not to return to work as a window washer and to seek an alternative and safer occupation.

The issue of restrictions regarding alcohol consumption after traumatic brain injury, specifically as it relates to those at high risk for post-traumatic seizures, is wrought with major misconceptions and medico-legal implications. Although it is a common perception that patients with epilepsy, regardless of etiology, experience problems with seizure control if they use alcohol, experimental studies testing this belief do not support it (Hauser, Ng, & Brust, 1988). Because the interaction of alcohol, seizures, and epilepsy is not yet completely clear, a more conservative approach to recommendations/restrictions on alcohol consumption following traumatic brain injury is indicated.

Driving can be important to work reentry. The medico-legal and social issues regarding PTE and driving capabilities are vast, but proper documentation of adequate seizure work-up, treatment, and patient/family education on seizure risk is essential regardless of state laws. Most states require a patient to be seizure free for 6 months before driving, and then only with medical clearance. Other deficits in brain injured patients that can affect driving skills include poor judgment of traffic situations, impulsiveness, and visuospatial impairments (Van Zomeren, Brouwer, & Minderhoud, 1987). Proper driver screening evaluations are essential for the brain injured person to guarantee personal safety and the safety of others. Various evaluative procedures, such as the Cognitive Behavioral Driver's Inventory (CBDI) (Engum, Cron, Hulse, Pendergrass, and Lambert, 1988), have been proposed to more critically and objectively assess driving skills after traumatic brain injury. Further critical assessment of the skills needed for successful and safe driving, however, is needed if we are to accurately decide who can and cannot drive after traumatic brain injury. In the meantime, we must err on the side of being overly conservative in restricting persons who possess questionable driving capabilities. Such restrictions protect the client and society, as well as, the rehabilitation team (Beresford, 1988).

The issue of restricted driving can present a major obstacle to work reentry unless alternative transportation can be provided, such as public transportation, family/friends, carpooling, or walking.

POST-TRAUMATIC HYDROCEPHALUS

Post-traumatic hydrocephalus (PTH), like PTE, is one of the few neurological conditions that can result in functional deterioration after traumatic brain injury. PTH patients typically had intraventricular or subarachnoid hemorrhages during the acute period. These hemorrhages may lead to aberrations in the absorption of cerebrospinal fluid (CSF) and resultant neurological deterioration. The typical presentation of PTH is normal pressure hydrocephalus (NPH) with gait apraxia, dementia, and urinary incontinence. Various diagnostic tests (such as the CSF tap test, CSF compliance studies, magnetic resonance imaging [MRI] with brain water mapping, serial brain scans, and cisternography) have been used to determine which patients with hydrocephalus might benefit from treatment via shunting procedures (Katz, Brander, & Sahgal, 1989). It is critical for the physiatrist to understand that PTH can present in many different ways (Beyerl & Black, 1984). Although its incidence is only 1 percent to 8 percent in traumatic brain injury (Grosswasser, Cohen, Reider-Grosswasser, & Stern, 1988; Gudeman et al., 1981), PTH should always be considered in the differential diagnosis of a patient who deteriorates neurologically or functionally at any time postinjury.

OLFACTORY DYSFUNCTION

The effect of cranial nerve injuries in traumatic brain injury is underestimated with regard to their potential functional consequences. Any cranial nerve can be damaged secondary to brain injury.

A common deficit resulting from cranial nerve injury is anosmia (loss of sense of smell), which may occur in as many as 25 percent of moderate to severe brain injuries. Sense of smell is mediated by the first cranial nerve that has its cortical representation in the frontal and temporal lobes. Anosmia can result from tearing of the olfactory nerves secondary to shearing forces or from frontal cortical injury secondary to focal contusion (Costanzo & Becker, 1986).

From a functional standpoint, anosmia can affect work reentry in terms of safety issues (i.e., the ability to smell chemical leaks, gas, or smoke), general hygiene, and ability to cook. In addition, post-traumatic anosmia is a strong clinical indicator of orbital frontal injury and can correlate with psychosocial deficits and poor vocational reintegration (Varney, 1988). Various artificial noses are being developed to help anosmic persons detect noxious odors (these are generally mediated via the fifth cranial nerve). Work reentry recommendations from the physiatrist need to consider the prognosis for recovery from anosmia (generally believed to be 50 percent) and the importance of intact olfaction in a job setting.

VISUAL DEFICITS

Visual problems, common after traumatic brain injury, can have a significant impact on the patient's ability to reintegrate into the workplace. Visual acuity can be compromised by injury to the second cranial nerve (the optic nerve) and usually occurs within the first week postinjury. An integrated visual rehabilitation program consisting of neuro-ophthalmologic, ophthalmologic, optometric, occupational therapy, and physiatric intervention is important considering the functional morbidity of such injuries (Gianutsos, Ramsey, & Perlin, 1988). Visual field deficits, such as homonymous hemianopsia (loss of half of each visual field), are common with temporal lobe and/or occipital lobe injuries due to interruption of the optic radiations. These deficits may not be appreciated by the brain injured person. Other visual deficits resulting from traumatic brain injury can include blindness, color vision problems, photophobia (sensitivity to light), scotomas (blind spots), and various eye movement disorders. All these deficits can potentially affect an individual's work performance, even compromising safety or work efficiency. The physiatrist should direct the visual rehabilitation of the patient, including optometric clinical management—low vision devices, polycarbonate lenses, absorptive lenses, or prismatic corrections (Tierney, 1988). For cranial nerves 3, 4, and 6, new ophthalmologic surgical techniques are being used to correct extraocular muscle imbalances secondary to post-traumatic neuropathy (nerve injury). The efficacy of botulinum toxin for treatment of post-traumatic extraocular imbalances remains experimental.

AUDIOVESTIBULAR DYSFUNCTION

Deficits in auditory and vestibular function are also common after head injury, especially with longitudinal fractures of temporal bones. Sequelae include sensorineural hearing loss, conductive hearing loss, tinnitus (not common in severe injuries), and post-traumatic vestibular dysfunction (Sakai & Mateer, 1984). Proper screening, diagnosis, and treatment of these deficits can be critical to work reentry success. Hearing aids may benefit certain patients, and education on noise level protection for the good ear is critical. Tinnitus has been treated with sound-masking devices and biofeedback. Dizziness secondary to vestibular dysfunction on a peripheral basis can be treated with pharmacological agents, such as meclizine, dimenhydrinate, and scopolamine. The physiatrist must be aware of the sedating properties of these medications and their potential for cognitive suppression. Physical therapy interventions, such as labyrinthine exercises, can also be incorporated into treatment. Traumatically brain injured patients often complain of balance problems, which are not always secondary to post-traumatic vestibular neuropathy. They may be due to dysfunction of the autonomic, proprioceptive, visual, and/or cerebellar systems or simply to the sensory integration of their summated input. Objective testing via posturography can clarify the cause of balance dysfunction via dynamic computerized multisystem tests and guide the physiatrist in physical therapy prescription (Tangeman & Wheeler, 1986) as it may pertain to balance function in the work place.

OROPHARYNGEAL DYSFUNCTION

Oropharyngeal control can be affected adversely secondary to injuring cranial nerves 9 and 10. Because most competitive employment requires the individual to communicate at work, the physiatrist may need to offer treatment options for the patient with communication/swallowing dysfunction. It should be noted that isolated injury to these nerves is rare and that sequelae like dysphonia (difficulty speaking) also can occur at a cortical level. Traumatic injury to the last four cranial nerves (Collet-Sicard syndrome) is generally associated with gunshot injuries (Mohanty, Barrios, Fishbone, & Khatib, 1973). These patients often will require intestinal feeding secondary to clinically significant aspiration risk. Prolonged oral transit times and delayed swallowing reflexes are common in severely injured patients (Field & Weiss, 1989). They may also have problems with excessive salivation and poor vocal cord closure. Excessive salivation can be treated with anticholinergics, but adverse cognitive side effects make them a last ditch effort. A patient's voice quality and airway protection can improve after injection of Gelfoam or Teflon into the paretic vocal cords. Dopamine agonists have been used to treat dysphagia (difficulty swallowing), but further controlled trials are needed in this treatment area (Rucker, Zasler, Narasimhachari, Biewen, & Cockrell, 1988). The physiatrist must understand pharmacologic and nonpharmacologic interventions and their recommended timing postinjury to maximize spontaneous recovery without compromising the patient's functional status for extended periods.

COMMUNICATION DEFICITS

Numerous other communication deficits aside from vocal cord dysfunction can adversely affect the brain injured person's ability to reenter the workplace. These include dysphasia (deficit in expressive/receptive language), dysprosody (deficit in ability to comprehend/express emotional content in language), dysarthria (unclear speech due to weakness of oral musculature), and oromotor dyspraxia (inability to properly coordinate the motor planning of movements related to speech). Many of these deficits will improve over time, but therapy by a speech-language pathologist can help support recovery and teach patients to compensate. Pharmacotherapy with dopamine agonists is a reported treatment of dysphasia, but further research is being conducted to clarify its role (Bachman & Morgan, 1988).

BOWEL AND BLADDER DYSFUNCTION

Bowel and bladder dysfunction can obviously impair one's ability for vocational reintegration. Persons with traumatic brain injury and associated frontal lobe injury commonly suffer from urinary urgency and incontinence secondary to disinhibition of detrusor musculature. Proper bowel management is important to avoid extremes of stool consistency (resulting in diarrhea or constipation). The physiatrist needs to be aware of appropriate treatment, including diet, fluid intake, defecation schedules, and pharmacologic intervention—hopefully coordinated so as to not interfere with vocational pursuits.

VISUOPERCEPTUAL DEFICITS

Visuoperceptual and attentional disorders resulting from traumatic brain injury can compromise an individual's capability to return to competitive employment. These attention disorders can interfere with timely recognition and processing of environmental cues, limiting work performance. Symptoms, appearing alone or in clusters, can represent involvement of the sensory/perceptual, motor/intentional, and attentional systems. The physiatrist and the rehabilitation team must know assessment techniques to prescribe appropriate remediation for these deficits. For assessment purposes, the categories are sensory losses and visual fields cuts, hemi-inattention and hemispatial neglect, hemiperceptual deficits, and gaze and visual pursuit problems.

Research on therapeutic interventions for hemi-inattention, conducted at the New York University Institute of Rehabilitation Medicine, has shown benefits to visual scanning training, cancellation training, and somatosensory awareness training (Gordon et al., 1985). Pharmacotherapy with dopamine agonists for hemi-inattention and neglect also have been reported (Fleet, Valenstein, Watson, & Heilman, 1987; Zasler & McNeny, 1989).

Finally, a study concluded that nonpharmacologic treatments of acquired visuoperceptual disorders can indeed result in functional improvements related to increased capability for independent living (Gouvier, Webster, & Warner, 1986). Various remediation programs have been developed for training attention to task in both the auditory and visual spheres (Wood, 1986) and for remediating higher order reasoning skills, constructional dyspraxias, topographical disorientation, and memory deficits (Jurko & Smith, 1981).

NEUROPSYCHOLOGICAL ISSUES

Ongoing neuropsychological intervention for cognitive deficits (such as memory and organization problems) resulting from traumatic brain injury should be considered for any patient with such persistent deficits that functionally compromise the potential for work reentry. A proliferation of clinical studies in recent years shows the efficacy of neuropsychological rehabilitation (Bleiberg, Cope, & Spector, 1989; Gordon, Hibbard, & Kreutzer, 1989). The physiatrist also can maximize cognitive performance by offering various pharmacologic interventions, including nonadrenergic agonists, dopaminergic agonists, cholinergic agonists, nootropics, and neuropeptides. There is probably no "magic bullet" as far as drug intervention. However, further research currently is underway to elucidate clinical parameters that may support use of particular agents for remediation of cognitive dysfunction.

In the workplace, compensatory strategies can maximize work performance with regard to cognitive skills. Simple measures such as keeping a memory log book can help those with memory dysfunction. Cognitive prostheses in the form of hand-held computers have also been used to help the patient reenter the work environment more easily. Research is ongoing to develop more advanced cognitive prostheses to aid individuals with memory, organization, initiation, learning, and other neurobehavioral skills (Conder & Allen, 1982). These miniature computers may eventually be integral to state-of-the-art cognitive remediation programs.

BEHAVIORAL DYSFUNCTION

Behavioral issues may adversely affect work reentry potential (Brooks, McKinlay, Symington, Beattie, & Campsie, 1987). Various behavioral management techniques are available. To maximize success of behavioral modification techniques used in the work setting, the rehabilitation team must integrate appropriate conditioning procedures into the process and fully recognize the patient's cognitive limits. To adequately treat unacceptable behavior, the treatment team must first identify all variables associated with the undesirable behavior, including frequency, triggering factors, temporal relationships, and consequences. Many pharmacologic agents have been used in attempts to control pathological behavioral disorders resulting from traumatic brain injury. While neuroleptics are agents of choice for managing behavioral problems associated with organic brain disease, much scientific data support the policy of avoiding these drugs in patients with traumatic brain injury. Neuroleptics' significant anticholinergic and dopaminergic antagonist activity, potential adverse effects on the quality of neural recovery after brain injury, and significant long-term side effects bespeak against their general use in this patient population. Other classes of drugs that show better promise for treatment of behavioral dysfunction after traumatic injury include stimulants, antidepressants, anticonvulsants, lithium carbonate, and atypical agents like beta-blockers, amino acids, hormonal agents, and calcium-channel blockers (Horn, 1987).

Proper pharmacologic management of behavioral disorders may be critical to successful vocational reintegration. Therefore, the physiatrist must have a firm grasp of principles of psychopharmacologic therapy and potential drug interactions and side effects. Numerous over-the-counter medications (cough and cold formulas being most notorious), alcohol, and tobacco can interact adversely with prescribed medications for behavioral dysfunctions to cause medical problems like seizures, sedation, cognitive dysfunction, and behavioral disruption. Patients and employers must be educated to such potential complications to avoid jeopardizing job security.

SEXUALITY ISSUES

Inappropriate sexual behavior is common after moderate to severe brain injury and is obviously unacceptable in the workplace. The literature on psychosexual dysfunction after traumatic brain injury is relatively scarce, although a recent study found a fairly high incidence of negative changes in sex drive, erectile function, and frequency of intercourse (Kreutzer & Zasler, 1989). Hyposexuality is more common than hypersexuality, but some patients are sexually inappropriate on the basis of disinhibition rather than true hypersexuality. Disinhibition is generally associated with frontal lobe injury; true hypersexuality is theorized to be related to limbic or diencephalic damage.

Social skills training and behavioral modification techniques can help diminish some of these inappropriate behaviors. Hormonal agents and serotonergic agonists can be utilized for treatment of libidinal changes.

NEUROPHYSICAL DEFICITS

Motor/coordination deficits that can occur are spasticity, ataxia, tremor, dyskinesias (abnormal movement), and dystonias (abnormal muscle tone). These neurophysical sequelae can markedly impair a traumatically brain injured individual's ability to reintegrate into the workforce. Spasticity, for example, can compromise the brain injured person's efficiency with ambulation, wheelchair mobility, and upper extremity function.

The physiatrist should play a major role in treatment, which should be algorithmic and include removal of nociceptive stimuli potentially exacerbating the spasticity, physical modalities, oral medications, chemical neurolysis (nerve blocks and motor point blocks), orthopedic procedures, and neurosurgical procedures.

Physical and occupational therapy staff can decrease the effects of neurophysical deficits through neurophysiological mechanisms including orthotic devices (Montgomery, 1987), compensatory strategies, and adaptive/assistive equipment. Pharmacological agents are being used to treat neurophysical sequelae, including ataxia, dystonia, tremor, myoclonus, and dyskinesias. This author has utilized 5-hydroxytryptophan with relatively good success for treatment of cerebellar ataxia in traumatic brain injured persons, and others have reported similar findings (Trouillas, Brudon, & Adeleine, 1988). The drug treatment of spasticity is still quite controversial. Most physiatrists avoid use of Valium because of sedating properties and resultant cognitive suppression and use baclofen sparingly because of its central action and potential for sedation. Dantrolene sodium, which is peripherally acting, may be a more appropriate agent in this patient population due to its relative lack of sedation. All antispasticity medications have side effects, both cognitive and otherwise, so it is critical for patients receiving such medications to obtain proper medical follow-up. Further research is needed on the clinical indications and contraindications for drug therapy of these numerous neurophysical deficits so that functional capabilities can be maximized and potential side effects minimized.

ORTHOPEDIC ISSUES

Because orthopedic sequelae of traumatic brain injury are quite common, any physiatrist should have a solid knowledge base in orthopedic rehabilitation (Botte & Moore, 1987). Management of orthopedic sequelae can be divided into three phases (Garland & Keenan, 1983). In the acute period, musculoskeletal injuries should be diagnosed and treated appropriately. Many fractures and peripheral nerve injuries may go undetected in the acute period postinjury, so adequate neuro-orthopedic assessment is critical. Results of fracture treatment may be complicated by comorbidity factors like spasticity and heterotopic ossification. The preferred method of treatment for long-bone fractures is open reduction and internal fixation. Open reduction and internal fixation is preferable due to potential complications of casting in patients who are at a relatively low neurologic level and/or are agitated.

The subacute period of ongoing neurological and functional recovery may last for several years postinjury, with the vast majority of improvement occurring in the first 18 months postinjury. During this phase, physicians try to avoid major orthopedic complications, such as myostatic contractures, that may later compromise mobility status and vocational reintegration. The incidence of contractures increases with longer duration of coma and typically occurs around the hips, shoulders, and ankles (Yarkony & Sahgal, 1987). Limb positioning and maintenance of range of motion are critical factors in preventing such complications. Physical therapy interventions—such as electrical stimulation of antagonistic muscles, functional electrical stimulation, inhibitive casting, serial casting, range of motion exercises, ultrasound, and icing—can minimize hypertonicity while preventing contractures. The discriminate use of anesthetic and phenol motor point and/or nerve blocks can serve both diagnostic and therapeutic purposes. Limited range of motion at a joint, assuming it is not due to bony ankylosis and/or heterotopic bone, may be due to either myostatic contracture, hypertonicity, or a combination of the two. Anesthetic blocks can allow the skilled physiatrist to assess the contribution of hypertonicity to the range of motion limitations. Such a procedure can help determine the appropriateness of nerve or motor point blocks with phenol for a more definitive and long-lasting diminution in local tone with a resultant increase in range of motion and function (Garland, Lucie, & Waters, 1982; Keenan, 1987). Discriminant use of antispasticity agents may also help (O'Shanick & Zasler, in press).

Once neurological recovery has plateaued, the chronic phase of orthopedic rehabilitation of the brain injured patient begins. More definitive and invasive orthopedic procedures are used for correcting residual limb deformities and excising heterotopic bone. It is felt that clinically significant neurogenic heterotopic ossification, ectopic bone causing pain, or decreased range of motion occurs in approximately 11 percent of traumatic brain injured patients (Garland, Blum, & Waters, 1980). The most common sites of occurrence are the hips, shoulders, elbows, and knees. A low rate of recurrence and good functional results can be expected in patients who have made "good" neurologic recovery at approximately 18 months postinjury

(Garland, 1988). Surgical intervention for spastic limb deformities or fixed contractures generally is not considered until neurologic recovery has plateaued and the patient is no longer making significant functional gains; it should be considered only after more conservative methods of management have failed. Surgery is indicated when there are correctable functional deficits or associated problems with skin care, such as pressure sores or hygiene. Surgical corrections generally consist of tendon release or lengthening procedures for spastic muscle limb deformities and soft tissue releases for fixed contractures. Tendon transfers are reserved for cases of peripheral nerve injury where the transfer involves nonspastic musculature. Transfer of spastic muscles has been found to result in unpredictable functional outcomes and is usually contraindicated (Botte & Keenan, 1987).

Lower extremity orthopedic surgical procedures can be divided into functional versus nonfunctional ones (Smith & Leventhal, 1987). Functional procedures might include hip adductor release, selective quadriceps release, selective hamstring release, and correction of equinovarus deformity; nonfunctional procedures would consist of hip and knee flexion contracture release.

SUMMARY

In conclusion, the physiatrist can and should play a major role in the long-term care of the traumatically brain injured individual. Such a conclusion is justified if one understands the unique holistic perspective that physiatrists have on the care of their patients, in addition to the uniqueness of their rehabilitative training. A skilled physiatrist can assist patients in gaining maximal functional independence through a variety of interventions, thereby optimizing their potential for vocational reintegration.

REFERENCES

Adams, J.H. (1894). Head injury. In J.G. Adams, J.A.N. Corsellis, & L.W. Cuchen (Eds.), *Greenfield's neuropathology* (pp. 85–124). New York: John Wiley.

Adams, J.H., Graham, D.I., Scott, G., Parker, L.S., & Doyle, A.P. (1980). Brain damage in fatal non-missile head injury. *Journal of Clinical Pathology, 33*, 1132–1145.

Auerbach, S.H. (1986). Neuroanatomical correlates of attention and memory disorders in traumatic brain injury: An application of neuro-behavioral subtypes. *The Journal of Head Trauma Rehabilitation, 1*, 1–12.

Bachman, D.L., & Morgan, A. (1988). The role of pharmacotherapy in the treatment of aphasia: Preliminary results. *Aphasiology, 2*, 225–228.

Becker, D.P., Miller, J.D., & Greenberg, R.P. (1982). Prognosis after head injury. In J.R. Youmans (Ed.), *Neurological surgery: A comprehensive reference guide to the diagnosis and management of neurosurgical problems* (pp. 2137–2174). Philadelphia: W.B. Saunders.

Bennett, T.L. (1987, September/October). Post-traumatic epilepsy: Its nature and implications for head injury recovery. *Cognitive Rehabilitation*, pp. 14–18.

Beresford, H.R. (1988). Legal implication of epilepsy. *Epilepsia*, *29*, S114–S121.

Beyerl, B., & Black, P.M. (1984). Post-traumatic hydrocephalus. *Neurosurgery*, *15*, 257–261.

Bleiberg, J., Cope, D.N., & Spector, J. (1989). Cognitive assessment and therapy in traumatic brain injury. *Physical Medicine and Rehabilitation, State of the Art Reviews*, *3*, 95–121.

Botte, M.J., & Keenan, M.A.E. (1987). Reconstructive surgery of the upper extremity in the patient with head trauma. *The Journal of Head Trauma Rehabilitation*, *2*, 34–45.

Botte, M.J., & Moore, T.J. (1987). The orthopedic management of extremity injuries in head trauma. *The Journal of Head Trauma Rehabilitation*, *2*, 13–27.

Brooks, N., McKinlay, W., Symington, C., Beattie, A., & Campsie, L. (1987). Return to work within the first seven years of severe head injury. *Brain Injury*, *1*, 5–19.

Conder, R.L., & Allen, L.M. (1982, November). Individualized memory prosthetic device. Project #R43NS26967-01, NIH Grant.

Cope, D.N., & Hall, K. (1982). Head injury rehabilitation: Benefit of early intervention. *Archives of Physical Medicine and Rehabilitation*, *63*, 433–436.

Costanzo, R.M., & Becker, D.P. (1986). Smell and taste disorders in head injury and neurosurgery patients. In H.L. Meiselman, & R.S. Rivlin (Eds.), *Clinical measurement of taste and smell* (pp. 34–50). New York: Macmillan.

Engum, E.S., Cron, L., Hulse, C.K., Pendergrass, T.M., & Lambert, W. (1988, September/October). Cognitive behavioral driver's inventory. *Cognitive Rehabilitation*, pp. 34–50.

Feeney, D.M., & Walker, A.E. (1979). The prediction of posttraumatic epilepsy. *Archives of Neurology*, *36*, 8–12.

Field, L.H., & Weiss, C.J. (1989). Dysphagia with head injury. *Brain Injury*, *3*, 19–26.

Fleet, W.S., Valenstein, E., Watson, R.T., & Heilman, K.M. (1987). Dopamine agonist therapy for neglect in humans. *Neurology*, *37*, 1765–1770.

Garland, D.E. (1988). Clinical observations on fractures and heterotopic ossification in the spinal cord and traumatic brain injured populations. *Clinical Orthopaedics*, *233*, 86–101.

Garland, D.E., Blum, C.E., & Waters, R.L. (1980). Periarticular heterotopic ossification in head injured adults: Incidence and location. *Journal of Bone Joint Surgery*, *62*, 1143.

Garland, D.E., & Keenan, M.A.E. (1983). Orthopedic strategies in the management of the adult head-injured patient. *Physical Therapy*, *63*, 2004–2009.

Garland, D.E., Lucie, R.S., & Waters, R.L. (1982). Current uses of open phenol nerve block for adult acquired spasticity. *Clinical Orthopaedics*, *165*, 217–222.

Gianutsos, R., Ramsey, G., & Perlin, R.R. (1988). Rehabilitative optometric services for survivors of acquired brain injury. *Archives of Physical Medicine and Rehabilitation*, *69*, 573–578.

Glenn, M.B. (1986). Update on pharmacology: Anticonvulsants for prophylaxis of post traumatic seizures. *The Journal of Head Trauma Rehabilitation*, *1*, 73–74.

Gordon, W.A., Hibbard, M., Egelko, S., Diller, L., Scotzin, M., Lieberman, A., & Ragnarsson, K.T. (1985). Perceptual remediation in patients with right brain damage: A comprehensive program. *Archives of Physical Medicine and Rehabilitation*, *66*, 353–359.

Gordon, W.A., Hibbard, M., & Kreutzer, J.S. (1989). Cognitive remediation: Issues in research and practice. *The Journal of Head Trauma Rehabilitation*, *4*, 3.

Gouvier, W.D., Webster, J.S., & Warner, M.S. (1986). Treatment of acquired visuoperceptual and hemiattentional disorders. *Annals of Behavioral Medicine*, *8*, 15–20.

Grosswasser, A., Cohen, M., Reider-Grosswasser, I., & Stern, M.J. (1988). Incidence, CT findings and rehabilitation outcome of patients with communicative hydrocephalus following severe head injury. *Brain Injury*, *2*, 267–272.

Gudeman, S.K., Kishore, P.R.S., Becker, D.P., Lipper, M.H., Girevendulis, A.K., Jeffries, B.F., & Butterworth, J.F. (1981). Computed tomography in the evaluation of incidence and significance of post-traumatic hydrocephalus. *Neuroradiology, 141*, 397–402.

Guidice, M.A., & Berchou, R.C. (1987). Post-traumatic epilepsy following head injury. *Brain Injury, 1*, 61–64.

Harvey, R.F., & Jellinek, H.M. (1981). Functional performance assessment: A program approach. *Archives of Physical and Medical Rehabilitation, 62*, 456–461.

Hauser, W.A., Ng, K.C., & Brust, J.C.M. (1988). Alcohol, seizures, and epilepsy. *Epilepsia, 29*, S66–S78.

Horn, L.J. (1987). Atypical medications for the treatment of disruptive, aggressive behavior in the brain-injured patient. *The Journal of Head Trauma Rehabilitation, 4*, 18–28.

Jennett, B. (1975). *Epilepsy after non-missile head injuries* (2nd ed.). Chicago: William Heinemann Medical Books.

Jennett, B. (1983). Posttraumatic epilepsy. In M. Rosenthal, E.R. Griffith, et al. (Eds.), *Rehabilitation of the head injured adult.* Philadelphia: F.A. Davis.

Jennett, B., & Bond, M. (1975). Assessment of outcome after severe brain damage. *Lancet, 1*, 480–484.

Jurko, M.F., & Smith, R.R. (1981). Recent developments in brain rehabilitation. *Southern Medical Journal, 74*, 727–730.

Katz, R.T., Brander, V., & Sahgal, V. (1989). Updates on the diagnosis and management of posttraumatic hydrocephalus. *American Journal of Physical Medicine and Rehabilitation, 68*, 91–96.

Keenan, M.A.E. (1987). The orthopedic management of spasticity. *The Journal of Head Trauma Rehabilitation, 2*, 62–71.

Krauss, J.F., Black, M.A., & Hessol, N. (1984). The incidence of acute brain injury and serious impairment in a defined population. *American Journal of Epidemiology, 2*, 186–201.

Kreutzer, J., & Zasler, N.D. (1989). Psychosexual consequences of traumatic brain injury: Methodology and preliminary findings. *Brain Injury, 3*, 177–186.

Kreutzer, J., Wehman, P., Morton, M.V., & Stonnington, H.H. (1988). Supported employment and compensatory strategies for enhancing vocational outcome following traumatic brain injury. *Brain Injury, 2*, 205–223.

Maas, A.I.R., Braakman, R., Schouten, H.J.A., Minderhoud, J.M., & Van Zomeren, A.H. (1983). Agreement between physicians on assessment of outcome following severe head injury. *Journal of Neurosurgery, 58*, 321–325.

Mohanty, S.K., Barrios, M., Fishbone, H., Khatib, R. (1973). Irreversible injury of cranial nerves 9 through 12 (Collet-Sicard syndrome). *Journal of Neurosurgery, 38*, 86–88.

Montgomery, J. (1987). Orthotic management of the lower limb in head injured adults. *The Journal of Head Trauma Rehabilitation, 2*, 57–61.

O'Shanick, G., & Zasler, N.D. (in press). Neuro-psychopharmacological approaches to traumatic brain injury. In J. Kreutzer & P. Wehman (Eds.), *Community integration after traumatic brain injury*. Baltimore: Paul H. Brookes.

Pellock, J.M. (1989). Editorial: Who should receive prophylactic antiepileptic drugs following head injury? *Brain Injury, 3*:107–108.

Rappaport, M., Hall, K.M., Hopkins, K., Belleza, T., & Cope, D.N. (1982). Disability rating scale for severe head trauma: Coma to community. *Archives of Physical Medicine and Rehabilitation, 63*, 118–123.

Reynolds, E.H. (1983). Mental effects of antiepileptic medication: A review. *Epilepsia, 23*, S85–S95.

Rucker, K.S., Zasler, N.D., Narasimhachari, N., Biewen, P.C., & Cockrell, J.L. (1988). Resolution of swallowing disorder with *L*-dopa and evaluation of CSF neurotransmitters in brain injury. *Archives of Physical Medicine and Rehabilitation, 69,* 734.

Sakai, C.S., & Mateer, C.A. (1984). Otological and audiological sequelae of closed head trauma. *Seminars in Hearing, 5,* 157–174.

Smith, C.W., & Leventhal, L. (1987). Surgical treatment of lower extremity deformities in adult head-injured patients. *The Journal of Head Trauma Rehabilitation, 2,* 53–56.

Tangeman, P.T., & Wheeler, J. (1986). Inner ear concussion syndrome: Vestibular implications and physical therapy treatment. *Topics in Acute Care Trauma Rehabilitation, 1,* 72–83.

Teasdale, G., & Jennett, B. (1974). Assessment of coma and impaired consciousness: A practical scale. *Lancet, 2,* 81–83.

Tierney, D.W. (1988). Visual dysfunction in closed head injury. *Journal of the American Optometric Association, 59,* 614–622.

Trimble, M.R. (1987). Anticonvulsant drugs and cognitive function: A review of the literature. *Epilepsia, 28,* S37–S45.

Trouillas, P., Brudon, F., & Adeleine, P. (1988). Improvement of cerebellar ataxia with levorotatory form of 5-hydroxytryptophan. *Archives of Neurology, 45,* 1217–1222.

Van Zomeren, H.H., Brouwer, W.H., & Minderhoud, J.M. (1987). Acquired brain damage and driving: A review. *Archives of Physical Medicine and Rehabilitation, 68,* 697–705.

Varney, N.R. (1988). Prognostic significance of anosmia in patients with closed-head trauma. *Journal of Clinical and Experimental Neuropsychology, 10,* 250–254.

Vogenthaler, D.R. (1987). An overview of head injury: Its consequences and rehabilitation. *Brain Injury, 1,* 113–127.

Weiss, G.H., Salazar, A.M., Vance, S.C., Grafman, J.H., & Jabbari, B. (1986). Predicting posttraumatic epilepsy in penetrating head injury. *Archives of Neurology, 43,* 771–773.

Wood, R.L.I. (1986). Rehabilitation of patients with disorders of attention. *The Journal of Head Trauma Rehabilitation, 3,* 43–53.

Yarkony, G.M., & Sahgal, V. (1987). Contractures. A major complication of craniocerebral trauma. *Clinical Orthopaedics, 219,* 93–96.

Zasler, N.D., & McNeny, R. (1989). Neuropharmacologic rehabilitation following TBI via dopamine agonists. *Archives of Physical Medicine and Rehabilitation.* Manuscript submitted for publication.

Chapter 5

Rehabilitation Engineering and Environmental Modifications

Kali Mallik

Rehabilitation engineering is an application of engineering to improve the quality of life for persons impaired with physical, mental, social, and cognitive disabilities through a rehabilitation team approach combining medical, engineering, counseling, and other related principles.

This field emerged from biomedical engineering because of demands for artificial limbs when soldiers with injuries returned home after World War II. These pioneering efforts resulted in new and improved prostheses (artificial limbs) designs with improved sockets, knee components, and better alignment and fitting practices. But, the application of rehabilitation engineering for persons with severe disabilities in the areas of therapeutic activity in daily living, vocational evaluation, training and job placement, did not start until passage of the 1973 Rehabilitation Act. There is no doubt that the Technology-Related Assistance for Individuals with Disabilities Act of 1988 will impact service delivery systems to optimize the productivity of persons with severe disabilities. This is a federal legislation to expand the availability of assistive technological services and devices for persons with disabilities.

Rehabilitation engineering services can be offered by persons with backgrounds such as industrial designing, carpentry, engineering (e.g., mechanical, electrical, industrial, etc.), occupational therapy, physical therapy, and speech/hearing. These professionals can aid in the rehabilitation process by providing

- a basic working knowledge of mechanical and electrical engineering
- an adequate knowledge of human engineering factors of persons with and without disabilities

- a creativity for cost-effectively solving specific physical, cognitive, and social problems
- a comprehension of aesthetics, so that adaptations, modifications, or custom designs maintain the image of a consumer product
- an ability to work cooperatively with the counselor, other rehabilitation professionals, and persons with disabilities
- a basic knowledge of safety while providing aids and devices

INTERVENTION FOR THERAPY AND EVALUATION

Through evaluation and therapeutic techniques, rehabilitation engineering intervention can have two basic goals: to prevent further deterioration of an individual's physical capabilities (this is reactive) and to enhance an individual's functionality (this is proactive). For example, tissue contractures need an early preventive intervention to make the individual more functional, while cognitive and other training may expedite the rehabilitation process.

Many individuals with traumatic head injury develop spasticity as a result of soft tissue contractures. Passive range-of-motion (ROM), exercise, positioning, and orthotic devices, may be inadequate for maintaining joint motion. Serial casts applied to ankles, elbows, or knees, increase ROM. Casts can be reapplied until an optimum result is achieved (Booth, Doyle, & Montgomery, 1983; Leahy, 1988). When the contracture resists ROM exercises or serial casting, functional surgery is most often directed, followed by serial casts and orthotic devices. Orthosis is mechanical support and bracing of weak or affected joints or muscles to maintain normal or usual position (Garland & Keenman, 1983).

Neuromuscular electrical stimulation (NMES) of a peripherally intact nerve with the subsequent muscle contraction can be an effective means of managing contractures at many joints. This stimulation technique augments the auditory and visual feedback mechanism of facilitating voluntary motor control. It also can temporarily relieve spastic tone.

The Rancho Los Amigo Rehabilitation Engineering Center in Downey, California, reported the following case history using NMES (Baker, Parker, & Sanderson, 1983).

Case Study

A.J., a 22-year-old man, sustained a head injury in a car accident in December 1979. Six months postinjury, he demonstrated a residual spastic left hemiplegia (paralysis of one side of the body) with heterotopic ossification of both hips and the left elbow, which resulted in the use of a wheelchair for his mobility. After attempts with drug therapy and singular lengthening of both the left hamstrings and left Achilles tendons in July 1981, A.J. still used a wheelchair for mobility. In March 1982, he was admitted to Rancho Los Amigos Hospital and testing revealed that he was cognitively alert and oriented, but impaired motor planning and severe ROM limitations interfered with functional activities.

In April, after surgery was performed, A.J. began intensive physical and occupational therapy programs in conjunction with NMES. NMES of the gluteus maximus and quadriceps femoris muscles was done during standing and standing up activities to promote increased hip and knee extension. As the dynamic balance improved, A.J. began to walk in the parallel bars and eventually progressed to a cane.

On September 21, 1982, A.J. was discharged from the hospital to home as an independent ambulator for 400 feet and classified as "independent-to-supervised in bed and transfer activities."

COGNITIVE-PHYSICAL: THE DUAL CHALLENGE

Objective vocational evaluation data of a person with brain injury are sometimes difficult to obtain. This task becomes more complex when a person sustains both cognitive and physical impairments. The evaluator must isolate the physical performance from cognitive and psychological influences. In 1988, the Brain Injury Task Force of the Wisconsin Department of Health and Social Services listed physical, cognitive, and psychosocial impairments that may be associated with persons with head injuries (see Table 5-1).

The Rehabilitation Research and Training Center of Emory University in Atlanta, Georgia, adopted an evaluation technique to measure physical performance of individuals with hemiplegia. The approach, called Methods-Time-Measurement (MTM), puts all physical tasks into the basic groups of grasp, position and release, reach and move, and records them in units of time. After a brief training session, the individuals in the Emory University study (Chyatte & Birdsong, 1971) were divided into four groups, and each one was asked to perform as follows:

- Group A: using the affected hand to perform the tasks
- Group B: using the unaffected hand to perform the tasks
- Group C: using both hands to perform the tasks
- Group D: analyzing the problem mentally, without manual contact

Table 5-1 Impairments Associated with Brain Injury

Physical	*Cognitive*	*Psychosocial*
Speech	Short/Long-Term Memory Loss	Fatigue
Vision	Poor Concentration	Mood Swings
Hearing	Slow Thinking	Denial
Other Sensory Impairments	Short Attention Span	Self-Centeredness/ Agitation
Headaches	Misperception	Anxiety
Lack of Coordination	Communication	Depression
Spasticity of Muscles	Reading Skills	Poor Self-Monitoring
Paralysis of One or Both Sides	Writing Skills	Emotional Lack of Control
	Planning	
Seizure Disorder	Sequencing	Sexual Dysfunction
	Impaired Judgment	
		Restlessness
		Lack of Motivation
		Inability to Cope
		Excessive Laughing or Crying
		Difficulty Relating to Others

Source: From *Final Report of Brain Injury Task Force* by S. Stoffels, 1988, Madison, WI: Department of Health and Human Services.

This comparative evaluation can help isolate specific deficiencies so that a proper engineering technique can be applied in providing aids and devices.

Persons with cognitive and perceptual deficits due to brain injury may need a comprehensive evaluation about their ability to operate an automobile safely. The Rehabilitation Engineering Center of the University of Michigan in Ann Arbor, Michigan, modified a standard electric AMIGO wheelchair to evaluate auditory-motor planning, visual-motor tracking, perceptual-motor planning, divided attention task, and such driving configurations as straightaway, S-curve, figure-eight, and serpentine. Thirteen persons with severe closed head injury were successfully evaluated with the AMIGO wheelchair after such installation as steering wheel, foot-operated acceleration and brake, electric horn, adjustable seat, anti–tip over device, etc. (Kewman & Seigerman, 1983).

All individuals, after eight 2-hour driving sessions, showed substantial improvement in the driving tasks. Preliminary results of the driver education teacher's rating of each individual's operation of an automobile in traffic indicated that three participants improved sufficiently to be recommended for a license.

Cognition Orthosis (COGORTH) is a computerized software medium that can be used for cognitive retraining of many brain injured individuals. COGORTH, a programming language for Apple II personal computers, provides sequential messages that are displayed on a video screen. This guides the individual in completing complex activities. It not only checks an individual's performance errors, but it helps to improve performance. It also provides audiovisual cues to request an individual's attention, as indicated in the following case history (Levine, Krishch, Krueger, & Jaros, 1984):

Case History

Judy, a 28-year-old woman with a wide range of neurocognitive deficits, including severe memory impairments, was evaluated through the use of COGORTH by the Rehabilitation Medical Staff of the University of Michigan in Ann Arbor. During initial trials, Judy was instructed to make two batches of cookies using sequential written instructions only. Judy made many errors during the first session, becoming completely confused. However, she performed the second session, which was based on COGORTH computerized instructional modules, without any errors. The sequential messages helped Judy to complete the step-by-step tasks.

ENVIRONMENTAL MODIFICATION

People whose functional limitations are severe face potential vocational barriers in environments in which they live. Environmental modification provides aids for people or alters their physical surroundings to produce many advantages, including improving their productivity, versatility, and adaptability. In the work environment, these improvements can allow the traumatic brain injured person to perform wider ranges of tasks with less fatigue. This simplification of perceptual, physical, and cognitive tasks also can reduce the time and motion required for job tasks.

Environmental modifications can increase opportunities for participation in the labor market for persons with severe disabilities. This section describes various methods by which people with severe disabilities can be competitively employed at home or at onsite jobs. Specific attention is paid to the use of low-cost, simple adaptations that enhance independent work functioning for gaining access to source documents, improving communications, using office and home equipment, increasing mobility, and easing other activities of daily living (Mallik, 1979). Some adaptive devices, many commercially available, are discussed with relation to specific functional impairments.

Gaining Access to Source Documents

Persons with severe physical impairments due to brain injury have limitations in reach, use wheelchairs for mobility, and must overcome man-made obstacles every day. In an office, such a person faces difficulties in using the surface of a desk and reaching files kept at various heights. The problem is more severe if individuals have limited or no use of their hands, arms, and shoulder muscles or have paralysis of all extremities. Because individuals in these disability groups are most likely to need desk jobs, the ability to reach source documents (the telephone directory, books explaining how to code information, office files, forms, reference books, reports, journal articles, and invoices) is crucial to their vocational success (Mallik & Sablowsky, 1975).

If necessary, suitable modifications should be made so that an individual can reach the documents easily, even with limited functional capabilities (Mallik & Mueller, 1975, 1977). Modifications may include placing file stacks at appropriate height and reach and reducing the height of file cabinets with easy-opening cabinet door mechanisms. Documents on microfilm provide access to information while eliminating the strength and precise manipulation required for lifting heavy documents and turning pages. Information can be programmed into a personal computer and retrieved by using keyboards, voice input devices, sip and puff devices, or an infraray control switch. Adjustable tables/desks can help individuals reach desk surfaces without fatiguing hand and shoulder muscles.

A simple aid for people with limited reach or grasp is an automatic page turner, which holds books or magazines at the proper reading angle and turns one page at a time (forward or backward) with the slightest touch. Once a book is slipped inside the device and the proper angle is adjusted, reading is feasible in bed, in a wheelchair, or at a table. A portable page turner with a rechargeable battery is also available.

Persons with visual impairment can get information through optical aids such as hand magnifying glasses with or without illumination, closed captioned reading machines, or raised letters on file cabinets. An Optacon (a device that scans the character while it outputs a number of pins, which vibrate on the finger tip in accordance to the pattern) has also been used to solve the source document access problems of people with no vision, provided they do not have any loss of tactile stimulation of their fingers. Voice output or Braille output computers may be a solution for many persons.

For people with cognitive limitation, access to documents can be improved through the use of various search techniques, which can be alphabetical, numerical, or chronological or can involve special symbols. For example, a person having problems in reading names or numbers could use various symbols or colors to recognize them.

Communication Aids

The telephone is one of the basic tools through which a person can maintain communication with the community, fellow workers and supervisors. Simple tasks, such as lifting and holding a telephone receiver while dialing, can present a problem for the person with minimal grasp, elbow extension and flexion, and finger strength. A flexible extension (gooseneck) attached to a Touch-Tone phone, which holds the receiver for the person, or a headphone set with a Touch-Tone phone can solve these problems. Communication control systems are available for people who have no use of hand, arm, and shoulder muscles. These systems give unaided access to a telephone, control of a television or radio, control of room lights, and a variety of other functions that can be selected by a tongue control switch, a voice input switch, or a puff/sip (breath control) mechanism.

A person with hearing impairments may face no problem in communicating with others through use of a TTY. With this device, messages are typewritten rather than audible.

Writing is another method of communication that should not be overlooked. If the individual is not able to write due to impaired hand function, then alternative approaches must be explored. The Tenodesis is a hand orthotic device that transfers the function of wrist flexion and extension to the fingers to facilitate pinching and grasping. So equipped, an individual can use electric typewriters (with or without a hand rest or keyboard guard), tape recorders with or without adaptation (which can be used as notebooks), and rubber stamps (which are useful if words need to be printed repeatedly).

Persons who cannot use handwriting as a mode of communication can frequently use a typewriter or word processing equipment. Word processing software with a dictionary helps individuals in checking and correcting spellings.

Many devices exist that can improve certain cognitive dysfunctions as a result of brain injury. Simple, low-cost electronic devices available in toy, electronics, and department stores are

- voice-activated pocket dictaphones—to record ideas and messages that are too important to forget
- electronic calendars—can be programmed to remind persons of special dates, important deadlines, and upcoming annual events

- Language Masters—can save time and effort by increasing accuracy and improving writing, spelling, and comprehension of anyone using the English language
- pocket computers—can remember hundreds of important names, phone numbers, and addresses and store messages
- automatic telephone dialers—can store and dial more than 50 telephone numbers
- rechargeable battery-operated electric razor-size copiers—can scan and copy printed materials (newspaper articles, recipes, job descriptions, etc.) on a two-inch-wide paper roll without toners and chemicals

Using Office and Home Equipment

Many jobs require equipment operation to accomplish one or more tasks, but performance features and control switches on such equipment are not designed for an operator with a disability. Small knobs, for example, are often difficult for an impaired hand to squeeze or turn. If this is the case, a small knob can be replaced by a lever that requires less than manipulation strength and dexterity. Switches can be modified to be activated with only a few ounces of force and can be placed in positions and marked with color codes that minimize fatigue, enhance productivity, and avoid confusion.

Various types of controllers for persons with disabilities are

- chin control (can be worn or fixed in the desired location)
- head control (left/right or forward/backward movement)
- joystick control (electric wheelchairs use this type of control)
- tongue control (activated by tongue movement)
- shoulder control (elevation and depression of shoulder)
- pneumatic control (puff/sip)
- eyelid control (microswitch is mounted on spectacles)
- voice control (unit is trained on individual's voice frequency)
- ultrasonic control (operates remotely by a sound)
- radio control (similar to garage door opener)
- infraray control (operated by infraray light beam)

A pneumatic holding device, for example, can grasp and release a piece that is otherwise difficult for an individual with hemiplegia to hold while operating a drill press. "Hold" and "release" modes can be activated by a microswitch placed at the best location for the worker.

A commercially available environmental control unit permits individuals to operate or control common electrical appliances located in the hospital, home, or office. Wheelchair-based environmental control is also feasible to operate the wheelchair, an orthotic device, a lapboard-mounted tape recorder, a powered recliner, a radio, a respirator, a door opener, or other equipment.

The Speech and Talking Calculator, a hand-held or tabletop electronic calculator that provides audio output for persons with visual impairment, is now available commercially. Persons with visual impairment may find it useful at home, in the classroom, and at work.

Persons who misplace keys can have problems getting to work on time. An electronic keyfinder can help if the miniature receiver is secured to the keychain. One can find the misplaced keychain, within a range of 50 feet, by pressing a little button on a small transmitter. The receiver attached to the keychain signals by beeping.

Mobility

Problems in mobility for persons with physical disabilities vary greatly according to the degree of impairments, but must be overcome for successful work reentry. Deep pile carpeting may make the use of crutches and walkers difficult. The solution to this problem is to cover rugs with plastic mats or get rid of carpeting altogether. Doorway access and doorknob manipulation problems can be solved by widening doorways, reducing door tension, installing an electric door opening/closing mechanism, or replacing doorknobs with levers.

If stair climbing is a problem, then an elevator may be a home solution. A stair glider, an electrically driven chair that glides on a rail installed on one side of a staircase, may be a solution in the environment.

A few steps in front of a house or a building may pose an architectural barrier for a person using a walker, crutches, or a wheelchair. The solution to this problem may be a ramp or a wheelchair lift.

Without the proper selection of a wheelchair, a person may find it difficult to move at work and home. Proper selection not only aids in comfort, but also helps to increase mobility. Variables to consider are diameter of the front wheels, chair size (adult, narrow adult, junior), arm type (fixed, detachable, adjustable, rotating, armless), frame construction (light, heavy, indoor, outdoor), back style (upright, semireclining, full reclining, zipper back, safety belt), foot and leg support (swinging, detachable, permanent, adjustable, ankle strap, toe strap, heel strap), drive (manual, power drive—proportional or microswitch), and wheels (pneumatic, semipneumatic, handrims, plastic-coated handrims).

The individual's need is based on the nature of the impairment, an analysis of how greatly movement is limited, and such problems as susceptibility of skin to breakdown, limited balance, bed sores, or other pain. Persons using wheelchairs may find sitting for a long time on any wheelchair cushion uncomfortable and, therefore, distracting. Many types of commercial wheelchair cushions are available:

- Checker board T-Foam Cushions
- T-Foam Cushions
- "Mud" Cushions
- "Gel" Pads
- "Flotation" Pads
- "ROHO" dry flotation Pads

Long-range mobility depends on the availability of accessible transportation systems. A cab may be used by many people who have manual wheelchairs. Powered wheelchairs, however, are not transported so easily. Persons requiring the use of powered wheelchairs should, if possible, purchase a specialized van equipped with a manual, hydraulic, or electric ramp or lift. Persons with physical impairments may drive a van or regular car using proper hand controls and hand orthotic devices to stabilize the forearm and hand. These devices also increase strength needed to operate the steering wheel and lever for acceleration and brakes. Many persons using manual wheelchairs may find it difficult to load and unload them. An electromechanical device, installed on the top of the car so it receives electrical power from the 12-volt car battery, allows a person to remove or replace a wheelchair without any assistance.

Activities of Daily Living

Activities of Daily Living (ADL) include training in self-care tasks like dressing, bathing, oral hygiene, eating manipulation, mobility, and communication. If a person spends a considerable amount of time and energy doing these activities, then less energy will be left for vocational pursuits. Such an uneven expenditure of energy deprives an individual of the chance to be a productive worker and threatens the success of work reentry. An evaluation of self-care activities assists the rehabilitation professional in determining the client's ability to adapt, compensate for, or perform job tasks optimally.

Many persons with spinal cord injury along with head trauma, may have little or no control of their bladder and use an external urinary catheter. The external male urinary catheter consists of a lightweight latex sheath, secured to a universal connector and accompanied by a high-quality elastic foam strap, to direct urine into a urinary leg bag. External female urinary catheters are available, but require diligent attention to prevent rashes and other skin reactions. Most females use internal catherization.

Persons in wheelchairs having impaired upper extremities find difficulties in transferring from wheelchair to bed, to car, to bathtub, to swimming pool, to and from commode, and so on. Lifts can assist such transfers with minimum assistance.

There are many other commercially available devices that can assist people to be self-sufficient in activities of daily living. Minor modifications or adjustments to these devices to meet individual need can be made by an occupational therapist, a physical therapist, an engineer, a designer, a handyman, or even a family member. The opinions and suggestions of the individual who requires special help are vital in helping to resolve a particular difficulty.

CASE HISTORIES: ILLUSTRATIONS OF RETURN TO WORK

The following brief case histories are examples of solutions that involved extraordinarily simple modifications to help people become productive after their traumatic brain injuries.

1. Bob is a vice president of an instrument company. After his head injury, he has significant difficulty in remembering names of many of his staff, but he knows the people by physical appearance. To initiate telephone communication, pictures of his staff were mounted next to his telephone intercom switches. Bob no longer has difficulty with communications via the telephone. Of course, the perception of accessing information may differ from person to person.

2. Rick is a 29-year-old male who sustained head injury due to a motorcycle accident, which left him paralyzed on the right side. Cognitively, his attention span is slow and he has difficulties remembering telephone numbers. Rick was placed in a reprographics job, where he duplicates, collates, and staples documents. He also is required to place telephone calls when machine servicing is necessary. Using his left functional hand and an electric stapler, he staples documents. For remembering telephone numbers, he uses an electronic phone dialer that stores telephone numbers. He only needs to know which knob to push to make a call.

3. Joe is a 42-year-old male who was hit by a car in 1950. He has been diagnosed as having a closed head injury accompanied by seizure disorders. Joe works at Marriott Inn as a buffet attendant. Due to his memory problems, he sometimes must be told several times about certain duties. Marriott has been very helpful in that respect and has assisted him in

completing his responsibilities with the help of a coworker who acts as a buddy. His seizures are controlled by medication.

4. Darlene is a 32-year-old who sustained spinal cord and head injury due to a diving accident. She uses a wheelchair for mobility. Darlene was offered a position in data entry operations at the U.S. Civil Service Commission. Although the restroom was accessible to her wheelchair, she lacked strength and stamina to transfer to the commode. Commercial transfer aids were inadequate and hand-held urine containers were inappropriate for the sitting position. After exploration of available containers, a laundry detergent bottle was modified for easy use and emptying from the sitting position. The shape of the bottle is an ideal fit with the body contour, after tapering off one side.

SAFETY ENGINEERING

Safety is the major factor that can reduce, if not eliminate, traumatic injuries. Proper use of helmets for motorcycle users and sports players; use of safety belts and installation of air bags in automobiles; safe driving speeds; and diving only in deep water may reduce traumatic brain injury. For some persons with brain injury, precautions may need to be taken to avoid further head injury. The following example will demonstrate the importance of a consumer's input into developing a product to do just this without drawing excessive or disruptive attention to preventing head injury in work and community settings.

The Job Development Laboratory of George Washington (GW) University in Washington, DC, conducted a research project on suitable head protection for persons suffering with seizures or with self-abusive behavior (Mueller, 1980). The investigation found a hockey helmet is well suited. It is washable, well-balanced, provides full protection to the head, and has a hinged face shield to make feeding easier than with conventional fixed-shield helmets. However, this hockey helmet still has the drawback of being quite conspicuous. For noninstitutionalized, seizure-prone persons, especially in the workplace, appearance is a major consideration. Many choose to risk head injury rather than wear an attention-drawing sports helmet. They bear the scars of repeated injuries from falling.

The GW investigators set out to develop a thin, lightweight helmet that could be concealed beneath a cap, wig, or other inconspicuous headgear. The design was intended to alleviate the following problems common to conventional protective headgear:

- excessive weight compounding balance and fatigue problems
- excessive size and unnatural appearance

- poor ventilation
- poor fit, especially for children or persons with abnormally shaped heads
- difficulty keeping the helmet clean

The first step in developing the new helmet was to find a suitable material that could provide adequate protection from head injuries. The laboratory staff experimented with various lightweight and high-shock absorption materials. The most appropriate materials seem to be Temper Foam (T-Foam) and Pelite high-density polyethylene foam. T-Foam, a NASA-developed, resin-impregnated foam, has excellent shock absorption but is relatively sensitive to moisture and chafing. Pelite polyethylene foam, on the other hand, is well suited for long-term skin contact and is often used as a socket liner in lightweight prostheses. A logical combination, then, seemed to be to sandwich T-Foam within layers of Pelite polyethylene foam. Various densities were than compared.

Having arrived at a sandwich using quarter-inch T-50 Foam within inner and outer layers of quarter-inch A-20 Pelite polythylene foam, the laboratory examined fabrication techniques. Because good fit is essential to appearance and protection, each helmet was vacuum-formed on an individually made plaster head form for custom fit. Several three-eighth-inch rubber strips were added to the form to provide ventilation tunnels. The Pelite inner liner of the helmet was then vacuum-formed over the head form and rubber strips and trimmed to the hair line. Pads of T-Foam were then glued to the inner Pelite liner between the ventilation tunnels. The outer layer of Pelite was vacuum-formed over the other builtup layers, trimmed to the hair line, and all edges were contact-cemented. Finally, the top section was removed for ventilation and this edge was also contact-cemented. The completed helmet was about .50 of an inch thick and weighed about 2 ounces; this compares to a commercial helmet of approximately .75 of an inch thick and 14 ounces.

Individuals wore the helmets under wigs and fitted into a golf cap intermittently for more than 6 months. The results have been very promising. None of these individuals has suffered head injury while wearing the helmet, although all have had seizures, many of which occurred in potentially hazardous areas, such as on concrete steps.

As an additional benefit, two of the subjects experienced a marked decrease in the frequency of seizures while wearing the helmets. Neurologists have noted a direct relationship between reduced anxiety and frequency of seizures.

PRODUCT SOURCES

Information on many of the aids and devices described in this chapter is shown below.

1. Abledata (Information available on more than 15,000 products from 1,900 manufacturers)
   Newington Children's Hospital
   Adaptive Equipment Center
   181 East Cedar Street
   Newington, Connecticut 06111
   (800) 344-5405 voice/TDD
   (203) 667-5405 voice/TDD

2. Accent On Living
   Box 700
   Bloomington, Illinois 61702

3. American Trauma Society
   P.O. Box 13526
   Baltimore, Maryland 21203
   (301) 528-6304

4. Emory University Research & Training Center on Head Trauma and Stroke
   1441 Clifton Road, NE
   Atlanta, Georgia 30322
   (404) 727-5486

5. Job Accommodation Network (JAN)
   P.O. Box 468
   Morgantown, West Virginia 26505
   (800) 526-7234

6. National Rehabilitation Information Center (NARIC)
   8455 Colesville Road, Suite 935
   Silver Spring, Maryland 20910-3319
   (800) 346-2742

7. Research and Training Center on Brain Trauma and Stroke
   Northwestern University
   Department of Rehabilitation Medicine
   633 Clark Street
   Evanston, Illinois 60201
   (312) 908-6017

8. Rehabilitation Research on Brain Trauma and Stroke
   University of Washington

Department of Rehabilitation Medicine
Seattle, Washington 98195
(206) 543-3600

9. Research and Training Center for Head Injury and Stroke
New York University Medical Center
400 East 36th Street
New York, New York 10016
(212) 340-6161

SUMMARY

Rehabilitation engineering is becoming an integral part of the rehabilitation process, particularly for persons with severe disabilities. Persons with traumatic brain injury have multiple disabilities and very often will benefit from engineering resources. This chapter illustrates how environmental modifications, in terms of aids, devices, and techniques, can help in the rehabilitation process.

Many adaptations, though simple, often require creativity to recognize that completely new functioning capabilities are being opened for persons with brain injuries. This is also illustrated through case histories.

There are many commercially available aids and devices that could have a direct impact on individual needs. Occasionally, these aids and devices may require some modifications to optimize individual needs. In some cases, one may need to design and fabricate a new device where nothing exists in accordance to an individual's need.

At the end of the chapter, resources are listed where rehabilitation professionals and persons with disabilities can benefit through inquiry.

REFERENCES

Baker, L., Parker, K., & Sanderson, D. (1983, December). Neuromuscular electric stimulation for the head injured patient. *Physical Therapy, 63*(12), 1950–1956.

Booth, B.J., Doyle, M., & Montgomery, J. (1983, December). Serial casting for the management of spasticity in the head-injured adult. *Physical Therapy, 63*(12), 1960–1966.

Chyatte, S.B., & Birdsong, J.H. (1971, January). Assessment of motor performance in brain injury. *American Journal of Physical Medicine, 50*(1), 17–30.

Garland, D., & Keenman, M.A.E. (1983, October). Orthopedic strategies in the management of the adult head-injured patient. *Physical Therapy, 63*(12), 2004–2009.

Kewman, D.G., & Seigerman, C. (1983, January). Driver readiness training for persons with brain damage. Sixth Annual Conference on Rehabilitation Engineering, San Diego, CA, p. 96–98.

Leahy, P. (1988, January). Precasting work sheet—an assessment tool. *Physical Therapy, 68*(1), 72–74.

Levine, S.P., Krishch, N.L., Krueger, M.F., & Jaros, L.A. (1984, June). The microcomputer as an "orthotic" device for cognitive disorders. Proceedings of the 2nd International Conference on Rehabilitation Engineering, Ottawa, Canada, p. 130–131.

Mallik, K. (1979). Job accommodations through job restructuring and environmental modification. In D. Vandergoot & J. D. Worrall (Eds.), *Placement in rehabilitation: A career development perspective* (pp. 143–165). Baltimore, MD: University Park Press.

Mallik, K., & Mueller, J. (1977). A practical design approach to rehabilitation products. *Proceedings of Systems and Devices for the Disabled*, Vol. 4, p. 36–39.

Mallik, K., & Mueller, J. (1975). Vocational aids and enhanced productivity of the severely disabled. *Proceedings of Systems and Devices for the Disabled*, Vol. 2, p. 203–207.

Mallik, K., & Sablowsky, R. (1975). Models for placement—job laboratory approach. *Journal of Rehabilitation, 42*(6), 14–21.

Mueller, J. (1980, June). Concealable helmet for seizure-prone individuals. In K. Mallik & E. Shaver (Eds.). *Job and self-sufficiency* (pp. 95–100). Washington, DC: The George Washington University.

Chapter 6

Development of a Work Reentry Program

David A. Ellerd

The purpose of this chapter is to follow the development of an actual work reentry program for persons with traumatic brain injury. Information is drawn heavily from development and operation of Project Re-Entry, funded by the California Department of Rehabilitation. The complexity of such a program needs to be emphasized from the beginning; it is clear that there are many crucial variables that profoundly affect employment outcome.

Step 1 is to clarify program goals and services. Start with a goal-directed statement such as

> Project Re-Entry will provide employment and related support services for persons with traumatic brain injury.

The statement presented can, and most likely will, be subjected to a variety of definitions. Therefore, develop a clear definition of the services to be provided before someone else does.

What are "Employment Support Services?" Basically, these are to find the person a job of interest within his/her skill capability and provide direct training and resources to facilitate a positive employment experience that presents options.

What is a "Traumatic Brain Injury?" At this point, it may be useful to differentiate between a medical diagnosis and a rehabilitation problem.

The medical diagnosis will give the physiological description and classification of the injury. For example:

> The client sustained a non-depressed skull fracture; basilar skull fracture; early hydrocephalus that was measured on CT scan as enlargements of the temporal horns of the lateral ventricles; and a subarachnoid hemorrhage associated with the basilar skull fracture.

A rehabilitation problem statement should indicate the functional impairments that are the outcome of the injury. For example,

> She has significant motor problems that include difficulty walking, poor balance, limited use of her right arm; she shows severe deficits in memory, both short-term verbal and long-term verbal and visual; problems with judgment, planning, organizing, and speed of mental processing.

The formal definition of traumatic brain injury used by the California State Department of Rehabilitation is "Acquired Traumatic Brain Injury (ATBI) is an injury that is sustained after birth from an external force to the brain, or any of its parts, resulting in physiological or anatomical change in brain functions."

DESIGNING SERVICES

To positively affect employment outcome, the service design of the program needs to include a variety of interdisciplinary services. Project Re-Entry's nonfacility based model provides

- evaluation of employment interest in relationship to skill capabilities
- job development/job analysis
- therapeutic placement(s)
- direct on-the-job training
- Social Security Administration/long-term disability (SSA/LTD) advocacy
- evaluation and referral for additional therapeutic services

The identification of services (to be provided) will influence the entrance criteria of a program, and hence influence decisions on client assessment. Related to what California's Department of Rehabilitation can provide in services, we established these entrance criteria

- medically stable/current work release
- motivation to achieve employment
- tolerance for support of Re-Entry staff

- free from alcohol and/or chemical dependency (this criterion was initiated after the first year of program operation, so it did not affect the inclusion of clients in the reported group)

Part of the criteria for program inclusion may be a specific type of assessment or an agreement to be tested to ensure the client meets all the other criteria. The more information that is available about the individual—whether through historical reports, personal interviews, or testing from an independent clinician—the greater will be the program's ability to reduce the error factor related to a successful job match. It will also reduce the probability of your program attempting to provide a needed service to someone that it was not designed to provide.

The therapeutic model service design (Figure 6-1) is a realistic design that provides not only for job development, matching, and coaching, but for continuous iterations of these services. It does not assume the perfect-job-match-on-the-first-try approach, which puts undue pressure on clients and staff. We have worked with a lot of individuals that have waited many years for the perfect job.

This model reflects what we consider a comprehensive employment process, not just a placement. The design allows for situational employment assessment and follows persons as they go through what appears to be a period of self-awareness related to their actual performance skills and difficulties. Key to this model is the presentation of realistic employment options. Unrealistic vocational expectations often occur. Our greatest success in dealing with them has been during the actual employment experience. Therefore, we include continual self-assessment within our job coaching and situational assessment goals.

DELIVERING SERVICES

Now that we have a design to reference, it's time to think about how to make it work (i.e., develop a service delivery system). This process involves formulating related variables into a complex and functioning unit. The variables include staffing patterns; procedures for handling referrals, assessments, and problem solving; a battery of training techniques; information sources; strategies for finding and matching jobs and evaluating job performance; and a group of medical and service professionals for client referrals.

The remainder of this chapter will describe how Project Re-Entry approached these issues and the resulting outcomes.

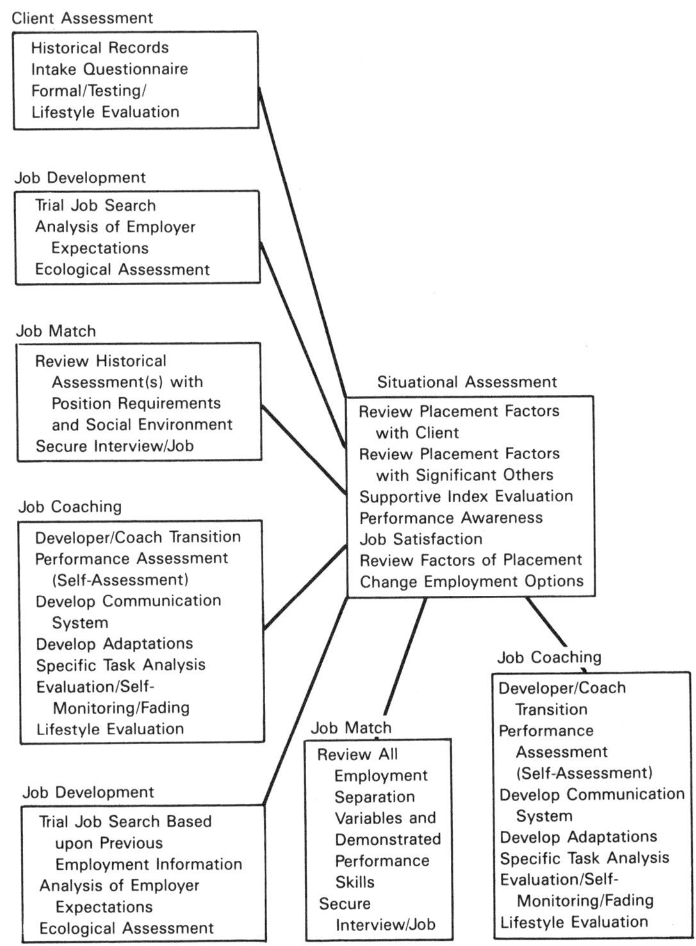

Figure 6-1 The Therapeutic Model

METHOD OF OPERATIONS IN PROJECT RE-ENTRY

Over a period of 12 months, 41 clients were referred for supported employment services. Because our services are funded by a Department of Rehabilitation Establishment Grant, all participants must first have an "open case" status with this agency. This requires a medical verification that the person is vocationally handicapped due to a disability and has potential for employment. The outcome goal for these individuals is competitive employment. Of the 41 referrals, we had 24 participants in the project. Tables 6-1 and 6-2 present their demographic profiles, educational backgrounds, and preinjury employment categories.

Table 6-1 Demographic Profile

Sex		*Age at Referral*	*Coma Period*	*Post-Trauma Period*	*Unemployment Period*
Male N = 17	Female N = 7	$\bar{x}$ = 31 Range = 19–56	$\bar{x}$ = 40.4 days Range = 8–118 days	$\bar{x}$ = 6.3 years Range = 7 mo.–17 yrs.	$\bar{x}$ = 5.3 years Range = 7 mo.–16.8 yrs.

Note: Mean age at the time of injury was 24.
N (number of participants) is 24.
$\bar{x}$ = statistical average

Table 6-2 Preinjury Educational Level and Employment Categories

Educational Level		*Employment Category*	
Non–High School Graduate	= 21%		
High School Graduate	= 42%	Unskilled Labor	= 59%
College Courses	= 25%	Skilled Labor	= 29%
College Graduate	= 12%	Technical/Management	= 12%

Note: N (number of participants) is 24.

There was a predominance of male participants (59 percent), with a mean age at referral of 31 (a range of 19 to 56). The mean age at the time of injury was 24 years with a coma period mean of 40.4 days (a range of 8 to 118 days). The post-trauma period time was 6.3 years (a range of 7 months to 17 years). This group had been unemployed a mean of 5.3 years (a range of 7 months to 16.8 years) before project involvement.

The information on the educational level for the group indicates that 42 percent were at the high school graduate level; 21 percent did not achieve this level; 25 percent were involved in college coursework; only 12 percent (number of people = 3) received a college graduation certificate. There may be a correlation between the age of injury ($\bar{x} = 24$ [$\bar{x}$ = statistical average]) and educational level, but our data did not indicate this. The data on preinjury jobs indicate that 59 percent were employed in unskilled labor positions (those that did not require any specialized skill or training to perform); 29 percent performed skilled labor duties; and 12 percent had technical or management positions requiring advanced skill performance.

Staffing Patterns

The staff-to-client ratio initially was set at one employment specialist to four employees. As the demands for client supervision/training changed, case assignments were adjusted. In addition, the need for a job developer position evolved several months into the project. This position accommodated our therapeutic placement model and relieved employment specialists from job development responsibilities. The total staffing pattern developed into 2.5 employment specialists, one job developer, one part-time secretary, and a director.

Employment specialist skills relate to situational observation and perception of the client (including lifestyle) and employment setting. The stated job responsibilities were job outline/task analysis, social skills counseling, SSA/LTD advocacy, employer and coworker interventions, money management, family counseling, and case management. Daily intervention time distribution (based on an 8-hour day) was on-site training (35 percent), on-site advocacy (20 percent), off-site travel/transportation (15 percent), off-site training and advocacy (20 percent), and program monitoring (10 percent).

The intervention time distribution is a guide for the daily delivery of services. However, variables that influence time distribution and possible case assignment are

- new client inclusion
- crisis intervention
- integration (acceptance) of employment specialist into employment setting
- client response to employment specialist
- employment changes
- geographical location of employment sites
- intervention time fading

Although the stated variables can influence time distribution, they should not influence the systematic delivery of services or fading procedures for clients. Nor should they affect decisions related to job matching or employment placements.

Intake

At the time of referral, we gave a written request for all historical records to each client. After receipt of records, the rehabilitation counselor and client met to discuss services and possible program inclusion. During this meeting (which may include significant others), specific services were discussed, the entrance criteria were reviewed, and the client's participation responsibilities were clarified. If the consensus was to proceed, an intake evaluation meeting was scheduled with the individual to gather information about preinjury/postinjury activities and current lifestyle. We covered

- identification information
- financial support status
- living arrangement
- education
- work history (pre/postinjury)
- disability (medical diagnosis/functional limitations)
- evaluations (neuropsychological; work evaluations; etc.)
- current activities
- behavioral/employment-related observations
- support system (social)
- rehabilitative services (current or prior)

- placement possibilities
- medical status checklist

The information received is compared with historical records and reports from significant others involved in the case. Just as important as objective/factual information are subjective reports related to the clients' perceptions of their lifestyle. Insight should be sought as to why the individual wants to work and selects certain types of employment and how the person feels about the "meaning" or "value" of work. Employment will often relate to lifestyle variables, such as self-worth, social status, interpersonal relationships, social integration, and financial independence. The focus should also be directed at perceptions of current skill capabilities and functional impairments. Employment will not provide a cure or make their lives perfect, but it can help clients face and overcome functional impairments, feel better about themselves, and be productive. It is important to communicate at this time that there is no such thing as the "perfect job" and we do not have a "magic wand" to wave and make everything better for them.

While the tendencies in these meetings are to spend time on evaluating employment settings and observable performance measures, more telling factors are the individual's self-evaluation and perception of his or her lifestyle. The point here is not to lose sight of the person for whom you are working.

Data Collection

A trial job search is initiated to identify types of positions that are of interest to the client and within his/her skill capability. For each potential job, data are collected on requirements, responsibilities, working conditions, and social environment using a job analysis format, which is then used to evaluate both the client and the placement.

The job developer works with the employment specialist and client (and significant others) to match areas of probable performance with a specific position. A job analysis form should include

- physical demands
- environmental conditions
- job materials
- work situation (repetitive/varied)
- task sequence
- aptitudes
- performance pace
- communication required

- interactions necessary (coworkers/supervisors)
- interactions necessary (general public)
- behavior acceptance range
- appearance requirements

If the comparison reflects a positive match, the position is a possible employment option. A meeting is set up among the job developer, the client, and potential employer. The interview should occur after the employer has been educated about the project and the employment specialist has assessed the job environment to be supportive. If the position is secured, a job outline is completed to use as a tool to collect actual performance data related to proficiency, rate, endurance, and quality. The rehabilitation team also assesses the need for adaptations and identifies potential obstacles.

The parts of the job that present difficulties are isolated in a specific task analysis. This analysis breaks down the performance aspects of a task into trainable components based on the individual's learning style. Task training is then performed and data collected based on specific needs and frequency of a task's performance. The job outline should be reviewed monthly and revised as indicated due to possible changes in performance or duties.

Frequency data related to nonskill types of behavior (e.g., timely attendance, inappropriate communication) are collected using a behavior data chart (see Figure 6-2).

Within 30 days of the employment start date, all these data are consolidated into an Individual Service Plan that identifies all goals for competitive employment related to skill performance and behavioral considerations. The plan includes specific objectives, baseline data, completion criteria, target dates, methods of training to be used, and types of measurements to be performed.

Social validation measures are used related to employer/employee work satisfaction and a supportive placement index that is conducted by the employment specialist. Basically, the employer rates the client, the client rates the job, and the employment specialist rates the environment. Each index reflects characteristics which are ordered from positive to negative with numerical rankings assigned from one to five. Although the data are subjective and the numbers assigned have no statistical validity, we have found the information directly relates to employment stability and helps focus intervention efforts.

Program Outcomes: An Interim Report

The outcome data are reflected in Table 6-3 for all 24 participants. The individual competitive employment placements are listed by case, including

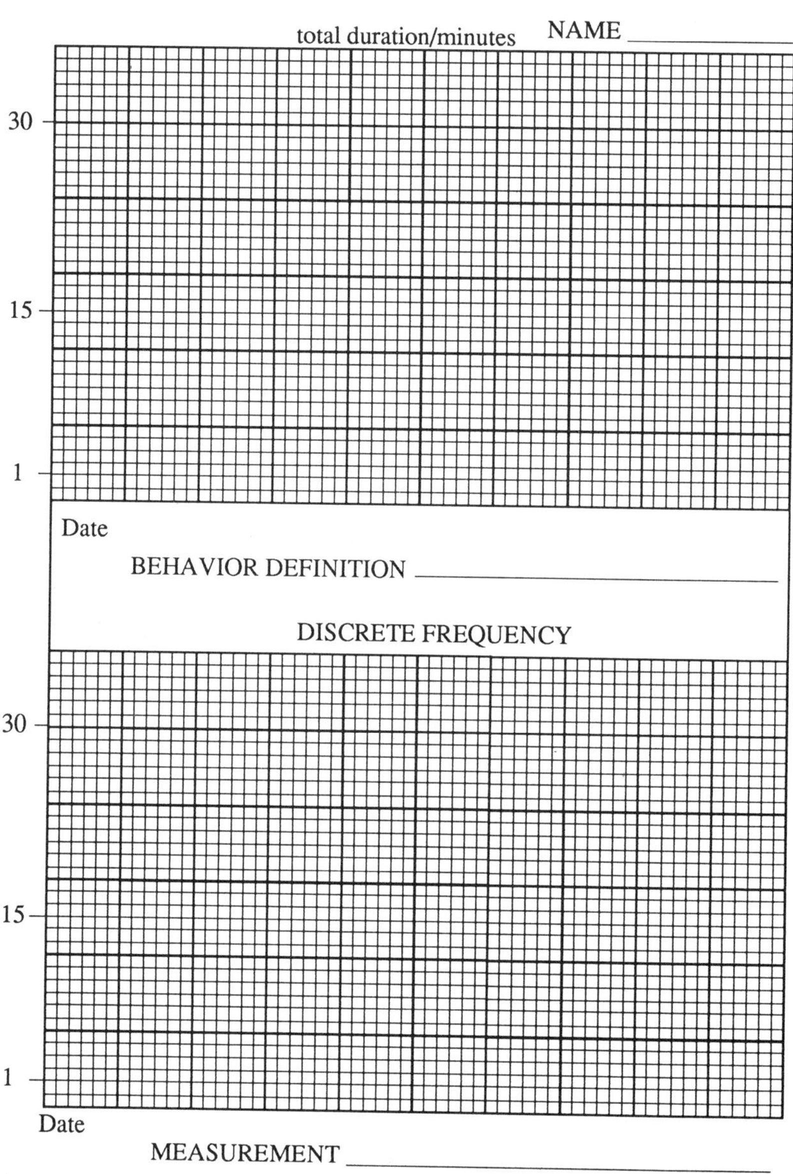

Figure 6-2 Sample Behavior Data Chart

hours worked per week and hourly rate of pay. The mean average for the group indicates 33 hours worked per week (a range of 20 to 40 hours) with an average wage of $5.19 per hour (a range of $3.35 to $9.89). The collective total of days worked was 2,086, with a mean of 86.9 days worked per client.

The data reflect that, after supported employment services, 17 individuals were employed out of the initial 24 participants, indicating an employment retention rate of 71 percent. The reasons for employment separation include alcohol and substance abuse (n = 2), medical problems (n = 2), low motivation (n = 1), being laid off (n = 1), and psychotic symptoms (n = 1).

The types of positions are categorized in Table 6-4 and compared with preinjury employment data. As indicated, 58 percent were employed in unskilled labor positions compared to 59 percent preinjury; 34 percent were in skilled labor positions compared to 29 percent preinjury; and 8 percent were in technical/management positions compared to 12 percent preinjury.

Due to the nature of the therapeutic placement model, which results in multiple placements, it is significant to compare productive work behavior postinjury with work behavior during project participation. The data (Table 6-5) indicate that the postinjury group worked a collective 18.4 years (only 14 percent) of their total opportunity period (after medical stabilization) or 139.4 years. These figures were markedly different during project participation, when the group worked 10.7 years (77 percent) out of a total opportunity period of 14 years.

SUMMARY

We came away with several lessons learned during development of Project Re-Entry. Initially, all referrals made to the project were accepted for services, and those who did not participate were not excluded by the project. Also, the entrance criteria did not require any formal testing or evaluation, and we did not state an exclusion based on alcohol/drug abuse problems.

As is the case for many new programs, the staff was anxious to begin placement efforts and therefore accepted referrals that needed services beyond our domain. For example, we found issues arising related to alcohol/substance abuse and medical problems, with which we were unprepared to deal. Fortunately, we were able quickly to locate resources to accommodate these needs. It should be noted that these resources were available to the general public and not specifically developed for individuals with a traumatic brain injury. We learned that identifying services that the program can provide and developing resources earlier, then proceeding at a gradual rate, will allow for more flexibility.

The therapeutic model evolved as a way to work with a person's unrealistic vocational expectations, to provide staff with actual employment perfor-

Table 6-3 Employment Status of Supported Employment Placements

Case	Job Title	Hour/Wage	Hire Date	Days Worked	Current Status
(01)	Mechanic helper	40/$4.00	04/29/88	16	Terminated—increased duties
	Stockroom helper	40/$4.25	07/06/88	04	Resigned—did not like job
	Utility man	30/$5.00	07/25/88	98	Resigned—did not like supervisor
	Repair assistant	20/$5.00	02/01/89	05	Laid off (job search)
(02)	Telemarketing representative	20/$4.25	04/24/89	14	Employed
(03)	General worker	40/$5.00	05/09/88	141	Terminated—alcohol abuse
	Furniture refinisher	40/$5.00	03/01/89	39	Employed (return from detox)
(04)	Office clerk	20/$5.50	05/09/88	67	Employment transfer
	Customer service	20/$4.25	06/27/88	04	Terminated—poor attendance
	Nursing assistant	40/$4.90	08/11/88	120	Employed
	Recreation assistant	40/$5.06	02/01/89	71	" (same employer as above)
(05)	General worker	40/$4.75	03/17/89	41	Employed
(06)	Shop helper	20/$3.35	05/16/88	29	Terminated—poor performance
	Stablekeeper	30/$4.60	07/05/88	15	Terminated—drug abuse (referred—out)
(07)	Service representative	20/$7.00	03/01/89	48	Employed
(08)	Food preparer	25/$4.25	05/22/88	45	Resigned—poor performance/reduced hours
	Kitchen helper	40/$4.75	09/06/88	03	Terminated—drug abuse (referred—out)
(09)	Kitchen helper	40/$3.35	05/23/88	11	Employment transfer
	Kitchen helper	40/$4.75	06/23/88	47	Medical leave—resigned
	Shop helper	25/$5.00	09/26/88	80	Medical leave—position open
	Shop helper	25/$6.00	01/01/89		(need physician's work release)
(10)	Administrative assistant	40/$6.73	07/05/88	196	Employed
(11)	Child caretaker	25/$5.00	09/13/88	72	Resigned—medical problems/motivational problems (job search)

Table 6-3 continued

(12)	Electronic assembler	40/$4.25	03/20/89	29	Employed
(13)	Yard man	40/$5.00	09/15/88	38	Medical leave—terminated
	Driver/maintenance	40/$5.00	01/11/89	1.5	Terminated—aberrant behavior
	Resource clerk	20/$9.89	02/04/89	54	Employed
(14)	Office clerk	25/$5.00	09/16/88	19	Terminated—poor performance
	Receptionist	20/$4.50	02/13/89	39	Terminated—poor performance/motivation
(15)	Sales representative	40/$7.50	04/10/89	23	Employed
(16)	Secretary	20/$5.55	08/22/88	200	Employed
	Secretary	30/$6.05	04/06/89		" (same employer as above)
(17)	Library assistant	20/$4.92	10/03/88	81	Employed (return from detox)
(18)	Nursing assistant	40/$4.90	10/07/88	2.5	Terminated—psychotic symptoms
(19)	Receptionist	25/$5.50	04/24/89	14	Employed
(20)	Animal caretaker	40/$4.50	11/11/89	11	Employment transfer
	Receptionist	40/$5.00	01/03/89	90	Employed
(21)	Painter's helper	40/$4.25	07/02/88	131	Terminated—poor performance (increased job duties)
	Auto shop assistant	40/$4.25			(Self-employment)
(22)	Mechanic assistant	40/$5.00	01/06/89	15	Terminated—poor performance (increased job duties)
	Owner—fruit stand				(Self-employment)
(23)	General worker	40/$5.00 40/$6.00 40/$7.00	11/03/88	95	Resigned—did not like job
	General warehouse worker	20/$5.00	05/01/89	17	Employed
(24)	Data entry person	40/$6.92	02/01/89	60	Employed
	Xs =	33/$5.19		TOTAL = 2,086 86.9 days	Employment Ratio 17/24 = 71%

Table 6-4 Employment Category Comparison Pre/Postinjury

Preinjury Employment Category		*Postinjury Employment Category*	
Unskilled Labor	= 59%	Unskilled Labor	= 58%
Skilled Labor	= 29%	Skilled Labor	= 34%
Technical/Management	= 12%	Technical/Management	= 8%

Table 6-5 Comparison of Productive Work Behavior Postinjury with Project Participation

Postinjury Activity		*Project Participation Activity*	
Employed	Work Opportunity	Employed	Work Opportunity
18.4 years	139.4 years	10.73 years	14 years
Work Behavior = 14%		Work Behavior = 77%	

Note: N (number of participants) is 24.

mance data, and to provide client options. The model does not reflect a "trial" or "temporary" employment position: Job placements are permanent and any changes are based on the client's actual performance and job satisfaction variables, not on time variables. A partial client commitment—"I'll try it for a while"—is not an acceptable attitude.

In the staffing pattern, we found the position of job developer, who relieves the employment specialist of development duties, is essential to this model. However, doing this means developing a method to transition the job developer out of the employment setting and the employment specialist in. Our job developer is also in a position to provide both backup support for crisis intervention and periodic evaluations of the environment, client, and employment specialist.

Two final lessons were learned. Although it is often stated by head injury providers of their clients that, "Because of the injury, they are a *totally* different person," we did not find this. Based on reports from significant others and despite obvious functional deficits, our group displayed as many similarities as differences in preinjury-postinjury personality/behavior. Finally, we learned that vocational success for persons with a traumatic brain injury requires constant training and guidance and support for the client, the employer, and significant others.

REFERENCE

California Department of Rehabilitation. (August 1, 1986). *Acquired Traumatic Brain Injury Position Paper*. Sacramento, CA: Office of the Director.

Chapter 7

Supported Employment Phase I: Job Placement

Pamela D. Sherron and Christine H. Groah

While there has been much discussion on the efficacy of supported employment programs for people with traumatic brain injury who are unable to gain employment (e.g., Wehman & Moon, 1989), there are few published efforts that describe in depth how to implement such programs. Hence, the next three chapters attempt to fill this need by detailing programmatic implementation guidelines. This chapter describes job development and placement techniques, Chapter 8 explains how to handle job site intervention, and Chapter 9 gives job retention strategies.

For job placement to occur, the employment specialist must simultaneously perform consumer assessment and job development. Consumer assessment is the process of gathering information about the abilities and interests of the individuals who the program is actively attempting to place. Job development is the process of identifying and assessing appropriate employment opportunities in the business community for those individuals. Job placement activities cannot begin until a program has generated an active pool of referrals.

Before generating an active pool of client referrals, a program should determine eligibility criteria for acceptance into the program. The following questions may assist in generating eligibility criteria.

- Who will be served by this program? How will you determine the target population, i.e., who is at risk of gaining or maintaining employment?
- What degree of injury will participants have sustained—mild, moderate, or severe? How will the degree of injury be measured—length of coma and/or Glasgow Coma Score upon emergency room admission?

- Will there be a restriction placed on the number of years postinjury?
- Is there an age range?
- What is the area in which services will be provided?
- Are individuals with a history of preinjury and/or postinjury alcohol/drug use excluded?

The supported employment program at the Medical College of Virginia uses the following eligibility criteria.

1. An individual must have sustained an open or closed moderate to severe traumatic head injury as indicated by one of the following:
   - record of coma greater than 24 hours
   - record of post-traumatic amnesia surpassing 24 hours
   - Glasgow Coma Score on initial admission of less than 13.
2. An individual with current ongoing substance abuse may be excluded initially and referred to a chemical dependence program.
3. An individual must not be competitively employed, except for individuals returning to preinjury employment, who may be provided with services if an assessment of their abilities and an analysis of the job indicate a likelihood of success.
4. An individual must live within a 30-mile radius of the service area.
5. An individual must be willing to work with the initial assistance and ongoing support of an employment specialist, but does not need to possess the precise skills for a given job.

SOURCES OF REFERRALS

The state Department of Rehabilitative Services is an excellent source of referrals. Meet with regional directors and counselors to explain the supported employment service. Hospitals and outpatient rehabilitation hospitals have social workers on staff who can make referrals; private rehabilitation providers and insurance carriers also can refer individuals.

State head injury foundations and local chapters are clearinghouses for information on traumatic brain injury and can be sources of referrals. Take advantage of this valuable resource. Employment specialists should meet with chapter presidents to present the supported employment service well in advance of its start-up date. This will allow the foundation to get the word out to its members, who are likely to be in prompt contact with the program. A foundation may also be able to provide a statewide directory of head injury services. If a chapter does not exist in your area, contact the National Head Injury Foundation to obtain information on how to get one started.

REFERRAL PACKAGE

A consumer referral packet given to individuals referred to the program can include a letter explaining eligibility criteria of the program, a fact sheet about supported employment services, and a three-part general health and history questionnaire. Part I of the questionnaire gathers information about date of injury, length of coma, current residence of the referral, current medications being taken, pre/postinjury work and history, current financial aid being received, and observed changes in the individual since injury. Physical, cognitive, behavior, communication, and social problems are indicated based on a frequency of occurrence—never to always. Part II of the questionnaire assesses a referral's pre/postinjury alcohol use, while Part III canvasses the individual's personal daily activities and sensory and physical abilities. At the end of each questionnaire part, the person filling out the forms is asked to indicate the accuracy of the information provided on a Likert scale ranging from 0 to 3, with 0 indicating not at all accurate and 3 indicating very accurate. See Appendix 7-A for a sample 3-part questionnaire.

CONSUMER EMPLOYMENT SCREENING

Individuals accepted into the program (active) referral pool are referred to as *consumers* and undergo a consumer employment screening. The screening consists of a home visit, a vocationally oriented neuropsychological evaluation, a career/interest inventory, and an assessment of source information. Employment specialists gather information from various sources about each consumer. It is best if at least two employment specialists are assigned to each new referral to maximize insight into consumer abilities and personalities.

Home Visit

The home visit should be scheduled within 2 weeks from the date of the referral. The two employment specialists, the consumer, and a significant other should be in attendance. Home visits allow employment specialists to establish rapport with consumers and families, gain insight into family dynamics, and to become familiar with consumer vocational interests and abilities. During the home visit, information is gathered using a Consumer Employment Screening Form, Mock Application Form, Release of Information to Other Sources Form, and the Financial Analysis Form.

Consumer Screening Form

On the Consumer Screening Form (Exhibit 7-1), the consumer is rated on 28 items ranging from availability and transportation to physical strength to unusual behavior. It is not enough to ask individuals if they can, for example, add or subtract; have them complete a written or oral mathematical equation. Extra space on the form for comments gives employment specialists room to record specific information. At a future time, the employment specialist will use the Consumer Screening Form to analyze the compatibility of job requirements and consumer abilities and interests.

Mock Application Form

The Mock Application Form reconstructs the individual's past work history. This historical review can informally assess the consumer's memory skills. It also can highlight preinjury work skills that may have been preserved, thus pointing to the types of job opportunities to seek during job development.

Unrealistic expectations may surface during this time. A consumer may insist on returning to former employment, despite evidence that this is not feasible. For example, a roofer may plan to return to previous employment when an unsteady and unbalanced gait is apparent. Due to the injury, diminished insight, poor self-awareness, and impaired problem-solving may instigate unrealistic expectations.

The employment specialist can assess the consumer's memory and ability to read, write, and follow instructions by how the individual fills out the Sample Application Form (see Exhibit 7-2). Personnel departments often require applications before scheduling an interview. It is helpful to have this mock information on file if an appropriate job opportunity arises that has a tight deadline and the employment specialist must complete the application. This form can also be used to develop a resume for the individual. Finally, filling out the mock application can stimulate conversation on current consumer interests, which can help assess suitability of a particular job match.

Releases of Information to Other Sources

Liability (e.g., transportation) releases and Release of Information Forms are signed during the home visit. The consumer should sign a release of information form for any source that may have valuable information on a consumer's vocational potential (see Exhibit 7-3). Sources may include

- state vocational rehabilitation
- social security administration
- medical facilities
- psychological services

- former employers
- educational institutions
- city or county court records
- department of motor vehicles

Financial Analysis Form

Of major concern to both consumers and families is the effect of employment on social security benefits. Although the exact ramifications of employment on financial status should be reviewed before placement, a general overview should be provided during the home visit. A Financial Analysis Form (Exhibit 7-4) may be partially completed at this time to help the employment specialist explain and document the effects of employment on the consumer's benefits. Current knowledge of federal benefit programs is critical so that an employment specialist can relay accurate information to the consumer and families. Contact your local Social Security Administration to get booklets/pamphlets with the most current information.

Information gathering is not a one-way process, however. The employment specialist should provide information to the consumer's family about supported employment services, including:

- The role of the employment specialist is to provide
  —100 percent service guarantee to employer if applicable
  —constant/consistent training to consumer
  —direct/honest/respectful feedback to consumer.
- The consumer does not have to be job ready, as training will take place on the job site.
- The employment specialist is available to assist the consumer with transportation training.
- The program does not operate on a first-referred, first-placed basis. Placements are made as the job match dictates.
- Individuals with realistic and varied interests may be placed sooner than individuals with unrealistic expectations or narrow career interests.

The home visit ends with the employment specialists scheduling a consumer to visit the supported employment program center for a career interest inventory. Career search programs, such as Virginia View, may help form a profile of an individual's interests and work environment preferences. These inventories are particularly helpful for individuals injured before establishing a work history or career, which is a common condition due to the frequency of traumatic head injury among young adults.

Exhibit 7-1 Sample Consumer Employment Screening Form

Consumer Employment Screening Form

Consumer:

Name: ______________________

SSN: ___/__/____

Staff member completing this form:

Name: ______________________

I.D. Code: ______________________

Date of screening (month/day/year): __/__/__

Type of screening: Initial ________ Ongoing/Employed ________ Ongoing/Unemployed ________

Total number of hours per week currently working: ________ Months per year: ________

General Directions: PLEASE DO NOT LEAVE ANY ITEM UNANSWERED

Indicate the most appropriate response for each item based on observations of the consumer and interviews with individuals who know the consumer (i.e., family members, adult service providers, school personnel, employers).

1. Availability: (Circle yes or no for each item)	Will Work Weekends	Will Work Evenings	Will Work Part-Time	Will Work Full-Time
	Yes / No	Yes / No	Yes / No	Yes / No

Specifics/Comments:

2. Transportation: (Circle yes or no for each item)	Transportation Available	Specialized Travel Services Accessible	Lives on Bus Route	Family Will Transport	Provides Own Transportation (Bike, Car, Walks, Etc.)
	Yes / No	Yes / No	Yes / No	Yes / No	Yes / No

Specifics/Comments:

3. Strength: Lifting and Carrying	Poor (< 10 lbs.)	Fair (10–30 lbs.)	Average (30–40 lbs.)	Strong (> 40 lbs.)
	________	________	________	________

Specifics/Comments:

4. Endurance: (without break)	Works < 2 hours ______	Works 2–3 hours ______	Works 3–4 hours ______	Works > 4 hours ______	
Specifics/Comments:					
5. Orienting:	Small Area Only ______	One Room ______	Several Rooms ______	Building-Wide ______	Building and Grounds ______
Specifics/Comments:					
6. Physical Mobility:	Sit/Stand in One Area ______	Fair Ambulation ______	Stairs/Minor Obstacles ______	Full Physical Abilities ______	
Specifics/Comments:					
7. Independent Work Rate: (no prompts)	Slow Pace ______	Steady/ Average Pace ______	Above Average/ Sometimes Fast Pace ______	Continual Fast Pace ______	
Specifics/Comments:					
8. Appearance:	Unkempt/ Poor Hygiene ______	Unkempt/ Clean ______	Neat/Clean but Clothing Unmatched ______	Neat/Clean and Clothing Matched ______	
Specifics/Comments:					
9. Communication:	Uses Sounds/ Gestures ______	Uses Key Words/Signs ______	Speaks Unclearly ______	Communicates Clearly, Intelligibly to Strangers ______	
Specifics/Comments:					

continues

Exhibit 7-1 continued

10. Appropriate Social Interactions:	Rarely Interacts Appropriately ______	Polite, Responds Appropriately ______	Initiates Social Interactions Infrequently ______	Initiates Social Interactions Frequently ______
Specifics/Comments:				
11. Unusual Behavior:	Many Unusual Behaviors ______	Few Unusual Behaviors ______		No Unusual Behaviors ______
Specifics/Comments:				
12. Attention to Task/ Perserverance:	Frequent Prompts Required ______	Intermittent Prompts/High Supervision Required ______	Intermittent Prompts/Low Supervision Required ______	Infrequent Prompts/Low Supervision Required ______
Specifics/Comments:				
13. Independent Sequencing of Job Duties:	Cannot Perform Tasks in Sequence ______	Performs 2–3 Tasks in Sequence ______	Performs 4–6 Tasks in Sequence ______	Performs 7 or More Tasks in Sequence ______
Specifics/Comments:				
14. Initiative/ Motivation:	Always Seeks Work ______	Sometimes Volunteers ______	Waits for Directions ______	Avoids Next Task ______
Specifics/Comments:				
15. Adapting to Change:	Adapts to Change ______	Adapts to Change with Some Difficulty ______	Adapts to Change with Great Difficulty ______	Rigid Routine Required ______
Specifics/Comments:				

16. Reinforcement Needs:	Frequently Required ______	Intermittent (daily) Sufficient ______	Infrequent (weekly) Sufficient ______	Paycheck Sufficient ______
Specifics/Comments:				
17. Family Support:	Very Supportive of Work ______	Supportive of Work with Reservations ______	Indifferent About Work ______	Negative About Work ______
Specifics/Comments:				
18. Consumer's Financial Situation:	Financial Ramifications No Obstacles ______	Requires Job with Benefits ______	Reduction of Financial Aid Is a Concern ______	Unwilling To Give Up Financial Aid ______
Specifics/Comments:				
19. Discrimination Skills:	Cannot Distinguish Among Work Supplies ______	Distinguishes Among Work Supplies with an External Cue ______		Distinguishes Among Work Supplies ______
Specifics/Comments:				
20. Time Awareness:	Unaware of Time and Clock Function ______	Identifies Breaks and Lunch ______	Can Tell Time to the Hour ______	Can Tell Time in Hours and Minutes ______
Specifics/Comments:				
21. Functional Reading:	None ______	Sight Words/ Symbols ______	Simple Reading ______	Fluent Reading ______
Specifics/Comments:				

continues

Exhibit 7-1 continued

22. Functional Math:	None ______	Simple Counting ______	Simple Addition/ Subtraction ______	Computational Skills ______	
Specifics/Comments:					
23. Independent Street Crossing:	None ______	Crosses Two Lane Street with Light ______	Crosses Two Lane Street without Light ______	Crosses Four Lane Street with Light ______	Crosses Four Lane Street without Light ______
Specifics/Comments:					
24. Handling Criticism/ Stress:	Resistive/ Argumentative ______	Withdraws into Silence ______	Accepts Criticism/ Does Not Change Behavior ______	Accepts Criticism/ Changes Behavior ______	
Specifics/Comments:					
25. Acts/Speaks Aggressively:	Hourly ______	Daily ______	Weekly ______	Monthly ______	Never ______
Specifics/Comments:					
26. Travel Skills: (Circle yes or no for each item)	Requires Bus Training Yes / No	Uses Bus Independently/ No Transfer Yes / No	Uses Bus Independently/ Makes Transfer Yes / No	Able To Make Own Travel Arrangements Yes / No	
Specifics/Comments:					

27. Benefits Consumer Needs (Circle yes or no for each choice):

Yes / No	0 = None	Yes / No	4 = Dental Benefits
Yes / No	1 = Sick Leave	Yes / No	5 = Employee Discounts
Yes / No	2 = Medical/Health Benefits	Yes / No	6 = Free or Reduced Meals
Yes / No	3 = Paid Vacation/Annual Leave	Yes / No	7 = Other (Specify): ______

28. CHECK ALL THAT CONSUMER HAS PERFORMED:

___ Bussing Tables	___ Sweeping	___ Using Dishwasher	___ Keeping Busy
___ Food Preparation	___ Assembly	___ Mopping (Indust.)	___ Clerical Work
___ Buffing	___ Vacuuming	___ Food Line Supply	___ Pot Scrubbing
___ Dusting	___ Restroom Cleaning	___ Trash Disposal	___ Other
___ Stocking	___ Washing Equipment	___ Food Serving	______

Medications? ______

Medical Complications/Conditions? ______

Additional Comments: ______

Source: Form developed by the Rehabilitation Research and Training Center, Virginia Commonwealth University, in cooperation with the Virginia Departments of Mental Health and Mental Retardation and Rehabilitative Services (Revised 4/87).

Exhibit 7-2 Sample Application for Employment

APPLICATION FOR EMPLOYMENT

PERSONAL INFORMATION

DATE: ____________ SOCIAL SECURITY # ____ - ___ - ________

NAME: ____
Last First Middle

PRESENT ADDRESS: ______________________________________
Street City State Zip Code

PERMANENT ADDRESS: ____________________________________
Street City State Zip Code

TELEPHONE # (___)_____ OWN HOME: _____ RENT: _____ BOARD: _____

MARRIED __ SINGLE __ WIDOWED __ DIVORCED __ SEPARATED __

ARE YOU AN ILLEGAL ALIEN? Yes ________ No ________

Referred By: ____

EMPLOYMENT DESIRED

POSITION __________ DATE YOU CAN START _________ SALARY DESIRED $ __________

ARE YOU EMPLOYED NOW? ____ IF SO MAY WE INQUIRE OF YOUR PRESENT EMPLOYER? ______________

EVER APPLIED TO THIS COMPANY BEFORE? ________________________ WHERE? ________ WHEN? ________

Education	Name & Location of School	Years Attended	Date Graduated	Subjects Studied
Grammar School				
High School				
College				
Trade, Business, or Correspondence School				

SUBJECTS OF SPECIAL STUDY OR RESEARCH WORK: ______________________________

WHAT FOREIGN LANGUAGES DO YOU SPEAK FLUENTLY? READ WRITE

U.S. MILITARY OR NAVAL SERVICE RANK PRESENT MEMBERSHIP IN NATIONAL GUARD OR RESERVES

HAVE YOU EVER BEEN CONVICTED OF ANY FELONY OFFENSES? IF SO, WHAT?

Exhibit 7-2 continued

FORMER EMPLOYMENT

Please give accurate, complete employment record. Start with present/most recent employment.

1.	Company Name:	Telephone # ( ) -
	Address:	Employed (State Month & Year) From To
	Name of Supervisor:	Weekly Pay Start Last
	State Job Title & Description:	Reason for Leaving:
2.	Company Name:	Telephone # ( ) -
	Address:	Employed (State Month & Year) From To
	Name of Supervisor:	Weekly Pay Start Last
	State Job Title & Description:	Reason for Leaving:
3.	Company Name:	Telephone # ( ) -
	Address:	Employed (State Month & Year) From To
	Name of Supervisor:	Weekly Pay Start Last
	State Job Title & Description:	Reason for Leaving:
4.	Company Name:	Telephone # ( ) -
	Address:	Employed (State Month & Year) From To
	Name of Supervisor:	Weekly Pay Start Last
	State Job Title & Description:	Reason for Leaving:

Exhibit 7-3 Sample Authorization for Release of Information Form

Authorization for Release of Information

Date: ____________________

PART I	PART II
To: ____________________	Re: Name: ____________________
____________________	Address: ____________________
____________________	City/State: ____________________
____________________	SSN: ____________________
	DOB: ____________________

PART III

Application has been made to the Rehabilitation Research and Training Center (RRTC) for assistance with employment to the person named in PART II. Therefore, you are authorized to release to the RRTC representative listed in PART IV relevant information including medical, psychological, educational, and/or vocational records, which will be used to develop a comprehensive consumer profile that is necessary for quality supported employment services.

PART IV

To: ____________________

____

____

Thank you for your assistance. Original Authorization for Release of Information is on file at the Rehabilitation Research and Training Center.

Neuropsychological Evaluation

A vocationally oriented neuropsychological evaluation can assess cognitive, intellectual, and psychomotor functioning. Test results aid the employment specialist in selecting reasonable and appropriate employment. The evaluation may suggest instructional strategies to use with the consumer as well as indicate potential problems. It is imperative to choose an evaluator who can interpret the results in functional terms.

Other Sources of Information

The employment specialist also should now be reviewing the consumer's rehabilitation, medical, psychological, educational, and past employment records. At the state level, rehabilitation counselors can shed more light onto consumer interests, abilities, personalities, and learning potential. Obtaining permission to go through a state's vocational rehabilitation file on a consumer may save the employment specialist time in tracking down the in-

Exhibit 7-3 continued

Authorization for Release of Information

Date: ____________________________

To develop a comprehensive consumer profile that is necessary for quality supported employment services, I authorize the exchange of information between the Social Security Administration, Department of Motor Vehicles, city/county courthouse, physicians, rehabilitation counselors, former employers and other appropriate agencies with authorized individuals from the Rehabilitation Research and Training Center.

Agencies or individuals I do not want contacted are: ____________________________

____

The date and/or conditions under which this release expires are: ________________

____

This authorization may be revoked prior to the stated expiration date.

Release of Information Authorized by:

Signature: ____

Client or Guardian

Witnessed by:

Signature: ____

RRTC Staff

Source: Virginia Commonwealth University, Rehabilitation Research and Training Center, Richmond, VA.

formation from other sources. Be sure to note the dates of all information reviewed to avoid using inaccurate (outdated) information.

For information on an individual's current physical abilities and medications, physicians are often helpful. If the consumer has not had a physical/medical evaluation within the past year, have him or her schedule one. An evaluation written in vocational functional terms is most helpful; establish a relationship with a physician who is willing to do this.

If the consumer has or is in therapy or counseling, it will be of benefit to meet with the psychological professional. Among other insights, this person may offer the employment specialist client-specific suggestions about preventing problems, dealing with difficult situations, and consumer strengths and weaknesses that can impact work. For example, a consumer with a history of inappropriate social interactions may have a greater likelihood of success in a position requiring minimal contact with others. Establish communication with the psychological professional who may be of assistance in the future.

Consider level of education and training as an indicator of motivation, areas of interest, and types of jobs for which the person can be considered.

Exhibit 7-4 Financial Analysis Form

Financial Analysis

CONSUMER: ______________________ Date: ______________________

EXPENSES PER MONTH

A. Lodging .... __________
B. Utilities.. __________
C. Health/Medical Insurance.................................... __________
D. Health/Medical Expenses (include prescriptions, etc.) .... __________
E. Transportation.. __________
F. Food .... __________
G. Clothing .... __________
H. Taxes, F.I.C.A. .... __________
I. Other.. __________
TOTAL .... __________

SUPPLEMENTAL SECURITY DISABILITY INCOME/TRIAL WORK PERIOD (SSDI/TWP) MONTHLY STATUS

Month SSDI payments started .... __________
Number of months disability payments have been received............ __________
Number of months earned $75 or more per month (TWP month)...... __________
(competitive, workshop, etc.)
Number of trial work period months remaining .... __________

MONTHLY INCOME

	Pre-Employment	Through SSDI TWP months	After SSDI Stops Date
Earned Gross Income	__________	__________	__________
SSI	__________	__________(adjusted)	__________(adjusted)
Medicaid	yes no	yes no	yes no
SSDI	__________	__________	__________
Medicare	yes no	yes no	yes no
Other Income	__________	__________	__________
TOTAL	__________	__________	__________
MONTHLY EXPENSES	__________	__________	__________

To arrive at your new SSI payment resulting from going to work, as well as your *new total* monthly income, add in your figures where indicated.

$ __________ amount of your predicted *gross* monthly wages

- ____85.00____ exclusion (or $65.00 if your receive any other unearned income such as VA benefits or SSDI)

$ __________ remainder

One half of this remainder (above) is
$ __________ This is how much your usual SSI check will be reduced.
(Keep in mind that this change will show up in check form about 2 months after you report earnings.)

Exhibit 7-4 continued

NOW . . .
$ __________ amount of *current* (usual) SSI check
- __________ subtract reduction of check (from above)
$ __________ This is your *new* SSI payment amount after going to work.

To figure your *total new* monthly income . . .
$ __________ your new SSI payment amount
+__________ your monthly income from work (net)
$ __________ your *new* total monthly income

Past employers will be able to provide actual observations on consumer skills and abilities. If the consumer returned to work postinjury, but was unsuccessful, the employer may be able to explain the factors involved. This information helps when making a job match and in the job site training of the individual.

Throughout the assessment process, an employment specialist may occasionally meet a consumer for coffee, lunch, or a stroll in the park. This provides an opportunity to interact with consumers outside of the home environment and get to know them better. Finally, the employment specialist analyzes all the information collected during this phase and begins using it for job development.

JOB DEVELOPMENT

As employment specialists collect and study consumer assessment information, they are involved, simultaneously, in job development. Job development is the process of identifying and assessing appropriate employment opportunities in the business community for individuals with severe disabilities. It consists of four primary activities: (1) conducting a community job market screening, (2) developing a marketing strategy, (3) making specific employer contact, and (4) completing a job analysis.

Community Job Market Screening

Devote several weeks to determining the current hiring trends in the local business community and identifying appropriate job opportunities for individuals with traumatic brain injury. Because the persons can have diverse interests, experiences, and abilities, investigating a cross section of industries and positions within them will facilitate a successful job match.

This job market screening is especially helpful for employment specialists new to a geographic area or implementing a new program. Gathering information and identifying appropriate types of jobs, rather than finding a specific opening and placing an individual, are the goals of a community job market screening. (However, if screening uncovers an actual job opening that appears to match a consumer's requirements, the employment specialist may consider placement at this time.)

The Community Job Market Screening Form (Exhibit 7-5) is useful for compiling information on job possibilities and companies. It is a good idea to update screening every 6 to 12 months to monitor new trends. The following guidelines can be useful in conducting a Community Job Market Screening:

- Visit your local chamber of commerce and state employment commission for business listings and information on hiring trends.
- Read regularly the business section of the local newspaper for information on new and existing businesses.
- Take advantage of free company tours of their facilities to view employees working in a variety of positions.
- Scan the Yellow Pages and the newspaper classified ads for companies that look interesting and schedule appointments to visit them in person. During the visit, find out what types of positions exist, what the job requirements are, and which positions have a high rate of turnover.
- Always be clear about your purpose for requesting an appointment with an employer. You may be the first contact an employer has with a supported employment program, and you could be setting the tone for all subsequent contacts with the employer.
- Write a thank-you letter and store it on a computer if possible; then modify it and send it to all employers you visit.
- Network with rehabilitation personnel from other agencies to share job leads and information.

As you visit employers, record information such as name, title, and phone number of the contact person; requirements of the position; environmental characteristics; and your perceptions of the employer's interest in supported employment services. The Employer Contact Sheet (Exhibit 7-6) can be used for this purpose and will serve as a source of information for making further contact with the employer.

Developing a Marketing Strategy

Employment specialists should have a well-defined marketing strategy in place before they begin to contact employers about specific job openings. A marketing plan must respond to the needs of employers, consumers, and funding sources. It should include

Exhibit 7-5 Community Job Market Screening Form

Community Job Market Screening Form

Date Completed: ____________________ Completed by: ____________________

1. General Screening

List job openings that occur frequently (derive from classified ads, employment service listings, public service ads, etc.).

Job Title/Type of Work	*General Requirements*

2. Specific Screening

List potential appropriate companies or industry in this community to contact for job openings.

Current

Company/Contact	*Type of Work*	*Address/Phone*

Developing

Company/Contact	*Type of Work*	*Address/Phone*

- personalized business cards for employment specialists to identify the person and program name, mailing address, and telephone number
- an attractive brochure, outlining the components of the supported employment program, which can be given to employers
- training and simulated exercises for employment specialists on how to deliver an effective presentation to employers

Exhibit 7-6 Employer Contact Sheet

Employer Contact Sheet

Name of Company: ____________________

Type of Company: ____________________

Mailing Address: ____________________

Phone Number: ____________ On Bus Line: ____________

Name of Contact Person: ____________________

Title of Position: ____________________

Job Site Visit (Schedule date): ____________________

Direction to Site: ____________________

____

____

Phone Contacts:

Date	Time per Call	Emp. Spec.	Comments/Reactions

Initial On-Job Site Visit Date: ____________________

Employment Specialist(s): ____________________

Transition Time: ________ Mileage: ________ Time on Site: ________

Describe visit:

(Types of jobs, current openings, wages, applicant procedures to follow, etc.)

____

____

____

____

____

____

Additional Visits:

Date: ____________ Employment Specialist(s): ____________

Transportation Time: ________ Mileage: ________ Time on Site: ________

____

____

____

Source: Virginia Commonwealth University, Rehabilitation Research and Training Center, Richmond, VA.

- tasteful, good-quality letterhead and envelopes with the program's name and logo
- a program name that conveys a clear and positive image of the supported employment service

Specific Employer Contact

The next step is to identify and pursue specific job vacancies. Employment specialists can use

- classified ads
- city, county, and state vacancy listings
- job hotlines
- career planning and placement offices on college campuses
- state employment commission
- personal contacts
- referrals from other employers
- networking with other agencies
- job bulletins compiled and distributed by personnel offices of local companies
- "help wanted" signs posted in area businesses

Should these sources fail to turn up appropriate job opportunities, contact employers identified during the community job market screening to inquire about available positions. Employment specialists also may want to make presentations to professional and civic organizations to expand their program's visibility and establish new employer contacts.

Throughout job development, review and keep in mind the interests, abilities, and experiences of individuals in the program's referral pool. For example, pursuing an available landscaping position may be a waste of time if no one in the referral pool can lift more than 20 pounds or has interest in this type of work. To meet consumer needs effectively and efficiently, employment specialists may want to alternate between developing jobs with specific individuals in mind and uncovering job opportunities that generally match individuals in the referral pool. Keep in mind that some employers are willing to negotiate job responsibilities and this possibility may be worth investigating.

Making Initial Contact

When telephoning an employer to investigate a job lead, first find out the name of the appropriate person with whom to speak. This person may be a personnel representative, secretary, direct supervisor of the individual in the available position, or company president or owner, so it is important to be prepared to speak with any level of employee. To avoid having to repeat your request for information on job requirements, job openings, or for an appointment, identify yourself, your affiliation, and your purpose for calling so that you can be referred promptly to the correct person. (This is a somewhat controversial point. By divulging this information up front, you may be allowing yourself to be screened out. However, attempting to gain access to an employer by holding back information may create employer distrust and prevent you from establishing a good relationship with him or her.)

If a job opening exists, state your purpose for calling and gather general information about the position (i.e., job responsibilities, skill requirements, pay rate, hours, location, and benefits). If the job sounds appropriate, *briefly* explain your program and ask to set up an appointment with the employer so that you can explain your program more and view the requirements of the job. Log all telephone contact information collected from your conversation on a form such as the Employer Contact Sheet (Exhibit 7-6) for future reference.

Even the most seasoned employment specialists are sometimes reluctant to use the telephone for employer contacts for fear of receiving a negative response from an employer. To help prepare for successful telephone contact, employment specialists can

- develop and use a planned approach, even a script, so that you will feel confident and sound professional
- set aside a block of time each day for making phone calls
- go to a quiet room with no distractions to make your calls
- list the worst possible responses that you could get from an employer and the likelihood that each will occur; for example, the employer could insult you (unlikely to occur), the employer could say no (might occur), the employer may hang up on you (probably won't occur)
- have in mind a purpose for calling (to gather information about a specific job opening, to arrange an appointment with an employer, to determine whether a position exists within a company, etc.) and be clear about communicating that purpose
- establish a goal for the number of appointments you can reasonably expect to make and keep making calls until you reach the goal
- remember that your level of enthusiasm will be communicated in your voice; give yourself a "pep talk" before making your call
- don't tell the employer more than is necessary to get the appointment; if he or she insists on more information, explain briefly and honestly

Table 7-1 Ineffective Telephone Contact

Characteristic	*Communications to Employer*
Flat and unenthusiastic tone of voice	Employment specialist does not regard the purpose of the phone call as important
Purpose for calling is vague	Employer is likely to believe that his or her time is being wasted
Lengthy description of the cognitive and physical impairments of head injured people	Employer perceives that persons with traumatic brain injury are too impaired to fill any need in the organization
Employment specialist is passive participant in conversation	Employer recognizes quickly that the employment specialist is not likely to persist if the employer says no

how he or she can benefit from meeting with you (Payne, Miller, Hazlett, & Mercer, 1984)

- ask the employer open-ended questions as opposed to yes/no questions
- keep in mind that employers are busy people and be sensitive about the amount of time you request of them
- be prepared to respond to negative replies and be persistent, but courteous

Table 7-1 lists characteristics of ineffective telephone contact.

Cold Calls. Contacting employers through cold calls, or drop-in visits, can be an effective way to obtain an appointment or find out what positions are currently available in a company. Obviously, employment specialists using this method have already succeeded in getting "a foot in the door" and it is much more difficult for employers to turn them away. However, cold calls are appropriate only when visiting publicly visible employers, such as retail store managers or fast food restaurant managers, or when a "help wanted" sign or ad in the newspaper indicates that one should apply in person. Most employers who are not publicly visible expect to be contacted by telephone (McLoughlin, Garner, & Callahan, 1987). However, at times personnel directors may be available. If not, you can use this opportunity to set up an appointment.

Letters. Employment specialists who experience difficulty gaining access to an employer through telephone or cold calls may want to send employers a brief letter introducing the supported employment program and enclose their program's brochure with a business card attached. Employers may be more receptive to a follow-up phone call if they have become familiar with what you have to offer.

Employer Presentation

As employment specialists prepare to meet with an employer, an obvious consideration is how to dress. As a representative of your program, the image that you project will reflect the quality of the service you provide. Besides conveying the message that you value the service you offer and the opportunity to meet with the employer, dressing in a businesslike manner will help boost your self-confidence and project a positive attitude. However, while a business suit may be appropriate to wear when meeting with a personnel director of a large company, such attire may appear out of place when meeting with a supervisor of an ice manufacturing company. Choose your dress according to the type of company you are visiting as well as the level of the person with whom you will be meeting. When in doubt, dress professionally.

Another key element in preparing to meet with an employer is organization. Take the time to collect program brochures; business cards; your Employer Contact Sheet, Employer Interview Form, and Job Screening Form (see Exhibits 7-6, 7-7, and 7-8 respectively); pens; and a notepad. Unless you are familiar with the location of the company you are visiting, obtain clear directions to the job site and take them with you. A detailed city map is a good investment for employment specialists who work in a medium to large city. Finally, always be on time for your appointment. If you are unavoidably delayed, call the employer and give him or her the option of rescheduling the appointment.

Just as no two employer presentations will ever be identical, employment specialists need to develop their own personal style for delivering an effective presentation. The following guidelines provide a framework for points you will want to include when meeting with an employer; however, adapt this information to meet your agency's needs.

Establish Rapport. Devote no more than a few minutes to engaging the employer in small talk to break the ice. Glance around the employer's office for any plaques, diplomas, photographs, or posters that might serve as the subject of some light conversation and comment on them. The key is to set the tone for getting to know the employer, but use good judgment in recognizing when it is time to move on to the purpose of your visit.

Introduce Your Agency. Establish the credibility of your program by briefly describing your agency's mission and role as a supported employment provider. Mention any relevant background information such as the number of years your agency has been providing services (if it is fairly well established), past and present populations of individuals it has served, and how it fits into the rehabilitation system.

Identify the Population. Avoiding technical jargon, explain that your program serves individuals who have sustained brian injuries, most com-

Exhibit 7-7 Sample Employer Interview Form

Employer Interview Form

Company: ______________________________ Date: ______________________

______________________________ Phone: ______________________

____

Person Interviewed: ______________________________

Title: ______________________________

Job Title: ______________________ Rate of Pay: ______________________

Work Schedule: ______________________________

____

____

Company Benefits: ______________________________

Size of Company (or number of employees): ______________________

Volume and/or pace of work:

Overall: ______________________ This position: ______________________

Number of employees in this position: ______________________

During the same hours: ______________________________

Written job description available: ______________________

Description of job duties: (Record on Sequence of Job Duties Form)

Availability of supervision (estimate percentage of time): ______________________

____

Availability of coworkers (direct or indirect): ______________________

____

Orientation skills needed (size and layout of work area): ______________________

____

What are important aspects of position:

Speed ________ vs. Thoroughness _____ Judgment _____ vs. Routine _____

Teamwork _____ vs. Independence _____ Repetition _____ vs. Variability ____

Other: ______________________________

What are absolute "don'ts" for employee in this position (e.g., manager's pet peeves, reasons for dismissal, etc.)? ______________________________

____

Describe any reading or math that is required: ______________________

____

What machinery or equipment will the employee need to operate? ______________

____

OBSERVATIONAL INFORMATION:

Appearance of employees: ______________________________

Atmosphere:

________ Friendly, cheerful ________ Aloof, indifferent

________ Busy, relaxed ________ Busy, tense

________ Slow, relaxed ________ Slow, tense

________ Structured, orderly ________ Unstructured, disorderly

Other: ______________________________

Environmental characteristics (physical barriers, extremes in temperature, etc.): ______

____

Comments: ______________________________

____

SIGNATURE/TITLE: ______________________________

Source: Virginia Commonwealth University, Rehabilitation Research and Training Center, Richmond, VA.

Exhibit 7-8 Sample Job Screening Form

Job Screening Form

Please complete one Job Screening Form for each job the consumer had during the period in question. All items refer to this particular position at this particular company for this particular location.

Consumer:
Name: ______________________
SSN: _ _ _ / _ _ / _ _ _ _

Staff member completing this form:
Name: ______________________
I.D. Code: ______________________

Company:
Name: ______________________
ID Code: ______________________

Screening Date: _ _ / _ _ / _ _
mo. day yr.

Type of service/employment for this report (Select one): __________
1 = Work activity or sheltered employment
2 = Entrepreneurial
3 = Mobile work crew
4 = Enclave
5 = Supported job
6 = Supported competitive employment
7 = Time-limited (No ongoing services anticipated)
8 = Other (Specify: ______________________

Type of screening: Initial __________ Ongoing __________ Final __________

Job title: ______________________

Current hourly wage (or wage at last date of employment in this position): __________

Did a wage change occur since the last job screening or job update? Yes ______ No ______
If yes, then complete this section:
Hourly rate changed from $______ to $______ on _ _ / _ _ / _ _
Hourly rate changed from $______ to $______ on _ _ / _ _ / _ _

Number of hours per week: ______ Months per year: ______

If less than 12 months per year, what months is the job not available? ______

Number of employees in this company at this location: ______

Number of employees without disabilities in immediate area (50 ft. radius): ______

Number of other employees with disabilities: ______

In immediate area (50 ft. radius): ______

Number of other employees in this position: ______

During the same hours: ______

General Directions: PLEASE DO NOT LEAVE ANY ITEM UNANSWERED

Indicate the most appropriate response for each item based on observations of the job and interviews with employers, supervisors, and coworkers. Also circle CI (critically important), I (important), LI (less important), or NI (not important) for each item to indicate its level of importance in *this position*.

1. Schedule: (Circle yes or no for each item) CI / I / LI / NI	Weekend Work Required Yes / No	Evening Work Required Yes / No	Part-Time Job Yes / No	Full-Time Job Yes / No
Specifics/Comments:				
2. Travel Location: (Circle yes or no for each item) CI / I / LI / NI	On Public Transportation Route Yes / No		On Handicapped Transportation Route Yes / No	
Specifics/Comments:				
3. Strength: Lifting and Carrying CI / I / LI / NI	Very Light Work (< 10 lbs) ______	Light Work (10–30 lbs) ______	Average Work (30–40 lbs) ______	Heavy Work (> 40 lbs) ______
Specifics/Comments:				

continues

Exhibit 7-8 continued

4. Endurance: (no breaks) CI / I / LI / NI Specifics/Comments:	Work Required for < 2 hours ________	Work Required for 2–3 hours ________	Work Required for 3–4 hours ________	Work Required for > 4 hours ________	
5. Orienting: CI / I / LI / NI Specifics/Comments:	Small Area Only ________	One Room ________	Several Rooms ________	Building-Wide ________	Building and Grounds ________
6. Physical Mobility: CI / I / LI / NI Specifics/Comments:	Sit/Stand in One Area ________	Fair Ambulation Required ________	Stairs/Minor Obstacles ________	Full Physical Requirements ________	
7. Work Pace: CI / I / LI / NI Specifics/Comments:	Slow Pace ________	Average Steady Pace ________	Sometimes Fast Pace ________	Continual Fast Pace ________	
8. Appearance Requirements: CI / I / LI / NI Specifics/Comments:	Grooming of Little Importance ________	Cleanliness Only Required ________	Neat and Clean Required ________	Grooming Very Important ________	
9. Communication Required: CI / I / LI / NI Specifics/Comments:	None/ Minimal ________	Key Words/ Signs Needed ________	Unclear Speech Accepted ________	Clear Speech in Sentences/Signs Needed ________	

10. Social Interactions:	Social Interactions Not Required ________	Appropriate Responses Required ________	Social Interactions Required Infrequently ________	Social Interactions Required Frequently ________
CI / I / LI / NI Specifics/Comments:				
11. Behavior Acceptance Range: CI / I / LI / NI Specifics/Comments:	Many Unusual Behaviors Accepted ________	Few Unusual Behaviors Accepted ________		No Unusual Behaviors Accepted ________
12. Attention to Task/ Perserverance: CI / I / LI / NI Specifics/Comments:	Frequent Prompts Available ________	Intermittent Prompts/High Supervision Available ________	Intermittent Prompts/Low Supervision Available ________	Infrequent Prompts/Low Supervision Available ________
13. Sequencing of Job Duties: CI / I / LI / NI Specifics/Comments:	Only One Task Required At a Time ________	2–3 Tasks Required in Sequence ________	4–6 Tasks Required in Sequence ________	7 or More Tasks Required in Sequence ________
14. Initiation of Work/ Motivation: CI / I / LI / NI Specifics/Comments:	Initiation of Work Required ________	Volunteering Helpful ________		Staff Will Prompt to Next Task ________
15. Daily Changes In Routine: Specifics/Comments:	7 or More Changes ________	4–6 Task Changes ________	2–3 Task Changes ________	No Task Changes ________

continues

Exhibit 7-8 continued

16. Reinforcement Available: CI / I / LI / NI Specifics/Comments:	Frequent Reinforcement ________	Reinforcement Intermittent (daily) ________	Reinforcement Infrequent (weekly) ________	Minimal Reinforcement (paycheck) ________
17. Employer Attitude: CI / I / LI / NI Specifics/Comments:	Very Supportive of Workers with Disabilities ________	Supportive with Reservations ________	Indifferent to Workers with Disabilities ________	Negative toward Workers with Disabilities ________
18. Employer's Financial Requirements: CI / I / LI / NI Specifics/Comments:	Financial Incentives Not Necessary ________	Tax Credit or Incentive (e.g., TJTC, OJT) ________		Subminimum Wage ________
19. Object Discrimination: CI / I / LI / NI Specifics/Comments:	Does Not Need To Distinguish Among Work Supplies ________	Must Distinguish Among Work Supplies with an External Cue ________		Must Distinguish Among Work Supplies ________
20. Time: CI / I / LI / NI Specifics/Comments:	Time Factors Not Important ________	Must Identify Breaks/Meals Etc. ________	Must Tell Time to the Hour ________	Must Tell Time to the Minute ________

21. Functional Reading: CI / I / LI / NI	None ________	Sight Words/ Symbols ________	Simple Reading ________	Fluent Reading ________
Specifics/Comments:				
22. Functional Math: CI / I / LI / NI	None ________	Simple Counting ________	Simple Addition/ Subtraction ________	Complex Computational Skills ________
Specifics/Comments:				
23. Street Crossing: None ____ CI / I / LI / NI	Must Cross 2 Lane Street with Light ________	Must Cross 2 Lane Street without Light ________	Must Cross 4 Lane Street with Light ________	Must Cross 4 Lane Street without Light ________
Specifics/Comments:				
24. Visibility to Public: CI / I / LI / NI	Consumer Not Visible ________	Occasionally Visible ________	Regularly Visible ________	Visible throughout the Day/Ongoing ________
Specifics/Comments:				

25. Benefits of Job:

Yes / No 0 = None	Yes / No 4 = Dental Benefits
Yes / No 1 = Sick Leave	Yes / No 5 = Employee Discounts
Yes / No 2 = Medical/Health Benefits	Yes / No 6 = Free or Reduced Meals
Yes / No 3 = Paid Vacation/Annual Leave	Yes / No 7 = Other (Specify): ____________

26. Level of Social Contact: (Circle one)

(0)—Employment in a segregated setting in which the majority of interactions with persons without disabilities are with caregivers or service providers. Example: Adult Activity Center Worker

(1)—Employment in an integrated environment in a shift or position that is isolated. Contact with coworkers without disabilities or supervisors is minimal. Example: Night Janitor

continues

Exhibit 7-8 continued

(2)—Employment in an integrated environment in a shift or position that is relatively isolated. Contact with coworkers without disabilities or supervisors is available at lunch or break. Example: Pot Scrubber

(3)—Employment in an integrated environment in a position requiring a moderate level of task dependency and coworker interaction. Example: Dishwasher required to keep plate supply stacked for cooks

(4)—Employment in an integrated environment in a position requiring a high degree of task dependency and coworker interaction and/or high level of contact with customers. Example: Busperson/Porter

---

27. CHECK ALL THAT APPLY TO POSITION:

___ Bussing Tables	___ Sweeping	___ Use Dishwasher	___ Keeping Busy
___ Food Preparation	___ Assembly	___ Mopping (Indust.)	___ Clerical Work
___ Buffing	___ Vacuuming	___ Food Line Supply	___ Pot Scrubbing
___ Dusting	___ Restroom Cleaning	___ Trash Disposal	___ Other
___ Stocking	___ Washing Equipment	___ Food Serving	___________

COMMENTS:

Rate of employee turnover (annual percentage):

Overall: ___________ This position: ___________

Number of supervisors: ___________ Rate of supervisor turnover: ___________

Written job description available? ___________

What are absolute "don'ts" for an employee in this position (manager's pet peeves, reasons for dismissal, etc.)? ___________

Environmental characteristics (physical barriers, temperature extremes, etc.): ____________

Additional Comments: ____________

Source: Form developed by the Rehabilitation Research and Training Center, Virginia Commonwealth University, in cooperation with the Virginia Departments of Mental Health and Mental Retardation and Rehabilitative Services (Revised 9/87).

monly as a result of automobile accidents. Many times, employers will know of someone, either personally or professionally, who has experienced debilitating injuries in an automobile or other accident, thus lending an effective point of reference to the discussion.

Be prepared to provide, in functional terms, information on individuals with traumatic brain injury, emphasizing that each person is unique due to the specific nature of the injury. (It is helpful to consider, in advance of your meeting with an employer, how you will describe individuals with TBI.) Remember to be honest and accurate in your explanation, but do not focus excessively on the deficits associated with traumatic brain injury as this is likely to create the impression that the persons you are attempting to place are far too disabled to be employed.

Then, present information on some of your program's successful placements, including types of positions and names of employers. (You should previously have obtained permission from supervisors of individuals who are currently placed to use them as references with prospective employers.) If you are involved with a new program with no previous placements of traumatic brain injured individuals, cite successful placements your agency has made with other populations or refer to successful placements made by similar programs.

Explain the Supported Employment Model. For employers who are unfamiliar with supported employment, you will want to educate them on the components of the model. Using your program's brochure as you cover each component will serve as a visual aid for the employer. Be sure to address the components described below.

- Job Placement—Explain that the analysis of job requirements made during job development is paired with information gathered on an individual's interests, abilities, and experience to make a successful job match. Emphasize that placement will not be pursued if an appropriate candidate for the job opening cannot be identified.
- Job Site Training—Establish the role of the employment specialist in accompanying the new employee to the job site, at no cost to the employer, to provide additional training and support. Make it clear that the employment specialist will actually contribute to completing the job duties if applicable while the individual develops the speed and endurance for completing the job.
- Ongoing Assessment and Follow-Along—Explain that when the individual can perform the job independently to the employer's satisfaction, the employment specialist will begin to gradually and systematically fade his or her presence from the job site. Emphasize, however, that the employment specialist will continue to monitor the individual's performance as long as he or she is employed to be proac-

tive in addressing any problems or issues that may arise as well as retraining or learning a new job responsibility.

Appeal to Vested Interests. Be sure to tell the employer about financial incentives, such as the Targeted Jobs Tax Credit (TJTC), which are available for hiring employees with disabilities. Stress that the ultimate goal in placing individuals in employment is to assist them in regaining their position in society as independent, contributing, and tax-paying citizens.

Another important point to mention is that research and experience have shown employees with disabilities to be motivated, dependable workers who tend to remain in their positions longer than non-disabled workers. This point is especially appealing to employers with a high rate of turnover.

Wrap-Up. Close your presentation by answering any questions the employer may have and use open-ended questions and diplomacy to get a verbal indication from the employer of his or her interest in working with your program. If the employer appears interested, find out whether there are any current job openings; if so, ask for the job requirements of any that sound appropriate and record the information on the Employer Interview Form (Exhibit 7-7). Arrange to observe the work area when it is convenient so that you can analyze the position in depth.

If no job openings are available, establish guidelines for further communication with the employer. Determine the application procedures should an appropriate position become available and, if possible, obtain an application for your files.

Always thank the employer, regardless of his or her interest, for taking the time to meet with you. Then, follow up with a thank-you letter.

It goes without saying that employer presentations do not always run smoothly. Refer to Exhibit 7-9 for a list of problems that employment specialists may encounter when meeting with employers and some recommended employment specialist responses.

Job Analysis

If it appears that an appropriate job opening exists, the employment specialist asks to observe or even shadow an employee working in that position so that the specific requirements of the job can be analyzed. Employment specialists assess the job in terms of such factors as productivity, endurance, strength, appearance, physical mobility, and communication skills. The aim of job analysis is to collect as much detailed information as possible that can be used, in combination with consumer assessment information, to make a placement decision.

Exhibit 7-9 Employer Contact Problems

Problem: The employer has had a "bad experience" with a "disabled person" in the past, so he or she is reluctant to hire another such employee.

Employment Specialist's Response: Find out what the specific problems were that he or she experienced with the employee and describe strategies you would use to address such problems. If the previous employee had not been involved with a supported employment program, emphasize that your role is proactive and ongoing in assisting an individual with successfully maintaining employment.

Problem: The employer is hesitant to interview an individual whom you have identified as appropriate for an available position because he or she does not want to disappoint the individual if it "doesn't work out."

Employment Specialist's Response: Emphasize that it would be very helpful for the individual to experience a job interview even if he or she is not offered the position. Remind the employer that you would like to participate in the interview and, thus, will be available to assist with any "rough spots" that may arise.

Problem: You have uncovered a job opening that sounds appropriate except that one of the job requirements is washing windows. No one in your referral pool is able to climb a ladder.

Employment Specialist's Response: Try to substitute another job duty for washing windows. For example, find out whether a job duty exists that the employer has difficulty getting completed and suggest that he or she incorporate this duty (if appropriate) into the available position.

Problem: You are delivering a presentation to an employer who has various openings for security guards. The employer, referring to a position at a construction site, responds that he or she doesn't know if he or she could hire someone with a disability because that person might fall in a piece of machinery and get "ground up," thus forcing the company to pay workers' compensation.

Employment Specialist's Response: Stress that, in a case such as this one, you would do a detailed assessment of the job requirements as well as the individual's abilities and deficits before you would consider placing someone in this position. Investigate other, more appropriate sites at which a security guard might be assigned.

In addition, explain that the company would not be responsible for paying workers' compensation as long as the injury sustained on the job is a manifestation of the individual's brain injury.

JOB PLACEMENT

To identify candidates from a referral pool for an available job opening, do a compatibility analysis integrating and comparing consumer assessment and job analysis information. The employment specialist should refer to neuropsychological reports, vocational evaluations, and previous educational or work history in the consumer file to assist in the decision-making process. When the employment specialist determines which candidate is the best match for the job, the consumer is notified of a possible job opportunity.

If the consumer is interested in the position, the employment specialist arranges a job interview for the consumer with the employer. Employment specialists frequently participate in the interview to support a consumer. If a start date is established during the interview, the employment specialist may take on the role of a case manager, coordinating transportation, working out the effects of employment on social security benefits, and obtaining the necessary paperwork for the Targeted Jobs Tax Credit (TJTC).

With much of the major job development behind you, specific job-site training and orientation is the next step. What follows is a complete description of training strategies.

SUMMARY

In summary, the end result of consumer assessment and job development is job placement. An employment specialist cannot get to know a consumer well enough or obtain too much information regarding the individual. As the employment specialist spends more time with the consumer and gathers information, the greater the likelihood of a successful job match. It is imperative that the consumer be involved in decisions regarding what types of jobs the employment specialist should pursue as potential placement.

Job development requires that an employment specialist become a professional sales person. By performing an ongoing thorough consumer assessment, the scope of job development can be reduced. As obvious as it may sound, remember if job development does not occur there will not be a placement.

With the job placement process behind you, job-site training and orientation is the next step. What follows is a complete description of training strategies.

REFERENCES

McLoughlin, C., Garner, J., & Callahan, M. (1987). *Getting Employed Staying Employed*. Baltimore: Paul H. Brookes.

Payne, J., Miller, A., Hazlett, R., & Mercer, C. (1984). *Rehabilitation on Techniques*. New York: Human Sciences Press, Inc.

Wehman, P., & Moon, S. (1988). *Vocational Rehabilitation and Supported Employment*. Baltimore: Paul H. Brookes.

Appendix 7-A

General Health and History Questionnaire Parts I–III

GENERAL HEALTH AND HISTORY QUESTIONNAIRE PART I

DIRECTIONS: We are interested in how the client has changed because of his/her head injury. Your answers to this form will help us understand problems related to the client's injury and provide the best treatment. All information will be kept confidential. Please answer **all** questions. We realize you may be uncertain about some of the information you provide. **Please be as accurate as possible.**

Your Name: ________________________________ Date _-_-_

Client's Name: ________________________________

Client's Address: ________________________________

____

Client's Phone Number: (_)________________________

Client's Social Security Number: _ _ _-_ _-_ _ _ _

1. **Your** relationship to the client: (circle one)
   mother father wife husband brother sister son daughter friend girl/boyfriend other ________________ (please write in)
2. What is **your** date of birth? (please write in)
   Month: ____________ Date: ____________ Year: 19___
3. **CURRENTLY**, are **you** working: (circle one)
   full time part time not working
   If Yes, please write in **your** occupation ____________________
4. **CURRENTLY**, are **you** in school? (circle one)

full time part time not in school

5. What is the highest grade **you** completed in school? (circle one)
   none / some college
   1-8 years / college graduate
   some high school / postgraduate
   high school graduate / unknown
6. Please indicate as accurately as possible the **date, month, and year** when the client was hurt:
   Month: ______________ Date: ______________ Year: 19___
7. What is the client's date of birth?
   Month: ______________ Date: ______________ Year: 19___
8. How long was the client unconscious or in coma? Please give your best estimate as to the number of minutes, days, hours or months:
   ___ Minutes ___ Hours ___ Days ___ Months
   ___ Never unconscious ___ Unknown
9. **CURRENTLY,** is the client taking medications for seizures? (circle one)
   Yes No
   If yes, please list **all** medications, including those for seizures, the client takes on a regular basis:
   1. ______________ 4. ______________
   2. ______________ 5. ______________
   3. ______________ 6. ______________
10. **CURRENTLY,** do you live with the client? (circle one)
    Yes No
11. **CURRENTLY,** where does the client live? (circle one)
    home/apartment hospital rehabilitation center/hospital
    nursing home adult home/transitional living center
    other ______________________________ (please write in)
12. **CURRENTLY,** who lives with the client? (circle all that apply)
    mother father wife husband brother sister son
    daughter friend girl/boyfriend other ______________
    (please write in)
13. If the client is **CURRENTLY** living at home, how **comfortable do you feel about leaving him/her at home alone?** (circle one)
    1 ——— 2 ——— 3 ——— 4 ——— 5
    very uncomfortable / a little uncomfortable / very comfortable
14. **CURRENTLY,** is the client medically restricted from driving? (circle one)
    Yes No
    If the client is not medically restricted from driving, does he/she have a valid drivers license? (circle one)
    Yes No

15. **CURRENTLY,** what is the client's marital status? (circle one)
    single | married
    steady relationship | separated
    engaged | divorced
    unmarried/living with mate | widowed
    If married, how many years has he/she been married? ___
16. **BEFORE** the injury, was the client working? (circle one)
    full time | 20–39 hours/week | 1–19 hours/week | not working
17. **BEFORE** the injury, was the client in school? (circle one)
    full time | part time | not in school
18. **CURRENTLY,** is the client in school? (circle one)
    full time | part time | not in school
19. **CURRENTLY,** is the client working? (circle one)
    full time | 20–39 hours/week | 1–19 hours/week | not working
20. What is the highest grade completed by the client? (circle one)
    none | some college
    1-8 years | college graduate
    some high school | postgraduate
    high school graduate | unknown
21. List the jobs the client held **BEFORE** the injury, the number of hours worked per week, and the starting and finishing dates of each job. If you are unsure of the exact dates, please give your **best estimate.** Where needed, describe the position held. Only include those jobs which the client earned at least minimum wage. **List his/her most recent job BEFORE the injury on line #1:**

	Type of Job	Average Number of Hours per Week	Month/Day/Year Started	Month/Day/Year Finished	Wages
1.	____________	_ hrs.	__/__/__	__/__/__	_________
2.	____________	_ hrs.	__/__/__	__/__/__	_________
3.	____________	_ hrs.	__/__/__	__/__/__	_________
4.	____________	_ hrs.	__/__/__	__/__/__	_________
5.	____________	_ hrs.	__/__/__	__/__/__	_________
6.	____________	_ hrs.	__/__/__	__/__/__	_________

22. List the jobs the client has held **SINCE** the injury, the number of hours worked per week, and the starting and finishing dates of each job. If you are unsure of the exact dates, please give your **best estimate.** Where needed, describe the position held by the client. Include only those jobs which the client earned at least minimum wage. List his/her most recent job **SINCE** the injury on line #1.

	Type of Job	Average Number of Hours per Week	Month/Day/Year Started	Month/Day/Year Finished	Wages
1.	____________	_ hrs.	__/__/__	__/__/__	_________

2. _____________ _ hrs. __/__/__ __/__/__ _________
3. _____________ _ hrs. __/__/__ __/__/__ _________
4. _____________ _ hrs. __/__/__ __/__/__ _________
5. _____________ _ hrs. __/__/__ __/__/__ _________
6. _____________ _ hrs. __/__/__ __/__/__ _________

23. **CURRENTLY,** is the client working in a sheltered workshop? (circle one)

Yes No

24. **Financial Aid:**

	Ever	In the Past Month	Current Payment per Month (if any)
a. SSI	Yes / No	Yes / No	____________
b. SSDI	Yes / No	Yes / No	____________
c. Medicaid	Yes / No	Yes / No	____________
d. Medicare	Yes / No	Yes / No	____________
e. Food Stamps	Yes / No	Yes / No	____________
f. Public Assistance (Welfare)	Yes / No	Yes / No	____________
g. Private Insurance	Yes / No	Yes / No	____________
h. Workers' Compensation	Yes / No	Yes / No	____________
i. Other ____________________	Yes / No	Yes / No	____________
j. Other lump sum financial settlements	Yes / No	Yes / No	____________

25. If the client is **not CURRENTLY** a full time student or is **not** working full time, which of the following **prevent or interfere** with employment. Put an "X" in the blank next to the items that apply:

___ no transportation
___ bad temper
___ no motivation/doesn't care
___ no pep or energy
___ can't walk/climb stairs
___ depression
___ poor vision
___ can't speak properly
___ can't understand speech
___ memory
___ seizures
___ medically ill, sick
___ thinking problems
___ trouble using hands, arms, legs

List any other problems that you feel get in the way:

____

____

26. **BEFORE** the injury, was the client a nondrinker (never drank alcoholic beverages)? (circle one)

Yes No

27. **BEFORE** the injury, did the client have a drinking problem? (circle one)

    Yes No

28. **CURRENTLY,** does the client drink alcohol? (circle one)

    Yes No

29. **CURRENTLY,** does the client have a drinking problem? (circle one)

    Yes No

30. **BEFORE** the injury, did the client use illegal drugs? (circle one)

    Yes No

31. Please indicate the drugs that were used **BEFORE** the injury:

    marijuana cocaine other: ____________ please fill in

32. **CURRENTLY,** does the client use illegal drugs? (circle one)

    Yes No

33. Please indicate the drugs **CURRENTLY** being used:

    marijuana cocaine other: ____________ please fill in

34. **BEFORE** the injury, was the client ever arrested? (circle one)

    Yes No

    If Yes, please explain each arrest:

    ____
    ____
    ____
    ____

35. **BEFORE** the injury, was he/she convicted? (circle one)

    Yes No

    If Yes, please explain each conviction:

    ____
    ____
    ____

36. **SINCE** his/her injury, has the client been arrested? (circle one)

    Yes No

    If Yes, please explain each arrest:

    ____
    ____
    ____

37. **SINCE** the injury, has he/she ever been convicted? (circle one)

    Yes No

    If Yes, please explain each conviction:

    ____
    ____
    ____

38. Place an "X" next to the services listed below that the client is **CURRENTLY** receiving. If the client is not receiving any services, leave question blank:

___ physical therapy	___ occupational therapy
___ psychotherapy	___ transportation
___ Virginia Department of Rehabilitative Services (DRS)	___ speech therapy
___ cognitive retraining	___ work adjustment/hardening
___ vocational training	

other, please specify: ____

____

____

PROBLEM CHECKLIST

DIRECTIONS: We would like to know if the client **CURRENTLY** has any of the problems listed below, and if so, how often. Please place an "X" in the box under the label ("never," "sometimes," "often," or "always") which best describes how often each problem occurs. **PLEASE ANSWER ALL ITEMS.**

SOMATIC	NEVER	SOMETIMES	OFTEN	ALWAYS	DOES NOT APPLY
01. Blackout spells ------------------------------------	[ ]	[ ]	[ ]	[ ]	
02. Difficulty lifting heavy objects -------------------	[ ]	[ ]	[ ]	[ ]	
03. Dizzy --	[ ]	[ ]	[ ]	[ ]	
04. Difficulty smelling things -------------------------	[ ]	[ ]	[ ]	[ ]	
05. Double vision --------------------------------------	[ ]	[ ]	[ ]	[ ]	[ ]
06. Drops things ---------------------------------------	[ ]	[ ]	[ ]	[ ]	
07. Eats too much --------------------------------------	[ ]	[ ]	[ ]	[ ]	
08. Food doesn't taste right ---------------------------	[ ]	[ ]	[ ]	[ ]	
09. Headaches --	[ ]	[ ]	[ ]	[ ]	
10. Loses balance --------------------------------------	[ ]	[ ]	[ ]	[ ]	[ ]
11. Moves slowly ---------------------------------------	[ ]	[ ]	[ ]	[ ]	
12. Muscles ache ---------------------------------------	[ ]	[ ]	[ ]	[ ]	
13. Muscles numb ---------------------------------------	[ ]	[ ]	[ ]	[ ]	
14. Muscles tingle or twitch ---------------------------	[ ]	[ ]	[ ]	[ ]	
15. Nauseous ---	[ ]	[ ]	[ ]	[ ]	
16. Nightmares ---	[ ]	[ ]	[ ]	[ ]	

17. Poor appetite	[ ]	[ ]	[ ]	[ ]	
18. Picks nose or skin	[ ]	[ ]	[ ]	[ ]	
19. Ringing in ears	[ ]	[ ]	[ ]	[ ]	
20. Seizures	[ ]	[ ]	[ ]	[ ]	
21. Stomach bloated or gassy	[ ]	[ ]	[ ]	[ ]	
22. Stomach hurts	[ ]	[ ]	[ ]	[ ]	
23. Tired	[ ]	[ ]	[ ]	[ ]	
24. Trips over things	[ ]	[ ]	[ ]	[ ]	
25. Trouble falling asleep	[ ]	[ ]	[ ]	[ ]	
26. Trouble hearing	[ ]	[ ]	[ ]	[ ]	
27. Trouble staying awake	[ ]	[ ]	[ ]	[ ]	
28. Trouble waking up	[ ]	[ ]	[ ]	[ ]	
29. Vision blurred	[ ]	[ ]	[ ]	[ ]	[ ]
30. Weak	[ ]	[ ]	[ ]	[ ]	

THINKING	NEVER	SOMETIMES	OFTEN	ALWAYS	DOES NOT APPLY
31. Difficulty handling money	[ ]	[ ]	[ ]	[ ]	[ ]
32. Can't get mind off certain thoughts	[ ]	[ ]	[ ]	[ ]	
33. Difficulty performing chores	[ ]	[ ]	[ ]	[ ]	[ ]
34. Difficulty attending work or school	[ ]	[ ]	[ ]	[ ]	[ ]
35. Concentration is poor	[ ]	[ ]	[ ]	[ ]	
36. Confused	[ ]	[ ]	[ ]	[ ]	
37. Drives dangerously	[ ]	[ ]	[ ]	[ ]	[ ]
38. Easily distracted	[ ]	[ ]	[ ]	[ ]	
39. Forgets or misses appointments	[ ]	[ ]	[ ]	[ ]	[ ]
40. Forgets peoples names	[ ]	[ ]	[ ]	[ ]	
41. Forgets phone numbers	[ ]	[ ]	[ ]	[ ]	
42. Forgets to do chores or work	[ ]	[ ]	[ ]	[ ]	[ ]
43. Forgets to eat	[ ]	[ ]	[ ]	[ ]	
44. Forgets to take medications	[ ]	[ ]	[ ]	[ ]	[ ]
45. Forgets yesterday's events	[ ]	[ ]	[ ]	[ ]	
46. Forgets what he/she reads	[ ]	[ ]	[ ]	[ ]	[ ]
47. Friends or relatives are unfamiliar	[ ]	[ ]	[ ]	[ ]	[ ]
48. Late for appointments	[ ]	[ ]	[ ]	[ ]	[ ]
49. Learns slowly	[ ]	[ ]	[ ]	[ ]	
50. Loses track of time, day, or date	[ ]	[ ]	[ ]	[ ]	
51. Loses way, gets lost	[ ]	[ ]	[ ]	[ ]	[ ]
52. Makes mistakes doing arithmetic	[ ]	[ ]	[ ]	[ ]	[ ]
53. Misplaces things	[ ]	[ ]	[ ]	[ ]	
54. Reads slowly	[ ]	[ ]	[ ]	[ ]	
55. Thinks slowly	[ ]	[ ]	[ ]	[ ]	
56. Trouble making decisions	[ ]	[ ]	[ ]	[ ]	
57. Trouble following instructions	[ ]	[ ]	[ ]	[ ]	
58. Loses train of thought	[ ]	[ ]	[ ]	[ ]	

59. Forgets if he/she has done things	[]	[]	[]	[]
60. Forgets to turn off appliances	[]	[]	[]	[]

BEHAVIOR

	NEVER	SOMETIMES	OFTEN	ALWAYS
61. Bored	[]	[]	[]	[]
62. Breaks or throws things	[]	[]	[]	[]
63. Complains	[]	[]	[]	[]
64. Cries	[]	[]	[]	[]
65. Curses at others	[]	[]	[]	[]
66. Curses at self	[]	[]	[]	[]
67. Difficulty understanding jokes	[]	[]	[]	[]
68. Disorganized	[]	[]	[]	[]
69. Difficulty enjoying activities	[]	[]	[]	[]
70. Feels hopeless	[]	[]	[]	[]
71. Feels worthless	[]	[]	[]	[]
72. Frustrated	[]	[]	[]	[]
73. Hard to get started on things	[]	[]	[]	[]
74. Hits or pushes others	[]	[]	[]	[]
75. Impatient	[]	[]	[]	[]
76. Inappropriate comments/behavior	[]	[]	[]	[]
77. Jumpy, irritable	[]	[]	[]	[]
78. Laughs for no reason	[]	[]	[]	[]
79. Lonely	[]	[]	[]	[]
80. Misunderstood by others	[]	[]	[]	[]
81. Nervous	[]	[]	[]	[]
82. No confidence	[]	[]	[]	[]
83. Restless	[]	[]	[]	[]
84. Sad, blue	[]	[]	[]	[]
85. Scared or frightened	[]	[]	[]	[]
86. Screams or yells	[]	[]	[]	[]
87. Sits with nothing to do	[]	[]	[]	[]
88. Threatens to hurt others	[]	[]	[]	[]
89. Threatens to hurt self	[]	[]	[]	[]

COMMUNICATION

	NEVER	SOMETIMES	OFTEN	ALWAYS	DOES NOT APPLY
90. Difficulty thinking of right word	[]	[]	[]	[]	

91. Difficulty pronouncing words -------------------	[ ]	[ ]	[ ]	[ ]	
92. Difficulty making conversation -----------------	[ ]	[ ]	[ ]	[ ]	
93. Makes spelling mistakes -------------------------	[ ]	[ ]	[ ]	[ ]	[ ]
94. Repeats what others say -------------------------	[ ]	[ ]	[ ]	[ ]	
95. Speech doesn't make sense ----------------------	[ ]	[ ]	[ ]	[ ]	
96. Talks too fast or slow----------------------------	[ ]	[ ]	[ ]	[ ]	
97. Trouble understanding conversation -----------	[ ]	[ ]	[ ]	[ ]	
98. Writes slowly --------------------------------------	[ ]	[ ]	[ ]	[ ]	
99. (His/her) writing is hard to read----------------	[ ]	[ ]	[ ]	[ ]	

SOCIAL	NEVER	SOMETIMES	OFTEN	ALWAYS	DOES NOT APPLY
100. Argues --	[ ]	[ ]	[ ]	[ ]	
101. Avoids family members-------------------------	[ ]	[ ]	[ ]	[ ]	
102. Avoids friends -----------------------------------	[ ]	[ ]	[ ]	[ ]	
103. Doesn't participate in sports ------------------	[ ]	[ ]	[ ]	[ ]	
104. Rude to others-----------------------------------	[ ]	[ ]	[ ]	[ ]	
105. Uncomfortable around others -----------------	[ ]	[ ]	[ ]	[ ]	

106. How much stress have you felt because of the changes in your relative/friend since the injury? (circle one number)

0	1	2	3	4	5	6
No stress			Moderate Stress			Severe Stress

107. How accurate are your answers to this questionnaire? (circle one number)

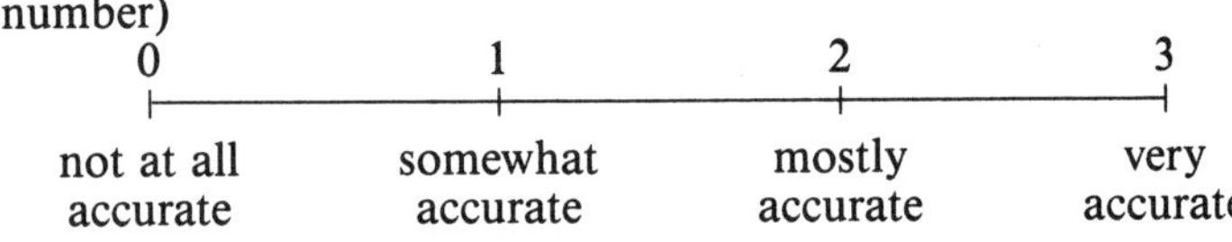

REMINDER: Please check to make sure that you have not skipped any items.

PART II

DIRECTIONS: We are interested in how the client has changed because of his/her head injury. Your answers to this form will help us understand problems related to the client's head injury and provide the best treatment. Please complete **all** questions. All information will be kept **confidential.** We realize you may be uncertain about some of the information you provide. **Please be as accurate as possible.**

Your Name: ______________________________ Date _-_-_
Address: ______________________________

____

Phone Number: ( )______________________________
Client's Name: ______________________________
Client's Social Security Number: _ _ _-_ _-_ _ _ _

1. **Your** relationship to the client: (circle one)
   mother father wife husband brother sister son
   daughter friend girl/boyfriend other ______________________
   (please write in)
2. **CURRENTLY,** do you live with the client? (circle one)
   Yes No
3. **BEFORE** the injury, did the client ever have any of the following medical problems? Please check all that apply:
   [ ] heart attack [ ] senility [ ] other
   [ ] stroke [ ] diabetes [ ] specify ____
4. **SINCE** the injury, has the client had any of the following medical problems? Please check all that apply:
   [ ] heart attack [ ] senility [ ] other
   [ ] stroke [ ] diabetes specify ____
5. For how many head injuries has the client received medical treatment? Be sure to include the client's most recent injury. (write in the number of head injuries)
   #______
6. **BEFORE** the injury, was the client ever treated by a psychiatrist or psychologist? (circle one)
   Yes No
   If yes, please check the following reasons that apply:
   [ ] depression [ ] schizophrenia [ ] nerves/tension
   [ ] drug/alcohol problem [ ] other ______________________
7. **SINCE** the injury, has the client been treated by a psychiatrist or psychologist? (circle one)
   Yes No
   If yes, please check the following reasons that apply:
   [ ] depression [ ] schizophrenia [ ] nerves/tension
   [ ] drug/alcohol problem [ ] other ______________________
8. **BEFORE** the injury, was the client ever held back a grade in school because of learning problems in reading, writing, and/or arithmetic? (circle one)
   Yes No
9. **SINCE** the injury, has the client been held back a grade in school because of learning problems in reading, writing, and/or arithmetic? (circle one)
   Yes No
10. **BEFORE** the injury, was the client ever placed in special classes for problems in reading, writing, and/or arithmetic? (circle one)
    Yes No
11. **SINCE** the injury, has the client been placed in special classes for problems in reading, writing, and/or arithmetic? (circle one)
    Yes No

DIRECTIONS: Please answer the following questions about the **client's CURRENT** alcohol use. **Please be as accurate as possible.**

To the best of your knowledge:

	Circle Correct Answer
1. Do you feel he/she is a normal drinker? **(if the client doesn't drink, circle Yes)**	Yes No
2. Do friends or relatives think he/she is a normal drinker? **(if the client doesn't drink, circle Yes)**	Yes No
3. Has he/she ever attended a meeting of Alcoholics Anonymous (AA)?	Yes No
4. Has he/she ever lost friends or girlfriends/boyfriends because of drinking?	Yes No
5. Has he/she ever gotten into trouble at work because of drinking?	Yes No
6. Has he/she ever neglected his/her obligations, his/her family, or his/her work for two or more days in a row because he/she was drinking?	Ye No
7. Has he/she ever had delirium tremens (DTs), severe shaking, heard voices or seen things that weren't there after heavy drinking?	Yes No
8. Has he/she ever gone to anyone for help about his/her drinking?	Yes No
9. Has he/she ever been in a hospital because of drinking?	Yes No
10. Has he/she ever been arrested for drunk driving or driving after drinking?	Yes No

DIRECTIONS: Please answer the questions below about the **client's** alcohol use. Questions 1 through 4 ask about the **client's** alcohol use **during the year BEFORE** the injury. Questions 5 through 8 ask about the **client's CURRENT** alcohol use. **Please be as accurate as possible.**

To the best of your knowledge:

1. **DURING THE YEAR BEFORE** the client's injury, how often did he/she have **one or more drinks** containing alcohol? (Check the category below that comes closest to the actual answer)

___ Three or more times per day
___ Two times per day
___ Once a day
___ Nearly every day
___ Three or four times a week
___ Once or twice a week
___ Two or three times a month
___ About once a month
___ Less than once a month but at least once a year
___ Less than once a year
___ He/she has never had any kind of beverage containing alcohol

DURING THE YEAR <u>BEFORE</u> THE CLIENT'S INJURY:

2. When the client drank alcohol, how often did he/she have **six or more** drinks? (Check the most appropriate category)

___ Nearly every time
___ More than half the time
___ Less than half the time
___ Once in a while
___ Never

DURING THE YEAR BEFORE THE CLIENT'S INJURY:

3. When the client drank alcohol, how often did he/she have just **four or five** drinks? (Check the most appropriate category)

___ Nearly every time
___ More than half the time
___ Less than half the time
___ Once in a while
___ Never

4. When the client drank alcohol, how often did he/she have just **one to three** drinks? (Check the most appropriate category)

___ Nearly every time
___ More than half the time
___ Less than half the time
___ Once in a while
___ Never

5. **DURING THE LAST 3 to 6 MONTHS,** how often did the client have **one or more** drinks containing alcohol? (Check the category below that comes closest to the actual answer)

___ Three or more times per day
___ Two times per day
___ Once a day
___ Nearly every day
___ Three or four times a week
___ Once or twice a week
___ Two or three times a month
___ About once a month
___ Less than once a month but at least once a year
___ Less than once a year
___ He/she has never had any kind of beverage containing alcohol

DURING THE LAST 3 TO 6 MONTHS:

6. When the client drank alcohol, how often did he/she have **six or more** drinks?

___ Nearly every time
___ More than half the time
___ Less than half the time
___ Once in a while
___ Never

7. When the client drank alcohol, how often did he/she have just **four or five** drinks?

___ Nearly every time
___ More than half the time
___ Less than half the time

___ Once in a while
___ Never

8. When the client drank alcohol, how often did he/she have just **one to three** drinks?

___ Nearly every time
___ More than half the time
___ Less than half the time
___ Once in a while
___ Never

9. How **accurate** are your answers to this questionnaire? (circle one number)

0	1	2	3
not at all accurate	somewhat accurate	mostly accurate	very accurate

PART III
Personal Activities of Daily Living

DIRECTIONS: We are interested in how the client has changed because of his/her head injury. Your answers to this form will help us understand problems related to the client's injury and provide the best treatment. All information will be kept **confidential**. Please answer **all** questions. We realize you may be uncertain about some of the information you provide. **Please be as accurate as possible.**

Your Name: ________________________________ Date __-__-__
Client's Name: ________________________________
Client's Address: ________________________________
____
Client's Phone Number: (__)________________________
Client's Social Security Number: _ _ _-_ _-_ _ _ _

1. **Your** relationship to the client: (circle one)
mother father wife husband brother sister son
daughter friend girl/boyfriend other ____________________
(please write in)

DIRECTIONS: Please answer the questions below as they apply to the client's **CURRENT** condition. Place an "X" in the box [X] to indicate the most appropriate answer.

1. **HEALTH** Because of health-related problems, how often is the client visiting or being visited by a physician or nurse? (do not include visits for physical or occupational therapy):

[ ] infrequently, no more than every 3 months
[ ] moderately frequently, at least every 3 months
[ ] very frequntly, at least once a week
[ ] client not in hospital, at least daily
[ ] client in hospital, seen daily

2. **SPEECH** When the client speaks to another person, does he/she speak:

[ ] without help from anyone and has no difficulty saying words

[ ] with some difficulty saying words, but without help from anyone else
[ ] with some help from another person (such as a coach or translator) or can communicate by using sign language or another symbolic equivalent (writing, communication board, etc.)
[ ] unable to communicate verbally, needing complete assistance from another person

3. **HEARING** When a person speaks to the client, does he/she hear:

[ ] normally, with both ears
[ ] with partial impairment or use of an assistive device (such as a hearing aid)
[ ] with some help from another person to speak extra loudly; or he/she can understand sign language, lip reading, or written communication
[ ] unable to hear and needing complete assistance from another person (meaning profoundly deaf and not able to understand sign language or lip reading)

4. **VISION** Does the client:

[ ] see normally with both eyes
[ ] see with partial impairment such as use of eyeglasses or eye medication
[ ] not see well due to either partial blindness or legal blindness and he/she uses a cane, guide dog, or some help from another person
[ ] not see at all due to blindness, with complete dependence on another person for assistance

5. **RIGHT UPPER LIMBS** Does the client's right shoulder, elbow, wrist, or fingers have:

[ ] normal strength including full coordinated and painless movement of joints
[ ] ordinary use in spite of some reduced strength or uncoordination
[ ] very limited use because of poor strength or uncoodination or else too much pain or stiffness to permit any more use than as a helping limb, OR if amputated, does he/she wear and use prosthesis daily
[ ] no use because of too much pain, OR if amputated, the client does not have to wear a prosthesis

6. **LEFT UPPER LIMBS** Does the client's left shoulder, elbow, wrist, or fingers have:

[ ] normal strength including full coordinated and painless movement of joints
[ ] ordinary use in spite of some reduced strength or uncoordination
[ ] very limited use because of poor strength or uncoordination or else too much pain or stiffness to permit any more use than as a helping limb, OR if amputated, does he/she wear and use prosthesis daily
[ ] no use because of too much pain, OR if amputated, the client does not have to wear a prosthesis

7. **RIGHT LOWER LIMBS** Does the client's right hip, knee, or ankle have:

[ ] normal strength including full coordinated and painless movement of joints
[ ] ordinary use in spite of some reduced strength or uncoordination
[ ] very limited use because of poor strength or uncoordination or else too much pain or stiffness to permit any more use than as a helping limb, OR if amputated, does he/she wear and use prosthesis daily
[ ] no use because of too much pain, OR if amputated, the client does not have to wear a prosthesis

8. **LEFT LOWER LIMBS** Does the client's left hip, knee or ankle have:
[ ] normal strength including full coordinated and painless movement of joints
[ ] ordinary use in spite of some reduced strength or uncoordination
[ ] very limited use because of poor strength or uncoordination or else too much pain or stiffness to permit any more use than as a helping limb, OR if amputated, does he/she wear and use prosthesis daily
[ ] no use because of too much pain, OR if amputated, the client does not have to wear a prosthesis

DIRECTIONS: For each task listed, please check one choice [X] that best describes how the client **CURRENTLY** performs the task.

9. **EATING** When the client eats and drinks, does he/she usually feed him/herself:
[ ] without use of assistive devices
[ ] with use of assistive devices such as spork, rocker knife, or extended straw

With help from another person (if so, which below):
[ ] helped by cutting meats, buttering bread, pouring liquids
[ ] helped with more than cutting meats, buttering bread, or pouring liquids, meaning that someone else helps bring food to the client's mouth
[ ] or the client is fed by a tube into the stomach

10. **DRESSING** Which choice best describes how the client usually gets dressed, including bra, slip, pull-overs, front-opening shirts and blouses, as well as undergarments, slacks, socks, nylons, and shoes, plus managing zippers?
[ ] by him/herself without the use of assistive devices
[ ] by him/herself with the use of assistive devices such as long-handled reachers, elastic laces, or Velcro closures
[ ] with some help from another person
[ ] or the client does not get dressed

11. **DON BRACE OR PROSTHESIS** Which choice best describes how the client usually puts on and takes off, if applicable, a prescribed sling, splint, brace (orthosis), corset, or artificial limb (prosthesis)?
[ ] not applicable because the client does not wear a brace or prosthesis
[ ] by him/herself with reasonable ease
[ ] by him/herself but taking a while to do it
[ ] with some help from another person

12. **GROOMING** How does the client generally take care of things such as brushing hair, shaving, cleaning teeth or dentures, and applying makeup?
[ ] by him/herself
[ ] by him/herself with the use of assistive devices
[ ] with some help from another person
[ ] with complete assistance from another person

13. **BATHING** How does the client bathe or take sponge baths?
[ ] able to wash and dry his/her entire body including back and feet by him/herself without the use of assistive devices
[ ] by him/herself with the use of assistive devices such as a long-handled brush or sponge
[ ] with some help from another person

[ ] with complete assistance from another person

14. **BLADDER CONTROL** With respect to bladder control, does the client usually:

[ ] have no accidents and have complete control
[ ] have no accidents but use special devices such as a catheter or urinary collecting device which he/she is able to clean and maintain him/herself
[ ] have occasional accidents or need some help from another person for any reason
[ ] have frequent accidents

15. **BOWEL CONTROL** With respect to bowel control, does the client usually:

[ ] have no accidents and have complete control
[ ] have no accidents but use special techniques such as stool softeners, suppository, enemas, or laxatives by him/herself
[ ] have occasional accidents or need some help from another person for any reason
[ ] have frequent accidents

16. **TOILETING** How well is the client able to clean him/herself and adjust his/her clothing after using the toilet?

[ ] by his/herself without the use of assistive devices
[ ] by his/herself with the use of assistive devices
[ ] with some help from another person
[ ] with complete assistance from another person

17. **HAND SKILLS** How well is the client able to write his/her name, turn a doorknob, turn a key in a lock, handle money, manipulate lamp and wall light switches, dial a telephone, turn a radio or TV on and off, turn a faucet handle, and open a jar?

[ ] by his/herself without difficulty with any of these
[ ] by his/herself with difficulty with some of these
[ ] with some help from another person
[ ] with complete assistance from another person

18. **TRANSFERRING: CHAIR** Which best describes how the client usually gets to and from a chair (including wheelchair if applicable) to a bed and returns or to stand and walk?

[ ] by his/herself without the use of assistive devices
[ ] by his/herself with the use of assistive devices
[ ] with some help from another person
[ ] with complete assistance from another person

19. **TRANSFERRING: TOILET** Which best describes how the client usually gets on and off a toilet?

[ ] he/she uses a toilet with fixed plumbing by his/herself and without the use of assistive devices
[ ] he/she uses a toilet by his/herself with the use of assistive devices (such as grab bars or an elevated seat) or else uses a commode which he/she empties his/herself
[ ] he/she uses either a toilet or commode with some help from another person
[ ] he/she is unable to use a toilet or commode

20. **TRANSFERRING: TUB/SHOWER** Which best describes how the client gets in and out of a tub or shower?

[ ] by his/herself without the use of assistive devices

[ ] by his/herself with the use of assistive devices (such as grab bars)
[ ] with some help from another person (includes supervision)
[ ] with complete assistance from another person
[ ] he/she is given sponge baths only

21. **TRANSFERRING: AUTOMOBILE** Which best describes how the client enters and leaves an automobile safely?

[ ] by his/herself without the use of assistive devices
[ ] by his/herself with the use of assistive devices such as a sliding board or a lift
[ ] with some help from another person
[ ] heavy lifting required or with complete assistance from another person

22. **AMBULATION: LEVEL SURFACE** How does the client walk on a level surface of 50 yards or more?

[ ] by his/herself without the use of assistive devices such as a cane or leg brace
[ ] by his/herself with the use of assistive devices such as a cane, walker, or leg brace
[ ] with some help from another person
[ ] not at all able to walk 50 yards or more (with or without help)

23. **AMBULATION: STAIRS** How does the client climb up and go down stairs (at least one full flight)?

[ ] by his/herself without the use of assistive devices or a handrail
[ ] by his/herself with the use of assistive devices (such as a cane or handrail)
[ ] with some help from another person
[ ] not able to climb a full flight of stairs

24. **AMBULATION: OUTDOORS** How does the client walk outdoors for a distance of 50 yards (about one block)?

[ ] by his/herself without the use of assistive devices such as a cane or leg brace
[ ] by his/herself with the use of assistive devices such as a cane, walker, or brace
[ ] with some help from another person
[ ] not at all able to walk as far as 50 yards with or without help

25. **WHEELCHAIR** How does the client usually propel and maneuver a wheelchair to turn corners or get close to the bed?

[ ] does not apply
[ ] by his/herself
[ ] by his/herself with the use of a power source such as a battery
[ ] with help from another person

26. If you reported that any of these problems are present, were the same problems present **BEFORE** the client's injury?

[ ] Yes
[ ] No

27. If you answered **yes** to question **26,** please write the numbers of the problems present **BEFORE** the injury in the space below.

Chapter 8

Supported Employment Phase II: Job-Site Training and Compensatory Strategies

Susan G. Killam, Joel F. Diambra, and Robyn Linn Fry

Job-site training is an important element in supported competitive employment and one of the characteristics that clearly differentiates it from traditional vocational rehabilitation approaches. An employment specialist or job coach is a pivotal person in job-site training. This person works one-on-one with the individual with a traumatic brain injury to provide individualized and consistent support services. Employment specialists play many roles and must be skilled job developers, job analyzers, job organizers, instructors, case managers, advocates, and more. This chapter will describe employment specialist job-site training activities using real cases to exemplify successful strategies.

When an employee with a traumatic brain injury begins a new job, the employment specialist accompanies the employee to the job site and stays with him or her until job performance is stabilized. Depending on the needs of the employee, employer, and job site, this may take weeks or even months of daily or weekly intervention. The employment specialist provides skill training to the new employee and also makes certain that all job duties are completed to company standards. This latter point is extremely important because, as part of supported competitive employment, employment specialists guarantee to an employer that job duties are completed to company standards from the first day of employment.

ORIENTATION AND ASSESSMENT

The initial period of job-site training is known as orientation and assessment. The employment specialist often drives the new employee to and from work for the first few days of this period. Although transportation training may be needed later, this initial travel support reduces the stress of having additional tasks to learn initially. Returning to work postinjury can be frightening and stressful for the new employee, and the employment specialist's job includes transitioning the worker from the home to work environment.

To familiarize the new employee with the work environment, the employment specialist and employee should also arrive early on the first day of employment. Time spent orienting the new worker to the layout of the work area, break room, and restrooms will help reduce feelings of disorganization for the worker.

On the first day, the employment specialist should assign the worker one or more tasks with which he or she is familiar or which require low supervision from the employment specialist. This will allow the worker to develop confidence in his or her abilities and to complete other job duties, and give the employment specialist time to reassess and modify the task analyses and work and training schedules. The employment specialist may need to reinforce the worker frequently to reduce the stress of learning new skills and beginning a new job.

Orient the Worker to the Work Environment

The employment specialist should organize a daily routine for the worker to follow at the job site, eliminating decisions such as which door should be used upon entering and leaving the job site and identifying times for breaks and lunch. Training the worker to follow this routine will reinforce time awareness and reduce disorientation and decision making. A job duties sequence form or checklist may be used to meet this need. Exhibit 8-1 is a morning checklist developed by one employment specialist for a worker. It provides the individual with an organized, sequenced routine to follow each morning while preparing for work. The procedure will help the individual arrive at the job site on time with the necessary materials to perform the job.

The employment specialist should diagram the work station, including maps outlining routes to surrounding areas such as staff restrooms, exits, supervisor's office, and lunch rooms. Figure 8-1 diagrams the work area of an employee who works as a pot scrubber in a large urban hospital. All areas in the kitchen have been included in the diagram, including areas in which the employee does not perform job tasks.

Diagraming the work area and related environments enables the employment specialist to identify orienting difficulties that may occur as a result of the layout. Although the specific work area may not present any orienting problems for the individual, the surrounding environments may. In Fig-

Exhibit 8-1 Morning Home Checklist

10:15 a.m.

	Sun	Mon	Tue	Wed	Thurs
1) Reset Alarm					
2) For Work: Hat					
Pencil					
Tablet					
Wallet					
Lunch Ticket					
Keys					
3) Turn off coffee pot					
4) Lock sliding glass door					
5) Shut windows					

LEAVE HOUSE AT **10:30 a.m.**

* **If you are late:** call 755-9333;
ask for the kitchen and tell them you are on your way

ure 8-1, the shaded area represents the employee's work area. The employee has the option of three kitchen exits to access surrounding pay phones, bank, gift shop, cafeteria, restrooms, payroll, waiting area, and outside exits and entrances. Identifying these possible orienting concerns during the initial stages of training allows the employment specialist to include route training in the overall orientation training program.

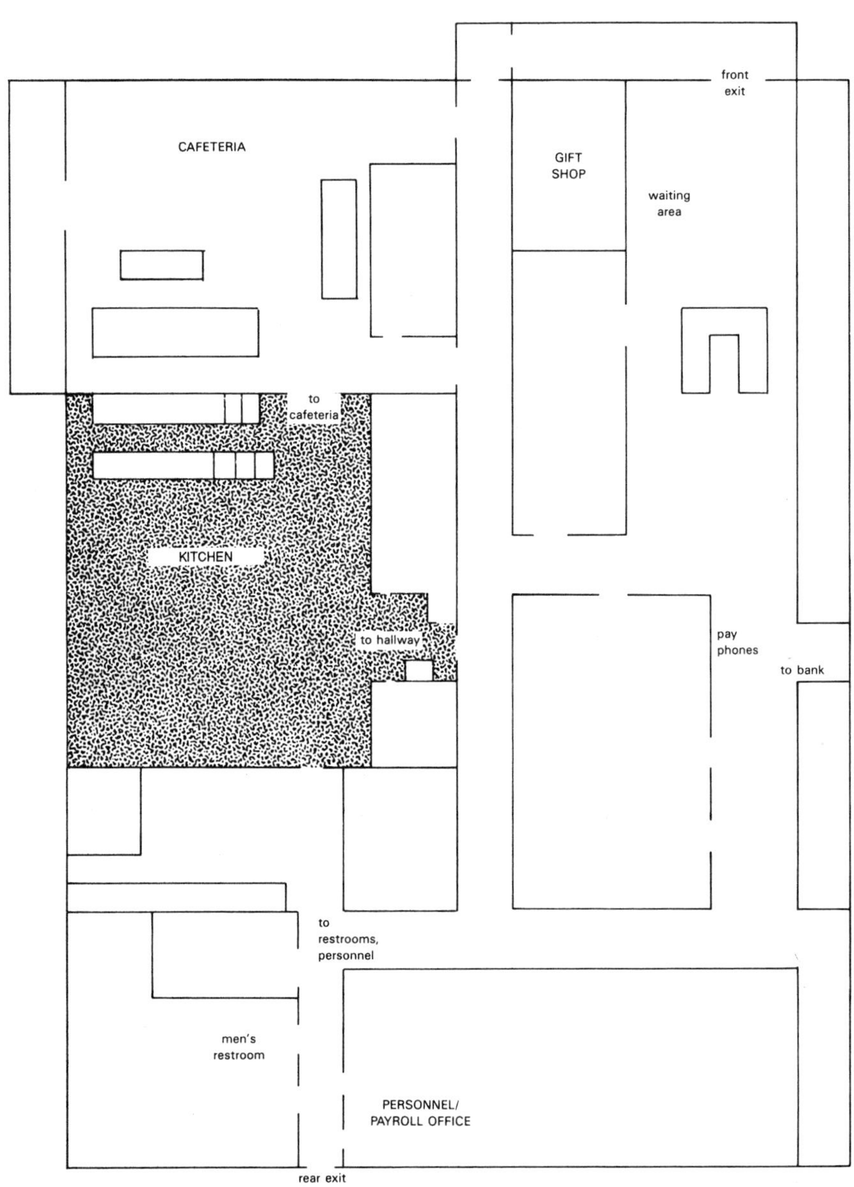

Figure 8-1 Diagram of Employee's Work Area

Orient Worker to the Community

If the worker does not drive, the employment specialist should discuss transportation options with the individual and, when appropriate, with the family. The pros and cons of each option should be discussed to select the one most appropriate for that individual. A transportation program should be designed to begin on the second or third day of employment.

Although some workers with traumatic brain injuries may drive, they may need transportation training to drive efficiently to and from the job site. This systematic training may involve the employment specialist transporting the worker the first week, following the worker the second week while he or she drives, and then meeting the worker at different landmarks or at the job site the third week. It may be helpful to provide written or pictorial directions to and from work. The directions may be attached to the dashboard of the worker's car, along with numbers to call if help is needed.

Before placement, the employment specialist should have spent 1 or 2 days shadowing a coworker or doing the job that the worker has been hired to complete. This gives the employment specialist hands-on experience in completing the job and an opportunity to develop a primary task analysis (Exhibit 8-2) and determine job duty sequence (Exhibit 8-3). During the critical first days of employment, this thorough preparation and organization by the employment specialist will reduce confusion and stress for the worker.

Modify/Adapt/Restructure

Before the individualized job duty task analyses are finalized, the employment specialist needs to assess and implement any necessary job modification/adaptations. Providing such modifications before the employee's first day on the job will eliminate one source of unnecessary frustration for the employee and provide an enhanced environment for skill training. Job modifications also must be related to task analyses. For example, if assessment information indicates that the individual is distractable, then the employment specialist can examine the environment with an eye toward reducing noise levels, work environment activity, and changes in routine and lighting that will hamper employee performance. Because it is not possible to foresee all necessary adaptations during the first few weeks of training, this need may surface later in the training process.

Task Analyze Job Duties

Task analysis is the process of breaking a task or job duty into smaller, discrete behaviors. A comprehensive task analysis is based on coworker ob-

Exhibit 8-2 Primary Task Analysis

Employee: Robert
Environment: Gayton Cafeteria
Instructional Cue: Prepare for Dinner

	6/14	6/15	6/16	6/19	6/20	6/21	6/22	6/23	6/26
1. Fill cart with ice and ice trays	+	+	+	+	+	+	+	+	+
2. Place ice in salad bar	+	+	+	+	+	+	+	+	+
3. Get salad bar cart from "walk-in"	+	V	+	+	+	+	+	+	+
4. Remove all lids in Kitchen	V	+	+	+	+	+	V	+	+
5. Place utensils on cart	+	+	+	+	+	+	+	+	+
6. Bring cart to dining room	+	+	+	+	+	+	+	+	+
7. Set up cart beside salad bar	+	+	+	+	+	+	+	+	+
8. Prepare soup tureen	V	+	+	+	V	+	+	+	+
9. Determine garnish for entrée	V	V	+	+	+	+	+	+	+
10. Place garnish on salad bar	+	+	+	+	+	+	+	+	+
11. Serve dinner	+	+	+	+	+	+	+	+	+
12. Clean up	V	+	+	+	+	+	+	+	+
13. Punch-out	+	+	+	+	+	+	+	+	+
Total Steps Correct	9/13	11/13	13/13	13/13	12/13	13/13	12/13	13/13	13/13
Percent Correct	69%	84%	100%	100%	92%	100%	92%	100%	100%

Instructional Code:

(+) = Correct   V = Verbal Prompt
(−) = Incorrect   M = Model/Gestural Prompt
P = Physical Prompt

Exhibit 8-3 Sequence of Job Duties

Daily

11:00 a.m.-noon	1) Punch in; get apron; wash hands
	2) Go to serving line to check: a. salad bowls b. plates c. napkins d. glasses
	3) Make decaf. coffee
	4) Set iced tea out—next to soda machine (refrigerator in buffet area)
	5) Get cart & load it up with . . . a. water glasses b. silverware c. coffee cups and saucers d. bread plates e. napkins
	6) Set up three tables for lunch
Noon-1:00 p.m.	7) Serve lunch, attend line, NOT DISHES!
1:00-1:30 p.m.	LUNCH
	8) Break down serving line
	9) Wash dishes
	10) Wash remaining dishes
	11) Fill up salad bar containers (make sure you can put lids on!) a. vegetables are rotated (old used first) every day! b. Tuesday and Thursday empty and clean all: 1) cottage cheese 2) pasta salad 3) cole slaw, etc. 4) salad dressings 5) yogurt
4:00 p.m.	12) Push finished cart into walk-in (refrigerator)
	13) Clean up area
	14) Fill salad bar with ice
	15) Take filled salad cart out of walk-in and set up salad bar
4:15-4:30 p.m.	Break, or after salad cart is finished
5:30-7:00 p.m.	DINNER 16) Set up garnishes—write down what garnish goes with what
7:00-7:30 p.m.	17) Clean up

servations, employer interviews, and employment specialist hands-on working in the specific job duties. The majority of task analytic development should occur before the first days of employee training, but task analyses will need to be rewritten and refined during the first few weeks of training.

All job duties for which the employee is to be trained should be task analyzed. The last step for each task should be the beginning or the set-up step for the next task in the sequence of job duties. This will enable the employment specialist to train the employee to sequence job duties. Omitting this link between individual tasks may result in acceptable skill acquisition and production standards on separate tasks but an inability of the employee to sequence work duties.

The employment specialist may not be able to obtain the pre-employment information needed to write a comprehensive task analysis before employment begins. At a minimum, major job tasks and duties, their sequencing, and the time alloted for their completion should be recorded before the first day. Identification of any changes in job duties throughout the day and use and care of equipment are also important information to record.

When the final job duty analysis has been completed, the employment specialist should meet with the supervisor to make sure it meets company approval. This will allow the employment specialist to make any changes in duties or routine early in the training phase. A set schedule will decrease confusion for the worker, who may experience difficulty with changes of routine (Gilbert, 1978).

After the worker has completed 2 weeks of employment, the employer should be asked to complete a supervisor evaluation (Exhibit 8-4). This evaluation gets the supervisor involved in the training process, provides the employment specialist and worker with a concrete tool to gauge progress, and identifies areas that need improvement. A worker self-evaluation can also be conducted at this time (Exhibit 8-5), which gives the worker a chance to evaluate his or her perception of job performance. The employment specialist and worker should discuss any discrepancies between the two evaluations.

The employment specialist then should complete a written progress report and review it as appropriate with the worker and family members. This allows for continual, proactive communication with all involved individuals.

INITIAL TRAINING AND SKILL ACQUISITION

The second phase of job site training is known as initial training and skill acquisition. By collecting baseline or test data on task performance before initiating formal skill instruction, the employment specialist can determine how

Exhibit 8-4 Supervisor Evaluation

Employee:
Name: ______________________
SSN: ___/__/____

Staff:
Name: ______________________
I.D. Code: ______________________

Company:
Name: ______________________
I.D. Code: ______________________

Date: __/__/__
mo. day yr.

How was this evaluation completed? ________ Personal Interview ________ Phone ________ Mail

Using the following scale, please check one number to the right of each question that best represents your opinion about this employee's present situation:

1	2	3	4	5
Extremely Dissatisfied	Somewhat Dissatisfied	Satisfied	Very Satisfied	Extremely Satisfied

How satisfied are you with this employee's . . .	1	2	3	4	5
1. . . . timeliness of arrival and departure from work?	___	___	___	___	___
2. . . . attendance?	___	___	___	___	___
3. . . . timeliness of breaks and lunch?	___	___	___	___	___
4. . . . appearance?	___	___	___	___	___
5. . . . general performance as compared to other workers?	___	___	___	___	___
6. . . . communication skills?	___	___	___	___	___
7. . . . consistency in task performance?	___	___	___	___	___
8. . . . work speed?	___	___	___	___	___
9. . . . quality of work?	___	___	___	___	___
10. . . . overall proficiency at this time?	___	___	___	___	___

11. Do you wish to meet with a representative from the program? Yes / No

Additional Comments: ____

____

Name (print): ______________________ Phone #: (____) ______________________

Signature: ____

Source: Form developed by the Rehabilitation Research and Training Center, Virginia Commonwealth University, in cooperation with the Virginia Departments of Mental Health and Mental Retardation and Rehabilitative Services (Revised 9/87).

much of each skill the employee can perform independently. If possible, baseline data should be collected for several days to ensure that they are stable. Besides providing the employment specialist with accurate task analyses of employee performance, baseline data can highlight the need for job restructuring or modification/adaptations that could lead to enhanced job performance.

Exhibit 8-5 Employee Self-Evaluation

Employee:
Name: ______________________
SSN: ___/__/____

Staff:
Name: ______________________
I.D. Code: ______________________

Company:
Name: ______________________
I.D. Code: ______________________

Date: __/__/__
mo. day yr.

How was this evaluation completed? ________ Personal Interview ________ Phone ________ Mail

Using the following scale, please check one number to the right of each question that best represents your opinion about your current work performance:

1	2	3	4	5
Extremely Dissatisfied	Somewhat Dissatisfied	Satisfied	Very Satisfied	Extremely Satisfied

How satisfied are you with this employee's . . .	1	2	3	4	5
1. . . . timeliness of arrival and departure from work?	___	___	___	___	___
2. . . . attendance?	___	___	___	___	___
3. . . . timeliness of breaks and lunch?	___	___	___	___	___
4. . . . appearance?	___	___	___	___	___
5. . . . general performance as compared to other workers?	___	___	___	___	___
6. . . . communication skills?	___	___	___	___	___
7. . . . consistency in task performance?	___	___	___	___	___
8. . . . work speed?	___	___	___	___	___
9. . . . quality of work?	___	___	___	___	___
10. . . . overall proficiency at this time?	___	___	___	___	___

Do you wish to meet with a representative from the program? Yes / No

Additional Comments: ____

____

Signature: ____

Source: Form developed by the Rehabilitation Research and Training Center, Virginia Commonwealth University.

To collect baseline data, the employment specialist uses the task analyses to observe and record initial employee performance on each of the job duties. After providing the work cue, the employment specialist should not provide any prompts or reinforcement. Moon, Goodall, Barcus, & Brooke (1986) outlined two methods that can be used to collect baseline data. The one selected should depend on the employee's learning style and the nature of the tasks. In the first method, initial performance is assessed on every step of the task analysis. If the step is completed correctly, a (+) is scored and the employee continues to work until an incorrect response is initiated. A (–) is recorded for an incorrect response and the employment specialist sets the worker up for the proceeding step in the task analysis. In this method the baseline is ended and training is initiated when all steps in the task analysis have been tested. In the second method, the baseline ends the first time the employee makes an error. This step and all remaining steps in the task analysis are scored (–). Training begins on the first missed step.

Establish a Training Schedule

Having determined the initial performance level of the employee, the employment specialist now decides the order in which the employee will be trained in job duties. During this initial training period, the employment specialist must ensure that company production standards are met. The employment specialist must select tasks that will enable him or her to provide training as well as maintain production standards by performing some of the tasks. A training schedule also assists the employment specialist with identifying peak time periods during the day for training and maintaining productivity.

Provide Systematic and Quality Instruction

The initial training and skill acquisition phase includes training on job tasks as well as training in related skill areas, including orientation (e.g., exits, cafeteria, vending machines, restrooms, personnel office, pay phones), social skills, and personal hygiene. Determining a training schedule for some of these skills will be difficult because instruction must occur as the situations arise. However, planning for these events in advance ensures that all skills will be taught in a systematic fashion.

The specialist can train employees in these related skills also by using a task analysis and systematic instructional techniques. Behavioral therapy methods also can be effective. This involves conducting a thorough behavioral analysis, closely monitoring progress, and applying behavioral therapy methods. Turkat and Behner (1989) have pointed out that these methods are not limited to reward systems.

Hegel (1988) demonstrated the utility of applied behavioral analysis in the rehabilitation of adults with head injuries. He reported improved compliance to rehabilitation therapies and decreased disruptive vocalizations in a subject by combining contingent reinforcement, goal-setting, and an extinction procedure. Cognitive behavioral methods, such as teaching, practice, reinforcement of appropriate responses, compensatory strategies, and overlearning of correct and incorrect responses, also have proven effective in remediating social interactional skill deficits in individuals who had sustained a traumatic brain injury (Giles, Fussey, & Burgess, 1988). Similar strategies should be explored and implemented by the employment specialist.

Choose Individualized Instructional Strategies

Individuals who sustain severe brain injury have a number of cognitive deficits (Conder et al., 1988). These deficits—which may include reductions in memory, reasoning, orientation, attention, visual perception and discrimination—vary among individuals and represent areas in which the employment specialist must provide individualized training. Selection of instructional strategies and prompts should be done using information from the neuropsychological evaluation, information obtained from the referral, initial intake information, and client preference.

Prompts and Cues

Use prompting and cueing strategies that take into account an individual's deficit areas and learning styles and will allow the worker to learn correctly from the beginning. Selected prompts should provide the necessary instructional assistance for the employee to achieve independent performance of the entire job. Exhibit 8-6 outlines general guidelines for delivering instructional prompts.

Prompt hierarchies consist of a sequence of two or more levels of prompts arranged systematically and delivered in either a least-to-most or most-to-least intrusive order (Snell & Zirpoli, 1987). Variations in prompting hierarchies may be appropriately developed using file assessment information for individuals who have sustained a traumatic brain injury.

Verbal prompts are generally considered least intrusive. However, this prompting style may not be suitable for some individuals who have sustained a traumatic brain injury. Kewman, Yanus, and Kirsch (1988) examined distractibility in auditory comprehension of traumatic brain injured individuals in everyday situations where competing or distracting auditory stimuli were present. Results showed that individuals who have sustained a traumatic brain injury have greater difficulty with an auditory comprehension task when distracting vocal stimuli are either present or absent.

The next level of prompt is generally a model. For some individuals, file assessment information may indicate that modeling may not be an appropriate strategy because the individual does not imitate well. The employment specialist must be creative and develop alternatives. Alternatives to model prompts can include specific task-related cues. For example, when prompting an individual to begin work at a computer terminal the employment specialist can begin with a verbal prompt by saying, "Turn the keyboard on." Or, the employment specialist can provide a less direct verbal

Exhibit 8-6 General Guidelines for Delivering Instructional Prompts

1. Peruse file information to determine cues and prompting strategies that respond to the individual's cognitive and sensory assets.
2. Model calm and appropriate behavior.
3. Arrange the environment to ensure that there is the least amount of stress possible.
4. Focus on a specific goal and discuss with the individual.
5. Reinforce.
6. In the event of confrontation or agitation, redirect and reinforce appropriate behavior.
7. Provide feedback to the individual and encourage feedback on the part of the individual.

Sources: From *Contemporary Challenges to the Rehabilitation Counseling Profession* (pp. 217–242) by S.E. Rubin and N.M. Rubin (Eds.), 1988, Baltimore: Paul H. Brookes Publishers. Copyright 1988 by Paul H. Brookes Publishers; and "Programme Description. An Interdisciplinary Programme for Cognitive Rehabilitation" by R. Conder et al., 1988, *Brain Injury, 2*(4), pp. 365–385. Copyright 1988 by Taylor & Francis, Inc.

prompt by asking, "What is next?" The next level of prompt might be a gesture toward the computer switch. Paraphrasing important instructions and prompts can facilitate the rehearsal process.

Seldom have intrusive prompts, such as physical prompting, been needed or proven useful for workers with traumatic brain injuries. Often the worker is resistant to being watched over and an employment specialist must recognize this and choose appropriate prompts. Richard, for example, uses an executive pocketbook developed by his employment specialist. This pocketsized notebook provides a permanent record of his sequence of job duties and the tasks involved in each duty. This strategy assists him with memory and sequencing difficulties while accommodating his preference for learning independently.

Memory impairment, a common and enduring consequence of severe, closed head injury, has been found to be resistant to many cognitive rehabilitation strategies (Godfrey & Knight, 1988). Long-term cues such as Richard's executive pocketbook often must be left in place to effectively deal with these memory impairments on job sites. The employment specialist must be cognizant of the individual's memory impairment while planning prompts and cues and training tasks.

Use Rationales

Systematic training coupled with an explanation or rationale often enhances learning by heightening attention and raising awareness. This strategy can arrest, correct, and/or disallow for rehearsal of an incorrect technique and can provide replicable instructional strategies. Using rationales, the employment specialist not only makes the employee aware of what he or she is expected to do, but also explains the method that he or she should use and why.

Incorporating an explanation in the instructional format was used with David in his porter position at a bowling alley. Although he reached skill acquisition on nearly all tasks during the first week of employment, he still had difficulty with dry mopping. David could move the mop from side to side but did not overlap the paths that he mopped. As a result, streaks were left where the mop had not reached. File information indicated that before his injury, David had owned a home. So the employment specialist asked David if he had ever mowed a lawn. David responded that he had mowed his lawn numerous times. Using this information, the employment specialist explained to David that the overlapping skill required for thorough dry mopping was identical to the overlapping skill required to thoroughly mow a lawn. If the paths of the lawn mower did not overlap, then tufts of grass were left behind exactly as dust and dirt would be missed if the dry mopping paths did not overlap. This explanation enabled David to perform the dry mopping task without error.

Select Reinforcements

Reinforcement is anything that increases the likelihood of a behavior occurring or increasing. Reinforcement should be given frequently at first and thinned out as the job placement proceeds. The employment specialist must be certain that any reinforcement chosen is actually reinforcing to the worker. Determining elements in the work environment that are natural reinforcements (e.g., paycheck, paid vacation, and supervisor and coworker praise) might eliminate the need to introduce secondary reinforcements.

However, if there are not enough naturally occurring reinforcers to maintain job performance during the initial training phase, the employment specialist may need to introduce secondary (artificial) reinforcers (e.g., taking the employee out to dinner or providing movie and theater tickets) or may have to program more frequently occurring natural reinforcement. Asking a coworker or supervisor to provide feedback to the employee for a completed job is one example of programming natural reinforcers. Although reinforcers that occur naturally are considered the best reinforcement method, programming reinforcement can be useful also and can teach coworkers when and how to deliver praise as a reinforcement.

The employment specialist must monitor the amount of reinforcement because it can lose its value if used too often. The employment specialist should determine an optimum range and pairing of reinforcers. For example, Ronald, a hospital employee, was required to stand while he performed his job. Although a rubberized mat had been added as a cushion, Ronald found that standing for long periods was tiring. Therefore, he found breaks and the opportunity to sit down and smoke a cigarette very reinforcing. The work schedule allowed for a naturally occurring 15-minute break in the morning and again in the afternoon. To program these reinforcements more frequently, the employment specialist adjusted the daily work schedule to include two breaks in the morning and two breaks in the afternoon. Instead of two 15-minute breaks, Ronald takes four 7-minute breaks and has more opportunities to sit, rest, and smoke.

Use Contingency Contracts

One method for systematically delivering reinforcement is to develop a written contingency contract or agreement signed by the employee and the employment specialist. A contingency contract (Exhibit 8-7 is an example) provides a permanent written record of the actions required by the employee to receive the reinforcement. Contingency contracts can be valuable tools to assist with training if they are developed mutually by the employment specialist and the employee. This process enables employees to be active participants in the development of assistive learning strategies.

Regardless of the type of reinforcement used, the employment specialist should always label a reinforcement. This tells employees why they are being reinforced. For example, the comment, "Great job double checking your work, Rob" makes the employee understand the reason he received reinforcement.

Compensatory Strategies and Adaptations

Compensatory strategies have been defined as the deliberate self-initiated application of sometimes unconventional procedures to achieve desired goals (Ylvisaker & Holland, 1985). These are adjustments an individual makes to get around a problem and therefore succeed at the desired task.

Compensatory strategies and adaptations have been extremely effective in providing successful job-site training for persons with traumatic brain injuries. Developed as the individual encounters difficulty with issues or tasks associated with job success, compensatory strategies range from the simple to the complex and from the expensive to cost-free and can be taught to the employee or may develop spontaneously. Because of this variability, the worker should always be involved in developing compensatory strategies to increase their acceptance and likelihood of success.

Compensatory strategies include work environment modifications, adaptive equipment, and reorganization of business equipment. Self-recording checklists, picture cues, elevated tables, a magnifying glass, and adaptive

Exhibit 8-7 Employee Contingency Contract

IF I CLEAN UP MY WORK AREA AT THE

END OF THE DAY ACCORDING TO THE

PICTURE CHECKLIST FOR

FIVE (5) CONSECUTIVE DAYS. . .

I WILL RECEIVE

TWO TICKETS TO A

RICHMOND BRAVES BASEBALL GAME

April 7 George Pastor
Date Employee

April 7 Amy J. Moore
Date Employment Specialist

reaches for high shelves are examples of individualized modifications that may enable an individual to successfully perform a job task. Identical compensatory strategies used with individuals with similar deficits have proven to be differentially effective (Penn & Cleary, 1988).

The individual's postinjury work history may provide useful strategies in developing compensatory skills, or family members can often provide effective ways of dealing with specific disabilities. During home visits, the employment specialist can gather information from family members on strategies that may be in use at home.

Compensatory strategies are an effective and frequently necessary complement to job-site training. Appropriate adaptations allow the worker to be more independent, decrease the employment specialist's intrusive intervention, and allow more positive interactions between trainer and consumer.

Pietruski, Everson, Goodwyn, and Wehman (1987) encourage professionals to use standard, nonadapted work supplies and equipment and help the individual to adapt them. Many times a creative employment specialist can analyze a job-site situation and arrange an adaptation or compensatory strategy that is inexpensive, unobtrusive, and practical. Many individuals may require physical adaptations to perform their jobs successfully. Physical changes should be made to the environment, not to the individual, to increase independence in the workplace. If the individual is using a wheelchair, for example, the work station or desk/table may need to be raised and bookshelves redesigned to make them more accessible to the individual.

For complex modifications, consult with physical therapists, occupational therapists, and rehabilitation technologists to analyze and develop appropriate strategies. Kreutzer, Wehman, Morton, and Stonnington (1988) outlined a three-step process used to develop compensatory strategies: (1) neuropsychological evaluation to determine the person's strengths and weaknesses, (2) task analysis to evaluate the work setting and the step-by-step processes needed for job completion, and (3) development of a series of specific instructions or materials to be used at the work site.

Adaptations can compensate for a deficiency or lack of ability in three broad categories: cognitive, physical, and other.

Cognitive

Persons with brain injuries may have a variety of cognitive deficits. These problems include memory loss, inability to recall information, sequencing or organizational difficulties, slow processing of information, overload of stimulation/information, decrease in motivation, distractibility, lack of insight, inability to globalize, episodic dyscontrol syndrome, and difficulty planning and seeing cause and effect. These deficits may be present in a number of different combinations depending on the areas of brain damage and diffusion of the injury.

Cognitive deficits, whether organic or functional, are major obstacles for the head injured individual in community and work reintegration and should be addressed when adopting compensatory strategies for the worker. Organic disorders are caused by the injury itself, while functional disorders may come from the person adapting to the injury. Considerations that should be kept in mind when choosing compensatory stategies include:

- cognitive level of the individual
- utilization of the senses that are most functional
- severity of self-selected strategies
- effectiveness of self-selected strategies

- individual problem-solving ability
- effectiveness of compensatory strategies in a work setting

Physical

Physical injuries can be subcategorized as physical and neurophysical. Physical injuries may include broken bones, lacerations, and severed limbs. Neurophysical injuries, those resulting from the injured brain, may include ataxia; poor fine-motor coordination; weakness in one side; double or tunnel vision; spasticity; balance problems; deficiencies in olfactory, touch, taste, and hearing senses; and limited range of motion. These deficits, if not compensated, play a major role in employment problems.

Other

This category refers to deficits that are indirectly related to cognition, have an uncertain origin, or originate because of psychological problems due to the traumatic change in personality and lifestyle a brain injury causes. These problems might include episodic dyscontrol syndrome or behavioral problems.

Compensatory Strategy Case Study

Mark is a microfilm clerk in the accounts payable division for a national electronics and appliance retail company. He is a 34-year-old married man who was injured in a single-car accident at age 30. He was driving his pickup truck home after drinking several beers, ran off a country road, and struck a tree. Mark sustained a severe brain injury, numerous lacerations, and a severe leg injury. Since his accident, he walks slowly with the aid of a leg brace, has static nerve palsy in his right leg, right-hand ataxia, and left eyelid droop. Mark complains of sun sensitivity and blurry vision in his left eye. His speech is slow and gruff but comprehensible.

Mark held a variety of preinjury jobs, including house painter, roofer, automobile body repair and painter, maintenance worker, and unit dietary clerk while in the Marines. Because of his physical limitations and his past work experience, Mark expressed interest in pursuing a clerical position. A position was found after several months of intense job development.

Mark's job duties as a microfilm clerk include boxing and organizing documents, pulling staples, straightening documents, microfilming all processed work, and filing and retrieving microfilm tapes. Initially, Mark had difficulty remembering the correct steps required to complete job tasks. For example, he would begin to photocopy documents but would forget to ensure checks were electronically marked using a switch on the microfilm machine.

His neuropsychological evaluation indicated that he retained information easier when it was presented in writing and it recommended using enlarged print due to Mark's blurry vision. Given this information, a task analysis was developed and implemented during training by the employment specialist. Mark was able to reach 100 percent acquisition rapidly using the task analysis. However, several weeks after reaching acquisition, he forgot several steps. Mark was retrained and provided with an enlarged copy of the task analysis, which was mounted on the wall in front of his work station. Mark quickly learned to use this compensatory strategy.

Mark's job required fine-motor skills when pulling staples, straightening documents, paper-clipping files, and fingering through stacks of papers. His fine-motor coordination and dexterity had been affected by his injury, resulting in low production rates causing him a great deal of frustration. The employment specialist and Mark created inexpensive, practical modifications that enabled him to increase his productivity to an acceptable rate and decrease his frustration. Modifications included a bowl in which to place paper clips, enabling him to dig for clips rather than struggle to pick one off the table top; butterfly clips and giant-size paper clips replaced the original smaller-size clips; textured rubber fingertips assisted him with filing through stacks of paper; and magic marker caps covered and protected critical switches that he would accidentally trip due to his ataxia. All these modifications combined cost less than $5.00 (see Table 8-1). The employer furnishes replacements when the paper clips run low or rubber fingertips wear out.

Table 8-1 Job Modifications and Costs for Mark

Description of Situation	*Modification*	*Application*	*Manufacturer*	*Approximate Cost*
Lost time in trying to pick up paper clips from table top	Giant-sized paper clips & bowl	Replaced all small paper clips with giant ones; implemented bowl for easier pick up	Giant clips; any plastic bowl of appropriate size	$1.00
Difficulty filing through stacks of papers	Rubber fingertips	Wears rubber fingertip on index finger to assist faster filing	Local office supply store	15 cents each
Accidentally tripping switches on microfilm machine/not aware of correct switch postures	Magic marker caps Notes	Placed caps over critical switches to prevent accidental tripping; placed notes on machine near corresponding switches to indicate proper positions	Employment specialist made	None

Train/Record/Revise

The employment specialist must first train for skill mastery, then for production proficiency. Revisions to instructional strategies should be based on employee progress evidenced in direct observations and data collection. Changes should be undertaken only after conferring with the employee. Data collection identifies emerging patterns and potentially troublesome areas that may surface in the fading and follow-along phases. In some situations, the employment specialist can assist the individual in the learning process by reanalyzing a difficult task analysis step and breaking it down further or, if appropriate, removing the step and selecting another method.

Or, instructional strategies may need revision because the employee may demonstrate during training an alternate method to accomplish the task. If this method accomplishes the same result and is efficient, then the employment specialist will need to revise the program to accommodate this revision. Before introducing any modifications however, the employment specialist and the employee should consider all options and decide which is the best method.

Some production problems may be resolved with an adaptation. Sign in/out procedures for Ronald, for example, were identified as a problem. Limited vision and a physical disability allowed Ronald to use only one hand to find his name in a payroll book and then to record his time in/out. Ronald required approximately 15 to 20 minutes daily to complete this task. The employment specialist analyzed the problem and determined that by attaching a "binder clip" (Exhibit 8-8) to the appropriate payroll sheet, Ronald could more quickly find his name in the payroll book. A cup hook was placed on the bulletin board above the sign in/out table so that the clip could be placed there when the payroll sheets were sent to accounting. This adaptation considerably reduced the amount of time Ronald spent signing in/out, thus allowing more time for him to perform work duties.

At times, it may be appropriate for the employment specialist to discuss troublesome areas with the work-site supervisor. The supervisor may provide valuable input to resolve an issue or may decide that methods developed by the employment specialist are more efficient than current practices.

In this initial training and skill acquisition phase, then, the employment specialist must be aware of two essential steps: First, instructional prompts, cues, and compensatory strategies must be presented systematically to facilitate performance of required tasks; second, employees must be provided the opportunity and time to practice or rehearse skills. This will enable workers to improve their job performance quickly and efficiently.

STABILIZATION

Stabilization is the third and final phase of job site training. How can the employment specialist determine when the initial training period has been

Exhibit 8-8 Example of Job Modification

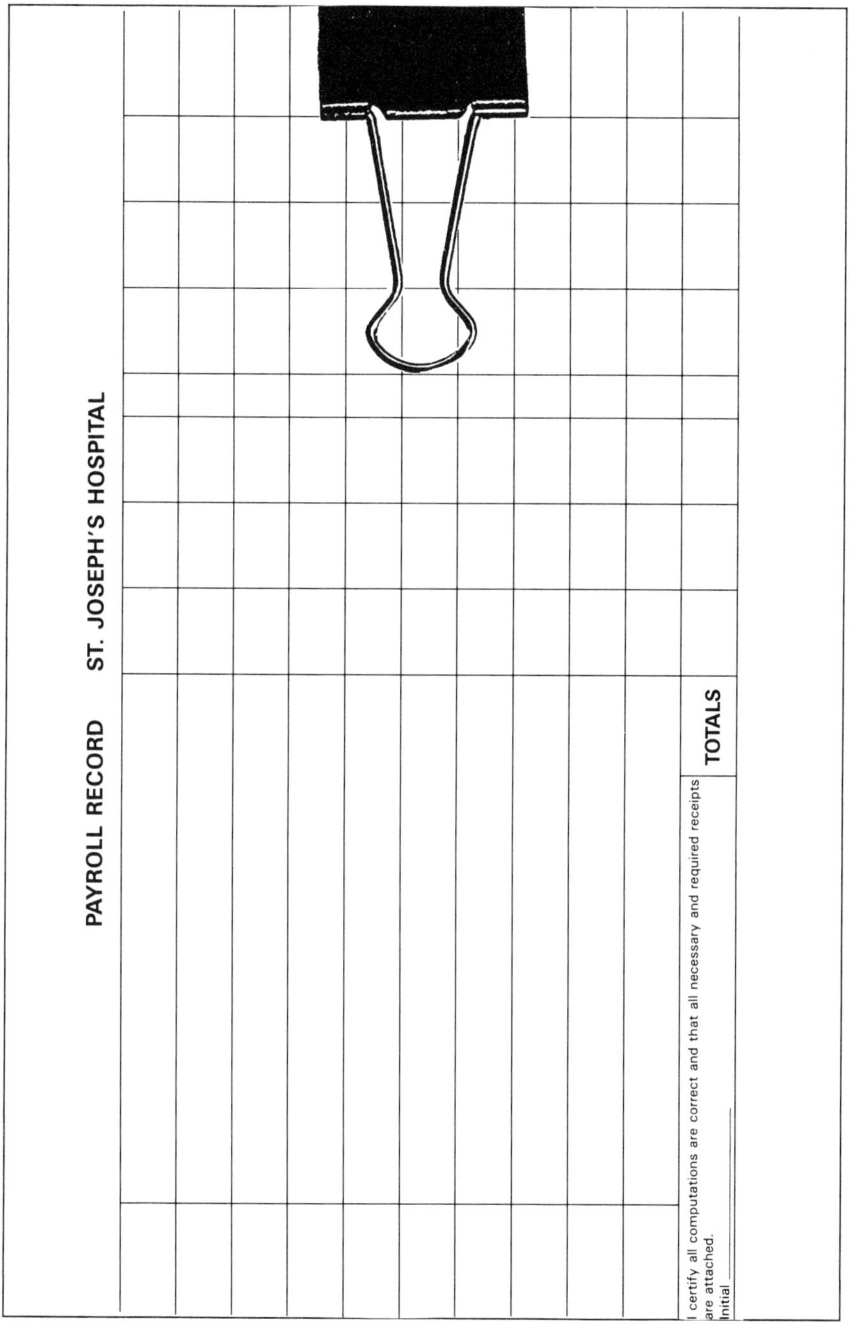

PAYROLL RECORD ST. JOSEPH'S HOSPITAL

TOTALS

I certify all computations are correct and that all necessary and required receipts are attached.
Initial ______

completed and an employee has stabilized? Stabilization, as defined by Hill (1987), occurs when the relative percentage of intervention time for the employee is less than 20 percent of actual work hours for 2 consecutive weeks. It is important to determine when stabilization has been reached so that the employment specialist can begin fading (i.e., limiting additional intervention). An employment specialist should consider skill acquisition, production rate, self-reinforcement and delayed gratification, on-site advocacy, medication stabilization, and emergency planning when planning fading.

Ensure All Tasks Are Trained

After Mark, the microfilm clerk in accounts payable, had reached 100 percent acquisition of skills and had increased his production rate to meet employer standards, the employment specialist began systematically fading from the site. As the employment specialist began to fade, boxes of already completed work began to pile in the microfilming office. A coworker asked Mark why he had not taken the boxes to storage. Mark responded that he had never been shown where these specific boxes were to be stored. Mark felt angry at the employment specialist for neglecting to show him the appropriate storage area and he felt embarrassed and inadequate in front of the coworker. The employment specialist had become so involved in training two more involved and difficult aspects of the job that he neglected to train for this seemingly minor duty. The employment specialist had been completing this task so that Mark could concentrate on the major duties of his job.

In this example, neglecting to train all job tasks created instability and required the employment specialist to return to the job site with Mark until he was able to complete all job duties independently. Ensuring that all job tasks are trained initially is a critical part of ensuring stabilization.

Ensure Production Rate

Once an individual is able to perform all the job duties, the employment specialist begins specific productivity interventions. Production rate will increase during initial training and skill acquisition with fluctuations from time to time. The employment specialist must verify an employee's productivity before beginning fading procedures.

Use Self-Monitoring and Self-Reporting

The employment specialist may determine that a self-monitoring procedure will ensure all tasks are performed productively. Priddy, Mattes, and

Lam (1988) and Burke, Smith, and Imhoff (1989) caution about using self-report assessments. Priddy et al. found that lack of orientation and memory deficits among brain injured adults can influence reliability of self-report assessments. Burke et al. (1989) found that cognitive deficits in comprehension, memory, and self-awareness after brain injury had a significant impact on self-report indices.

However, self-monitoring procedures have proven successful as both training and stabilization strategies for some individuals with traumatic brain injuries. Graphs and charts can assist workers with monitoring and assuming responsibility for maintaining their own job performance. For example, Mark had strict production quotas set by his employer. Mark did not realize his responsibility to meet these production standards because the employment specialist always completed the work Mark was unable to complete. Before fading, the employment specialist explained to Mark that he needed to process at least 250 checks per day to remain employed. The employment specialist used assessment graphs and showed Mark how to graph his daily performance (see Figure 8-2). After several weeks of self-monitoring, Mark graphed his progress and reached two of his preset goals, thus surpassing the employer's quota of 250 checks per day. For Mark, self-monitoring was an effective training strategy that was used to facilitate stabilization.

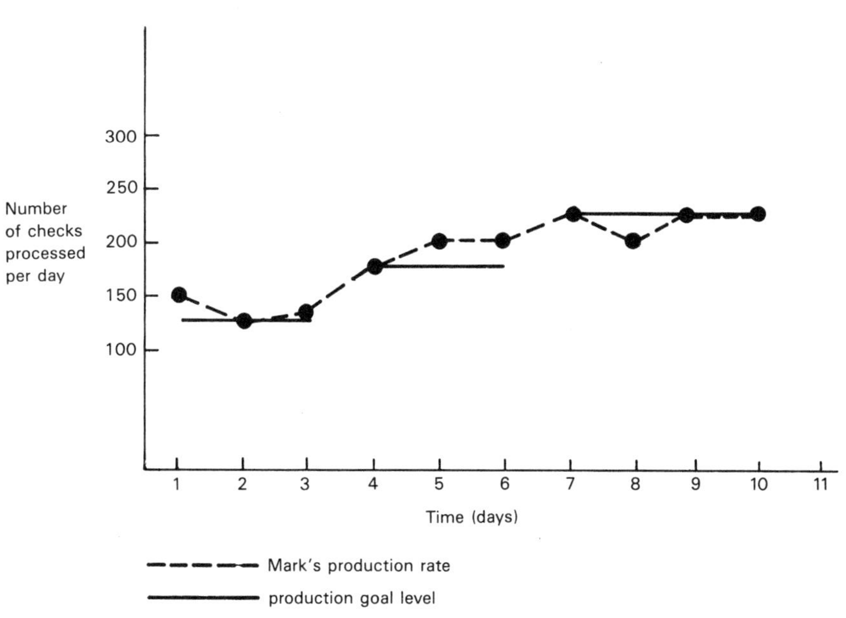

Figure 8-2 Example of Using Changing Criteria Design To Increase Employee Productivity

Use Self-Reinforcement

Teaching the employee self-reinforcement techniques facilitates stabilization and fading. For example, if the supervisor approves, the worker may be taught to self-initiate a break when he has completed a task ahead of schedule.

Self-reinforcement with delayed gratification may enable employees to realize they are in control of their own performance. This is also an appropriate stepping stone toward letting workers assume responsibility for their work success.

Use Advocacy

Advocacy does not occur at a specific time during the training process but is an ongoing role employment specialists assume during all phases of employment. Employee advocacy involves an active series of interventions by the employment specialist to enhance skill acquisition and maintenance of performance standards (Kreutzer et al., 1988).

During stabilization of employment for individuals with traumatic brain injuries, advocacy activities take many forms. Utilizing coworkers or supervisors as advocates at the job site is a critical component for successful employment for many individuals returning to work after sustaining brain damage.

Advocacy may include a coworker who is aware of any special situations with which the consumer may need assistance, a supervisor who has been given a list of steps to take in case of seizures, a store manager who has the employment specialist's phone number to use when problems arise, or a bus driver who prompts the employee to get off at a specific bus stop.

One part of advocacy is making sure employers are confident that they will be able to handle any issue if it arises. Although the employment specialist has shown coworkers and supervisors how to interact with the employee by effectively interacting with him or her in their presence, often coworkers feel hesitant to initiate interaction with the employee. If this interaction has not developed naturally, the employment specialist can arrange situations, such as eating lunch together, where the employee is likely to interact with coworkers. The employment specialist acts as a liaison between coworker and employee by actively participating in the interaction until rapport has been established and positive, appropriate interactions are taking place.

Coworkers often seek counsel from the employment specialist on interacting with the worker. Questions are typically directed at dispelling fears and discovering how to effectively interact with the worker—What should I do if . . . ? Is it O.K. to . . . ? Without infringing on the worker's confidentiality rights, the employment specialist can dispel unfound fears and suggest communication methods that have worked most effectively for them. It may be easier and more appropriate to direct the coworker to the employee to ask these questions. The employment specialist can again act as a liaison or buffer if the situation becomes uncomfortable.

Monitor Medication

It is not uncommon for persons who have sustained traumatic brain injuries to experience seizures or epilepsy after an accident. Taken on a regular and consistent basis, medications may stabilize or reduce the effects of seizures. However, workers must be able to manage these and other medications on and off the job site.

Employment specialists must be aware of these issues and assist with medication monitoring to ensure stable work performance. Close monitoring and prompting by the employment specialist help to ensure stabilization. First, the specialist must be sure the worker is able to determine the correct dosage to take. Second, the employment specialist needs to create a constant and continuous prompt that will continue after he or she has faded from the job site. One such technique is to purchase a wrist watch that sounds an alarm each time medication is to be taken and to pair the alarm with taking the appropriate dose of medication. Third, the employment specialist should monitor the worker's performance and ensure that he or she is able to manage the medication properly and consistently.

Ensure Emergency Planning

After training has been completed and fading has begun, the unexpected will occur: A car breaks down or medication runs out. Although it is impossible to foresee every circumstance that will affect work stabilization, proactive intervention can reduce their negative impact. For example, a list of steps, including the employer's phone number, could be placed in the glove compartment of the worker's car. In case of break down or minor accident, the worker would have a task analysis (list of steps) designed to walk him or her through the unforeseen crisis. Another example might be setting up a medical appointment before the worker's supply of medication expires or making a note for the worker to refill his or her prescription on a specified date. These types of interventions take foresight and planning by the employment specialist. However, they may be essential aspects of supported employment intervention to ensure stabilization at the job site.

Plan for Fading

Once all job tasks are stable or a compensatory strategy has been implemented, a specific fading schedule should be planned and scheduled. Two essential features should be considered in establishing a fading schedule: Fade slowly so that the worker gradually begins to perform the job independently and use data to determine particular tasks or times during which intervention may still be needed.

Fading of prompts is a gradual process in which prompts and reinforcement are reduced to less intrusive and more natural prompts and reinforcers. The employment specialist must monitor data during the fading process to ensure that the employee's performance does not decrease.

Although fading of prompts and cues is desirable, it may be necessary to keep some in place, especially if a sign, picture, or checklist corresponds to the individual's compensatory need and is not obtrusive in the environment.

Several factors support including the employee in the fading process. First, the employee may feel reinforced by the absence of the employment specialist because it indicates that the worker is performing successfully at the job. Allowing the worker to experience the decision-making process also may increase rapport and strengthen the employment specialist/worker relationship. Finally, the employment specialist can use this time to verbally reinforce the employee for hard work and effort and point out that the specialist will always be available to assist the employee with work-related issues.

On the other hand, trying to include an overly dependent employee in fading of the employment specialist may initiate new, undesirable behaviors by the employee. In this case, not including the employee in planning the fading schedule may be more beneficial to maintaining job performance.

During fading, use a calendar to highlight intervention. As time progresses, gradually decrease either the time of daily intervention or the amount of intervention days. The monthly planning calendar will enable a quick visualization of intervention reductions. It also will aid the employment specialist's supervisor in planning, the employer in facilitating communication with the specialist, and the employee in knowing when to expect the employment specialist.

SUMMARY

The use of individualized and systematic instructional and compensatory strategies throughout the intensive job-site training period is crucial for successful employment of individuals with traumatic brain injuries. The employment specialist, or job coach, is a pivotal person in providing these services. Working closely with employees, employers, coworkers, families, and other service providers enhances successful employment.

REFERENCES

Burke, J.M., Smith, S.A., & Imhoff, C.L. (1989). The response styles of post-acute traumatic brain-injured patients on the MMPI. *Brain Injury, 3*(1), 35–40.

Conder, R., Evans, D., Faulkner, P., Henley, K., Kreutzer, J., Lent, B., Maxwell, J., McNeny, R., Morrison, C., Pinter, B., Richardson, G., & Stith, F. (1988). Programme description. An interdisciplinary programme for cognitive rehabilitation. *Brain Injury, 2*(4), 365–385.

Gilbert, T.F. (1978). *Human competence: Engineering worthy performance.* New York: McGraw-Hill.

Giles, G.M., Fussey, I., & Burgess, P. (1988). The behavioral treatment of verbal interaction skills following severe head injury: A single case study. *Brain Injury, 2*(1), 75–79.

Godfrey, H.P.D., & Knight, R.G. (1988). Clinical notes. Memory training and behavioral rehabilitation of a severely head-injured adult. *Archives of Physical Medicine and Rehabilitation, 69*, 458–460.

Hegel, M.T. (1988). Application of a token economy with a non-compliant closed head-injured male. *Brain Injury, 2*(4), 333–338.

Hill, M. (1987). Interagency vendorization: Implementing and expanding supported employment services. Unpublished manuscript. Virginia Commonwealth University, Rehabilitation Research and Training Center, Richmond, VA.

Hill, M., Hill, J.W., Wehman, P., Revell, G., Dickerson, A., & Noble, J.H., Jr. (1987). Supported employment: An interagency funding model for persons with severe disabilities. *Journal of Rehabilitation, 53*, 13–21.

Kewman, D.G., Yanus, B., & Kirsch, N. (1988). Assessment of distractibility in auditory comprehension after traumatic brain injury. *Brain Injury, 2*(2), 131–138.

Kreutzer, J.S., Wehman, P., Morton, M.V., & Stonnington, H.H. (1988). Supported employment and compensatory strategies for enhancing vocational outcome following traumatic brain injury. *Brain Injury, 2*(3), 205–223.

Moon, S., Goodall, P., Barcus, M., & Brooke, V. (revised 1986). *The supported work model of competitive employment for citizens with severe handicaps: A guide for job trainers.* Richmond: Virginia Commonwealth University.

Penn, C., & Cleary, J. (1988). Compensatory strategies in the language of closed head-injured patients. *Brain Injury, 2*(1), 3–17.

Pietruski, W., Everson, J., Goodwyn, R., & Wehman, P. (1987). *Vocational training and curriculum for multihandicapped youth with cerebral palsy.* Richmond: Virginia Commonwealth University.

Priddy, D.A., Mattes, D., & Lam, C.S. (1988). Reliability of self-report among non-oriented head-injured adults. *Brain Injury, 3*(3), 249–254.

Snell, M.E., & Zirpoli, T.J. (1987). Intervention strategies. In M.E. Snell (Ed.), *Systematic instruction of persons with severe handicaps* (3rd ed.) (pp. 110–150). Columbus, OH: Charles E. Merrill.

Turkat, I.O., & Behner, G.W. (1989). Behavior therapy in the rehabilitation of brain-injured individuals. *Brain Injury, 3*(1), 101–102.

Ylvisaker, M., & Holland, A. (1985). Coaching self-coaching and rehabilitation of head injury. In F. Johns (Ed.), *Clinical management of neurogenic communicative disorders.* (chapter 5). Boston: Little, Brown.

Chapter 9

Supported Employment Phase III: Job Retention Techniques

Michael West and Trudie Hughes

Providing ongoing support services to promote job retention is an integral component of supported competitive employment for persons with traumatic brain injury. Because of the numerous problems experienced by these individuals and the continual threat of job termination, identifying and providing appropriate support services should be proactive rather than reactive (Kreutzer & Morton, 1988). Potential problem areas, antecedents, and consequences should be identified during the job stabilization phase, and a prescriptive, written follow-along plan developed by the employment specialist, the employer, coworkers, family members, the client, and any other concerned parties. For the benefit of both the client and the employer, response to crisis or requests for assistance should be immediate and according to the agreed plan.

The Rehabilitation Research and Training Center (RRTC) on Supported Employment at Virginia Commonwealth University has been providing supported employment services to persons with traumatic brain injury since 1985. The success of the RRTC supported employment follow-along initiative is evidenced by the fact that only 10.9 percent of all placements have ended by termination. This chapter will address strategies and techniques found effective in assisting traumatic brain injured individuals to maintain employment and will present two case studies illustrating the relationship between proactive follow-along services and job retention.

SUPPORTED VS. TIME-LIMITED EMPLOYMENT SERVICES

The distinguishing characteristic between supported employment and traditional time-limited vocational services is the provision of post-employment support services. While time-limited vocational services may incorporate supportive and follow-along methods, a supported employment program will by necessity include interventions at the job site due to the nature of its service consumers. The final regulations for the Rehabilitation Act Amendments of 1986 (*Federal Register*, August 14, 1987) differentiate the two:

> The need for job skills reinforcement under this program distinguishes supported employment from other rehabilitation programs where job accommodations or independent living services such as readers, transportation or housing may be the only needed post-employment services. . . . individuals with severe handicaps, with the exception of the chronically mentally ill, would be inappropriate candidates for supported employment if they do not need job skill training at least twice monthly (p. 30549).

Individuals targeted for supported employment programs would be expected to require ongoing support services for the duration of their employment, while traditional time-limited post-employment services by the federal statute do not extend beyond 18 months from the date of employment. While many individuals with even severe disabilities can obtain and sustain employment through time-limited services alone, many others cannot without regular intervention and support.

FUNDING OF FOLLOW-ALONG SERVICES

Time-limited vocational training services for supported employment consumers are generally funded by state vocational rehabilitation agencies, following the identification of an appropriate state or private nonprofit funding source for extended services (*Federal Register*, August 14, 1987, p. 30552). The coordination of funding from time-limited services to ongoing support has often been problematic for supported employment providers (Arkansas Research & Training Center, 1985), resulting in either the absence of follow-along or the abandonment of the supported employment concept.

Extended services funding may be even more problematic for the traumatic brain injured population, who may not fall under the traditional state mental health/mental retardation funding umbrella. In 1986 and 1987, 27 states were awarded systems change grants from the Rehabilitation Services Administration for the purpose of stimulating the development of supported employment. Kregel, Shafer, Wehman, and West (1989) found that only five of these states had identified funding sources for extended services for individuals with traumatic brain injury—and then only for those who also met the additional criteria of the state mental health, mental retardation, or developmental disability agency.

Supported employment provider agencies may need to approach nontraditional funding sources, such as head injury foundations, workmen's compensation or liability insurance carriers to obtain assurance of follow-along funding. Another alternative might be the setting aside of consumer resources for follow-along activities and utilizing the Plan for Achieving Self-support (PASS) income exclusion offered for SSI recipients (Nielson, 1986). Thus, consumers pay for their own follow-along services, but retain supplemental security income (SSI) cash benefits to offset their costs. Using the PASS exclusion has one serious drawback in that it can be extended for only 48 months. However, this strategy may give the program time to locate permanent funding for ongoing support.

COSTS RELATED TO FOLLOW-ALONG SERVICES

Funding formulas and costs for transitional and follow-along services vary tremendously from state to state (Wehman, Shafer, Kregel, & Twardzik, 1989). In Virginia, for example, job stabilization, and thus the termination of time-limited funding, occurs when average staff intervention time falls below 20 percent of the consumer's work hours for 30 days of employment (Rehabilitation Research and Training Center, 1988). Figure 9-1 shows the average amount of staff intervention per week as a percentage of work hours aggregated for all traumatic brain injury consumers served by the RRTC, beginning with the date of placement. Several assumptions may be made from these data:

- Traumatic brain injured consumers averaged about 22 weeks of transitional services before the stabilization period ended. It is interesting to note that this period is approximately 3 weeks longer than for all reported placed consumers in Virginia, a group comprised predominantly of individuals with mental retardation and chronic mental illness (Rehabilitation Research and Training Center, October, 1988).
- Consumers with traumatic brain injury averaged just under 2 hours of staff intervention time per week of extended services. At the RRTC's vendor rate of $26.92 per contact hour, the weekly cost of extended services has averaged approximately $54 per consumer.
- The mean length of employment at this writing is 36 weeks (and steadily increasing) for the 12 persons receiving follow-along services. The total cost for providing follow-along support services for 14 weeks (36 minus 22) is approximately $756 per placement.

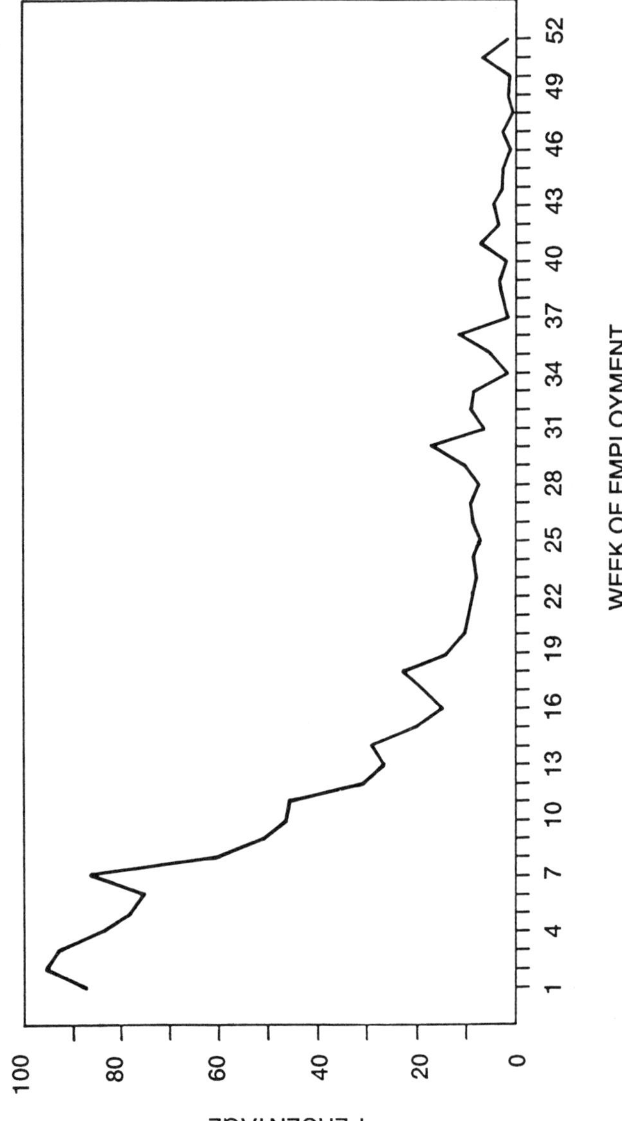

Figure 9-1 Staff Intervention Time As a Percentage of Work Time for Supported Employment Consumers with Severe Head Injuries

It should be noted that these are gross estimates of costs based on a limited number of placements by a university-supported demonstration project. However, the RRTC's vendor rate approximates those of other facility and nonfacility vendors. While the follow-along intervention time and costs for traumatic brain injured consumers compare favorably with those for other disability groups (Hill, Hill, Wehman, Revell, Dickerson, & Noble, 1985), we have yet to conduct true benefit/cost studies and alternative program cost comparisons because of the limited number of placements.

FAMILY INVOLVEMENT AND JOB RETENTION

Family involvement in job development, placement, and retention has long been recognized among service providers for consumers with developmental disabilities as essential for employment success. Without full support from the family, long-term job retention is unlikely (Kernan & Koegel, 1980; Kochany & Keller, 1981; Wehman, 1981). This support is usually manifested in agreements to provide transportation, to ensure that the consumer is adequately prepared to go to work, to monitor medication, to report health or psychological status, and to provide emotional support and encouragement. Depending on their age and levels of dependency, traumatic brain injured individuals also may need these home supports as part of a job retention plan. It is also helpful for family members to understand the difference between active involvement and overprotection. Untimely events, such as a parent calling or visiting an employer with complaints, have soured many employers on hiring workers with disabilities (Wehman, 1981).

Support programs for families of workers with traumatic brain injury will need to focus attention on three areas that directly influence job placement and retention: (1) helping the parents or spouse develop realistic vocational and independent living goals for the head injured person (Karpman, Wolfe, & Vargo, 1985; Schultz, 1986), (2) helping them develop mechanisms and skills for relieving family stress and dysfunction (Zarsky, Hall, & DePompei, 1987), and (3) helping family members understand and prepare for the financial implications of full-time or part-time employment, such as the loss or reduction of SSI, social security disability insurance (SSDI), Medicaid, or other entitlements (Noble & Collignon, 1987). The role of the employment specialist would be to help families obtain family-based therapy, not to provide it.

THE IMPORTANCE OF CHOICE

Although individuals who have sustained severe head injuries are aware often of the dissonance between their preinjury and postinjury status, including occupational levels, their expectations for recovery and return to work are often unrealistic (Nockleby & Deaton, 1987; Tyerman & Humphrey, 1984). Acceptance of the new self and its abilities and limitations is a critical antecedent of vocational adjustment. Employment specialists and counselors must balance the self-perceptions and interests of the head injured client against the real demands of the work world and present reasonable, obtainable career choices and goals. Mutual participation in identifying and making vocational choices during the placement phase is the first step towards long-term retention (Kreutzer & Morton, 1988).

The decision to remain in a position also is a choice for the employee with disabilities. Like everyone, they need the opportunity to advance, to change jobs, or even to be unemployed without being perceived to be failures (Anthony & Blanch, 1987).

PLANNING SERVICES FOR ENHANCING JOB RETENTION POTENTIAL

The fading of the employment specialist from the job site is perhaps the most difficult adjustment for both the supported employee and the employer. Fading too rapidly may result in a loss of skill and behavioral gains; fading too slowly may increase employee and employer dependence on the employment specialist. Determining the rate of fading must be made on an individual basis, using available client data (i.e., supervisor's evaluations and production rates) as guides (Wehman, 1981).

Fortunately, there are strategies for the employment specialist to mediate the effects of fading and, therefore, enhance job retention. Particularly relevant to follow-along services are self-management of behavior and the use of coworkers as cotherapists.

DEVELOPING SELF-MANAGEMENT STRATEGIES

The most powerful antecedents of and consequences to behavior occur in natural environments, be they vocational, social, or academic (Stokes & Baer, 1977). When the learner seems unable or unwilling to respond to natural antecedents and consequences, alternative strategies are in order. Self-administered cues and consequences have been successfully used in the instruction of children and adults with developmental disabilities in social, academic, daily living, and vocational applications (Crouch, Rusch, & Karlan, 1984; Karlan & Rusch, 1982; Wacker & Berg, 1983). Wacker and Berg (1986) describe the use of self-management within an employment situation. Although they specifically address strategies for workers with mental retardation, similar strategies may be useful for workers with traumatic brain injury who have deficits of memory, concentration, or disinhibition. By teaching self-control of behavior, the employment specialist is closer to ensuring that the worker can function in the workplace in the absence of external guidance and instruction.

Self-Administered Cues

Wacker and Berg (1986) describe three methods of self-cuing. The most frequently used form is *self-instruction*, in which the worker first is taught to perform the task and then to produce self-generated verbal prompts to initiate and complete the task. For example, after instructing a motel housekeeper on room cleaning tasks, the employment specialist might train the employee to initiate each task with an instruction (i.e., "First, clean the bathroom," "Next, dust the furniture") immediately before performance of each step. Self-instruction also might be used for initiating workplace social contacts at lunch or breaks, greeting the supervisor or coworkers, or responding appropriately to stressful situations.

In *verbal labeling*, tools, work pieces, or aspects of a job are made more concrete and salient by the worker verbalizing their names or labels. For example, in a data entry position that requires a unique entry format for each form or list, the employment specialist might instruct the worker to verbally name each form prior to entry. This verbal cue then triggers the appropriate response, in this case the selection of the appropriate format.

The third method of self-cuing is the use of a *permanent prompt*, such as a written list of duties or task sequences or picture prompts bound into a book. Another prompting system that might be less stigmatizing to the worker is the use of taped instructions and a portable cassette (Berg & Wacker, 1983). The worker is instructed to start and stop the tape at appropriate times to receive task or sequencing instructions.

Self-Administered Consequences

Training workers with disabilities to self-administer reinforcement and punishments has two potential benefits. First, the worker has the opportunity to receive greater amounts of reinforcement when natural reinforcement is scarce. Second, an employee who self-reinforces or punishes is less likely to be affected by disruptions at the job site, such as changes in supervision (Wacker & Berg, 1986).

Reinforcements and punishments to be self-administered at the job site should be based on the likes and dislikes of the worker and the level of tolerance at the work site. For example, a worker may be trained to allow himself a special treat at break periods for completing assignments or responding appropriately to coworkers. This type of self-reinforcement easily would be tolerated at most any job, whereas allowing extra break periods might not be.

PLANNING COWORKER INVOLVEMENT

One of the primary goals of integrated employment is development of friendships and social contacts between the worker with disabilities and coworkers. Coworkers also are resources for follow-along services. As passive resources, coworkers are: (1) normative references for assessing consumer work skills and behaviors and (2) subjective evaluators of consumer work performance (White, 1986). The use of coworkers as active change agents has been suggested as a means of controlling program costs (Hill & Wehman, 1983) and maintaining job performance through daily contact (Rusch, Martin, & White, 1985; Wehman, 1981).

Shafer (1986) describes three active functions that coworkers can perform as part of a job retention plan. The first is that of *advocates* for the supported employee, ensuring that he or she is treated fairly and with dignity while at work. Second, coworkers can be active *observers* and *reporters* of job performance and potential problems that may be developing. Finally, coworkers may function as *trainers*, providing instruction in new work tasks or periodic reinforcement for correct performance or appropriate behaviors. It is important in planning coworker involvement that individuals are selected who are willing and able to perform the duties as instructed by the employment specialist, and that their involvement with the supported employee will only minimally intrude upon their own job duties.

PLANNING AND IMPLEMENTING EXTENDED SERVICES

Effective follow-along uses formal and informal problem analysis and data collection strategies. Informal methods include initiating discussions with the supervisor, coworkers, or family members; accessing community support services; and supporting other client-related activities. Formal methods collect outcome data for ongoing assessment of work performance or program effectiveness.

On-Site Interventions

Following job stabilization, contacts with employers will typically involve site visits or telephone contacts about the employee's job performance. In most cases, the site visit is most useful in judging the employee's adjustment to the workplace, the supervisor, and coworkers (Hill, Cleveland, Pendleton, & Wehman, 1982). The employment specialist may also need to return to the job site for retraining activities in the event that the employee's work quality or speed diminishes over time or if job duties change (Moon, Goodall, Barcus, & Brooke, 1986).

Another vital concern may be monitoring the emotional stability of the employee. Disinhibition, temper outbursts, and other inappropriate behaviors are often latent responses to employment stress (Kreutzer & Morton, 1988) and may not be predictable, especially if the consumer has had no other postinjury employment. Employers will need to be informed of any known symptoms of an impending flare-up and appropriate means of supervisory response, including timeout procedures, suspensions, or calling the employment specialist for crisis intervention. Some initial negotiations between the employer and employment specialist may provide for "psychosocial first aid" (Isbister & Donaldson, 1987) to be administered at the job site by the employment specialist or qualified therapist if the employee's behaviors escalate beyond the supervisor's control.

It should be evident from the preceding discussion that many individuals with traumatic brain injury will require a sympathetic and understanding employer for placement to be successful. It is vital they know what to expect from the employee, both in productivity and behavior, and the degree to which professionals may be used as resources in correcting problems in either area.

Off-Site Interventions

The employment specialist should initiate ongoing contact with family members to discuss aspects of home life that could impinge on the work environment: the consumer's emotional stability, use or abuse of prescription and nonprescription drugs or alcohol, and problems related to finances, health, and family functioning. The employment specialist should refer as necessary the consumer and family members to treatment programs (e.g., Alcoholics Anonymous) and other services and entitlements (e.g., SSI, SSDI) and help them access these services (Kreutzer & Morton, 1988).

A comprehensive retention plan will also include varied advocacy efforts on behalf of the consumer. This might include progress or status reports to the consumer's vocational rehabilitation counselor, neuropsychologist, or physician; communicating changes in work schedule or problems with dress, medication, or finances to the staff of supervised apartments or groups homes; or dealing with a landlord or creditor for a worker who lives independently or semi-independently. In short, any problem that may affect the individual's job retention becomes the concern of the employment specialist.

Exhibit 9-1 Levels of Job Site Follow-Along Contacts

Level III	A minimum of two contacts per week with the client and employer. This schedule is followed immediately after job stabilization and during crisis periods.
Level II	A minimum of one contact per week. This is intended as an interim schedule during the fading process or following crisis resolution.
Level I	The legal and clinical minimum of one contact every 2 weeks.

Factors for determining an appropriate level of follow-along:

(a) the point from job stabilization
(b) any difficulties experienced during the job-site training phase
(c) changes in medication or health status
(d) changes in supervision or job duties
(e) particular behavioral characteristics of the individual
(f) periods of personal crisis, depression, stress, or alcohol or substance abuse that are likely to affect work performance
(g) the amount of intrusiveness that can be tolerated by the consumer and the employer

Scheduling Follow-Along Contacts

Little direction has been given as to the frequency and intensity of follow-along contacts. The determination of what is sufficient or necessary to maintain employment has generally been left to the discretion of the employment specialist, provided that legal minimum levels are met.

Rusch (1986) describes two types of schedules, the *adjusted* schedule and the *fixed* schedule. The adjusted schedule varies with the consumer's success in meeting the employer's expectations and in ratings of progress. If an employer cannot tolerate this arrangement, then a predetermined, or fixed, schedule of follow-along contacts is negotiated.

With consumers of the RRTC project, we are exploring more planned and systematic methods of scheduling follow-along contacts at the job site that meet individual needs for flexibility, crisis intervention, and frequency of contacts. Three levels of follow-along intensity have been identified. These are presented along with decision rules in Exhibit 9-1.

Using the follow-along scheduling form (Exhibit 9-2), the employment specialist plans dates to make job site contacts and submits a copy of the form to the program coordinator for monitoring implementation. The purpose of this procedure is not to scrutinize the activities of the employment specialist, but to ensure that other daily activities do not interfere with this vital program component. The employment specialist also may schedule off-site contacts as determined by collected data and the needs of the individual.

Exhibit 9-2 The Biweekly Follow-Along Planning Chart

Consumer	Staff Person	Week of	Sun	Mon	Tue	Wed	Thu	Fri	Sat
Consumer #1 [1 contact per 2 weeks]		10/16							
		10/23							
Consumer #2 [1 contact per week]		10/16							
		10/23							
Consumer #3 [1 contact per 2 weeks]		10/16							
		10/23							
Consumer #4 [1 contact per week]		10/16							
		10/23							
Consumer #5 [2 contacts per week]		10/16							
		10/23							
Consumer #6 [2 contacts per week]		10/16							
		10/23							
Consumer #7 [1 contact per week]		10/16							
		10/23							
Consumer #8 [1 contact per 2 weeks]		10/16							
		10/23							

Code:

E = Employer or coworker contact
C = Consumer-only contact
F = Family contact
O = Other contact

We have yet to determine if this system of follow-along planning is more effective in enhancing job retention than the more traditional discretionary methods of making job site follow-along contacts. However, we believe it affords a greater likelihood of detecting problem situations before they become job threatening and therefore enhances job retention potential.

The Support Group

The support group described for workers with psychosocial disabilities by Isbister and Donaldson (1987) can be a valuable medium for monitoring

Exhibit 9-3 Supervisor's Evaluation Form

Using the following scale, please check one number to the right of each question that best represents your opinion about this employee's present situation:

1	2	3	4	5
Extremely Dissatisfied	Somewhat Dissatisfied	Satisfied	Very Satisfied	Extremely Satisfied

How satisfied are you with this employee's . . .	1	2	3	4	5
1. timeliness of arrival and departure from work?	___	___	___	___	___
2. attendance?	___	___	___	___	___
3. timeliness of breaks and lunch?	___	___	___	___	___
4. appearance?	___	___	___	___	___
5. general performance as compared to other workers?	___	___	___	___	___
6. communication skills?	___	___	___	___	___
7. consistency in task performance?	___	___	___	___	___
8. work speed?	___	___	___	___	___
9. quality of work?	___	___	___	___	___
10. overall proficiency at this time?	___	___	___	___	___

Additional Comments:

ongoing adjustment to employment. A support group of consumers and employment specialists meets voluntarily to discuss problems or stresses associated with work and provide mutual emotional support. The supported employment staff are also able to monitor the emotional stability of group members and identify potential problem areas at the job site or home. A separate support group may be formed for families.

Supervisor's Evaluations

Formal supervisor evaluations provide insight not only into the work performance of the head injured employee, but also the expectations and priorities of the supervisor. For example, Shafer, Kregel, Banks, and Hill (1988) examined scores on the RRTC's Supervisor's Evaluation Form (see Exhibit 9-3) for initial and terminal evaluations for 125 workers with mental retardation. They found that employees who eventually were separated from their job tended to score lower than successful placements in the areas of attendance, punctuality, and timeliness of lunch and breaks. They conclude that employers may be willing to lower performance standards of speed and quality for a dependable, loyal worker. Although these findings have yet to be generalized to other disability groups, supervisor evaluation forms have utility for examining worker/supervisor relationships in both aggregated data and individual cases.

In the RRTC's data collection schedule, the Supervisor's Evaluation Form is completed by the employee's job site supervisor, ideally with the employment specialist and the employee present, at a minimum of 1 month, 3 months, and 6 months post-placement, and every 6 months after. Employment specialists may request evaluations from the supervisor on a more frequent schedule if deemed necessary and feasible. Because most performance evaluations used in business are not sufficiently expansive or behaviorally oriented for supported employment purposes (Rusch, 1986), employers are requested to use the RRTC's Supervisor's Evaluation Form in addition to any other method they would normally use.

Job Update Form

The Job Update Form (Exhibit 9-4) is used to collect data on job element changes, such as wages, work hours, and level of integration with customers or coworkers. This form is a shortened version of the RRTC's Job Screening Form, which also provides an analysis of job parameters, requirements, and expected competencies.

The Job Update Form is completed at 3 and 6 months post-placement, and every 6 months after.

Consumer Update Form

The Consumer Update Form (Exhibit 9-5) collects data on the supported employee's level of independence in the areas of: (1) the employee's vocational rehabilitation case status, (2) residential situation, (3) mode of transportation to and from work, and (4) the types and amounts of government financial aid and entitlements. The form is completed on the same schedule as the Job Update Form. Because this information is also collected before or at initial placement, changes in employee status as a direct result of employment can be tracked over time. Thus, this form provides a significant amount of information necessary for consumer-level benefit/cost analysis.

Consumer Self-Evaluation

When the supervisor completes a Supervisor's Evaluation Form, the consumer completes a similar form assessing his or her own work perform-

Exhibit 9-4 Job Update Form

1. Type of service/employment for this report (select one): ___________
   1 = Work activity or sheltered employment
   2 = Entrepreneurial
   3 = Mobile work crew
   4 = Enclave
   5 = Supported job
   6 = Supported competitive employment
   7 = Time-limited (no ongoing services anticipated)
   8 = Other (specify: ____)
2. Type of update: Ongoing ________________ Final ________________
3. Job title: ____
4. Current hourly wage (or last wage in this position): ______________________
5. Did a wage change occur since the last job screening or job update? __________
6. If yes, then complete this section:
   Hourly rate changed from $_______ to $_______ on __/__/__
   Hourly rate changed from $_______ to $_______ on __/__/__
7. Number of hours worked per week: _______ Months worked per year: _______
8. If less than 12 months per year, what months is the job not available?
9. Number of employees in this company at this location: ________________

Number without disabilities in immediate area (50 ft. radius): ________________
Number of other employees with disabilities: ______________________________
In immediate area (50 ft. radius): ______________________________________
Number of other employees in this position: _______________________________
During the same hours: ____

10. Level of social contact (circle one):
    0—Employment in a segregated setting in which the majority of interactions with persons without disabilities are with caregivers or service providers. Example: Adult Activity Center Worker

    1—Employment in an integrated environment on a shift or position that is isolated. Contact with coworkers without disabilities or supervisors is minimal. Example: Night Janitor

    2—Employment in an integrated environment on a shift or position that is relatively isolated. Contact with coworkers without disabilities is available at lunch or break. Example: Pot Scrubber

    3—Employment in an integrated environment in a position requiring a moderate level of task dependency and coworker interaction. Example: Dishwasher required to keep plate supply stacked for cooks

    4—Employment in an integrated environment in a position requiring a high degree of task dependency and coworker or customer interaction. Example: Busperson/Porter

Exhibit 9-5 Consumer Update Form

1. Current Department of Rehabilitative Services case status for this consumer (enter DRS code: ______________
   If never served by DRS, enter none in the space provided.

2. Current residential situation (select one only): ______________
   1 = Independent
   2 = Supported living arrangement
   3 = Sponsored placement (foster care)
   4 = Domiciliary care apartment (home for adults)
   5 = Supervised apartment
   6 = Parents
   7 = Other relatives
   8 = Group home/halfway house
   9 = Other (specify: ______________)

3. Current primary mode of transportation to work (select one only): ______________
   1 = Independent use of public transportation
   2 = Walks/rides bike or moped
   3 = Dependent use of public transportation (needed bus training)
   4 = Arranged car pool
   5 = Parent/friend drives
   6 = Handicapped transportation
   7 = Taxi
   8 = Drives own vehicle
   9 = Other (specify: ______________)

4. Financial aid received by consumer at present or as of last day of work. Circle yes or no for each selection. If yes, write the amount received to the left of the selection.
   ______ Yes / No None
   ______ Yes / No Supplemental Security Income
   ______ Yes / No Social Security Disability Insurance
   ______ Yes / No Medicaid
   ______ Yes / No Medicare
   ______ Yes / No Food Stamps
   ______ Yes / No Public Assistance (Welfare)
   ______ Yes / No Other (specify: ______________)

5. Total income from all government financial aid during the past month: ______

ance. This procedure gives the employment specialist insight into the consumer's perceptions of strengths and weaknesses, dissonance between consumer and supervisor perceptions, and areas in which to concentrate intervention.

CASE STUDY #1: DAVE

Consumer Characteristics

Dave sustained a Grade III head injury (Glasgow Coma Score of 9 or less at admission to intensive care) in a motorcycle accident at age 15 and was in a coma for 10 weeks. Residual symptoms of his injury include impaired right- and left-hand fine-motor dexterity, right-side spasticity, a stiff right knee, slurred speech, memory deficits, and a reduced tolerance for frustration.

Following graduation from high school, Dave worked as a porter, dishwasher, cashier, file clerk, and production worker in a sheltered workshop. According to Dave, he had difficulties relating to coworkers and supervisors in nearly every job that he held. He had also been arrested in 1984 for assault, trespassing, and disorderly conduct, and was sentenced to 13 months probation. Dave was unemployed at the time of his referral to the RRTC supported employment project, receiving SSI benefits totaling $340 per month, food stamps, and government subsidized housing. He self-reported that he had three or four drinks about four times a week.

Job Placement and Training

Dave and his employment specialist focused on three major concerns during the job development phase: Dave's occupational interests, neuropsychological and other assessment data, and his physical and behavioral limitations and problems. They agreed that Dave needed a tranquil, low-pressure work environment with few coworkers in the immediate vicinity. A part-time position was located as a warehouse worker, starting pay $3.90 per hour with benefits.

Dave's job duties involved locating stock within the warehouse, carting it from the storage area to a conveyor belt, and recording a 6-digit stock number on both a sheet and a computer. These duties required approximately 2 weeks of training to reach 100 percent proficiency. In addition, the employment specialist made several inexpensive adaptations in the work environment in response to persistent problems. For example, Dave repeatedly misplaced the pencil for recording stock numbers. The employment specialist purchased a pen with a Velcro fastener and attached this to Dave's clipboard. Dave also attempted to direct other new employees who were unfamiliar with procedures, which often resulted in outbursts of anger and frustration from Dave. The employment specialist made a permanent prompt—a laminated poster with detailed instructions—to which all new employees could refer, thus eliminating the need for them to ask directions from Dave.

Follow-Along Activities

Although Dave reached job stabilization in a relatively short period, the follow-along phase proved vital in keeping Dave on the job due to a number of problems and issues that later surfaced. The most serious problem was inappropriate responses to coworkers, such as yelling, threats, and occasionally, physical aggression. A self-monitoring system developed by the employment specialist was abandoned after 1 week because this in itself caused stress and anxiety for Dave. The employment specialist then used Dave's coworkers as cotherapists, instructing them in ways of reducing his frustration and anxiety levels, and leaving them detailed written instructions for reactions and consequences.

Dave exhibited other social problems that needed attention. For example, he went to his supervisor continually with work-related and personal problems, not only his own but also those of his coworkers. The employment specialist addressed this problem through counseling and role-playing exercises with Dave. In addition, Dave would become careless in performing his duties, resulting in inefficient work and occasional injuries to himself. The employment specialist developed a weekly feedback sheet for the supervisor to report to Dave and the employment specialist how Dave was performing his duties and responding to coworkers.

Off-site interventions were necessary with Dave as well, primarily in budgeting money, substance abuse, grooming and hygiene, and sexual dysfunction. The employment specialist addressed these problems through counseling.

Dave held his job for 14 months. His problems with injuries and aggression eventually resulted in his termination. In those 14 months, he earned $7,155 and received 293.5 hours of intervention time. Although his SSI cash benefits and food stamps were suspended during his employment, Dave continued to receive Medicare health coverage and housing assistance. He also reported that he had curtailed his excessive drinking. He was returned to the RRTC's referral pool for consideration for a second placement.

CASE STUDY #2: MATTHEW

Consumer Characteristics

Matthew received a Grade III head injury in an automobile accident at the age of 30 and was in a coma for 2 months. He previously had earned a general equivalency diploma (GED) and was employed at the time of his accident as a school maintenance assistant. As a result of the injury, he exhibited language, sight, and memory problems. Matthew also developed static nerve palsy in his right leg, resulting in difficulties walking and climbing stairs. He wears a leg brace and uses a cane for ambulation. He was 33 when referred to the RRTC and had not worked since his injury. He was separated from his wife and living with his sister and her family, receiving SSI benefits of $446 per month and Medicare coverage.

Job Placement and Training

Because of Matthew's physical problems and some past clerical experience and interest, job development efforts focused on office related occupations. A full-time position was located as a microfilm clerk in an office building, with a starting pay of $4.50 per hour with full benefits.

Matthew's primary job duties involved processing incoming checks and receipts by (1) stamping the receipts as paid, (2) balancing check totals to backup totals and correcting accounting errors, (3) microfilming checks and receipts, and (4) reboxing and shelving the work. Training in these skills was completed 3 weeks from the hire date, with Matthew able to complete 30 to 40 checks per hour with accuracy rates of 98 to 100 percent. Minor adaptations (e.g., written work sequences and reminders) at the work site helped Matthew maintain his work quality to the employer's specifications. In addition, the employment specialist purchased additional equipment (electric stapler, lower back cushion, work dividers) and raised Matthew's work table to compensate for his physical problems.

Follow-Along Services

Early in the follow-along phase, Matthew's supervisor requested assistance in improving his work speed. The employment specialist, therefore, initiated retraining activities to meet this need. He designated different intervals during work hours for Matthew to race the clock and graph his own performance levels. This procedure proved to be very reinforcing to Matthew: His speed improved without a decrease in work quality. Typed task analyses of Matthew's job duties were also left at the job site because he sometimes would forget steps of particular jobs.

Matthew has had recurrent problems with excessive drinking, resulting in a high absentee rate. On one occasion, he fell off his porch while drinking and bruised his ribs. He went to work the next day, but had to be sent home due to his pain. When discussions with Matthew about his drinking proved futile, the employment specialist and Matthew developed a written contract that called for Matthew to seek counseling to remain a supported employment client. In addition, Matthew's sister became involved in monitoring his alcohol intake and notifying the employment specialist whenever Matthew drank excessively.

Matthew has a goal of living independently. The employment specialist has worked with Matthew and the family to better budget his money and plan for that eventuality. Matthew still has some unrealistic expectations about his financial survival, which the employment specialist continues to address.

After 1 year, Matthew received a merit increase to $5.00 per hour. At this writing, he has remained in this position for 21 months and has earned $17,400. His SSI cash benefits have been halted, but he continues to receive Medicare health coverage. He also has received 688.5 hours of intervention time from his employment specialist.

SUMMARY

Several key points about the case studies are warranted.

- The two cases were selected to emphasize that the provision of systematic follow-along procedures involving the client, family, employer, and coworkers has resulted in long-term job retention for these individuals. Their earnings, while insufficient to sustain independence, have decreased their reliance on the social services system and their families and friends.
- Even though Dave was eventually terminated from his position, he was able to accumulate 14 months of continuous work experience in one position, $7,155 in earnings, and the self-confidence to pursue further employment. His supported employment experience, particularly in comparison with other persons with severe head trauma, can be characterized as nothing short of successful.
- Although many clients of supported competitive employment return sufficient tax revenue from their earnings to offset the cost of supported employment, these two individuals have not and perhaps never will. Yet both have become contributors to the economic system, rather than just consumers. Their contributions may be small in comparison to the cost of services, but they are significant in comparison to the economic and emotional impact of sporadic or no employment and custodial care.

REFERENCES

Anthony, W.A., & Blanch, A. (1987). Supported employment for persons who are psychiatrically disabled: An historical and conceptual perspective. *Psychosocial Rehabilitation Journal*, *11*(2), 5–23.

Arkansas Research & Training Center in Vocational Rehabilitation (1985). *Supported employment: Implications for rehabilitation services*. Little Rock, AR: University of Arkansas.

Berg, W., & Wacker, D. (1983). *Effects of permanent prompts on the vocational performance of severely handicapped individuals*. Paper presented at the Association for Behavior Analysis, Milwaukee, WI.

Crouch, K.P., Rusch, F.R., & Karlan, G.R. (1984). Competitive employment: Utilizing the correspondence training paradigm to enhance productivity. *Education and Training of the Mentally Retarded, 19*, 268–275.

Federal Register. (1987, August 14). Supported employment regulations for Vocational Rehabilitation Act Amendments.

Hill, J., Cleveland, P., Pendleton, P., & Wehman, P. (1982). Strategies in the follow-up of moderately and severely handicapped competitively employed workers. In P. Wehman & M. Hill (Eds.), *Vocational training and placement of severely disabled persons: Project Employability: Volume III* (pp. 160–171). Richmond, VA: Virginia Commonwealth University.

Hill, M., Hill, J.W., Wehman, P., Revell, G., Dickerson, A., & Noble, J. (1985).Time limited training and supported employment: A model for redistributing existing resources for persons with severe disabilities. In P. Wehman & J.W. Hill (Eds.), *Competitive employment for persons with mental retardation: From research to practice: Volume I* (pp. 132–168). Richmond, VA: Virginia Commonwealth University.

Hill, M., & Wehman, P. (1983). Cost-benefit analysis of placing moderately and severely handicapped individuals into competitive employment. *Journal of the Association for the Severely Handicapped, 8*(1), 30–38.

Isbister, F., & Donaldson, G. (1987). Supported employment for individuals who are mentally ill: Program development. *Psychosocial Rehabilitation Journal, 11*(2), 45–54.

Karlan, G., & Rusch, F. (1982). Correspondence between saying and doing: Some thoughts on defining correspondence and future directions for application. *Journal of Applied Behavior Analysis, 15*, 151–162.

Karpman, T., Wolfe, S., & Vargo, J.W. (1985). The psychological adjustment of adult clients and their parents following closed-head injury. *Journal of Applied Rehabilitation Counseling, 17*(1), 28–33.

Kernan, K., & Koegel, R. (1980). *Employment experiences of community-based mildly retarded adults*. Working paper No. 14, Sociobehavioral Group, Mental Retardation Research Center, School of Medicine, University of California, Los Angeles.

Kochany, L., & Keller, J. (1981). An analysis and evaluation of the failures of severely disabled individuals in competitive employment. In P. Wehman, *Competitive employment: New horizons for severely disabled individuals* (pp. 181–198). Baltimore: Paul H. Brookes.

Kregel, J., Shafer, M., Wehman, P., & West, M. (1989). Policy and program development in supported employment: Current strategies to promote statewide systems change. In P. Wehman, J. Kregel, & M. Shafer (Eds.), *Emerging trends in the national supported employment initiative: A preliminary analysis of 27 states* (pp. 15–45). Richmond, VA: Virginia Commonwealth University.

Kreutzer, J.S., & Morton, M.V. (1988). Traumatic brain injury: Supported employment and compensatory strategies for enhancing vocational outcomes. In P. Wehman & M.S. Moon (Eds.), *Vocational rehabilitation and supported employment* (pp. 291–311). Baltimore: Paul H. Brookes.

Moon, S., Goodall, P., Barcus, M., & Brooke, V. (1986). *The supported work model of competitive employment for citizens with severe handicaps: A guide for job trainers*. Richmond, VA: Virginia Commonwealth University.

Nielson, G.B. (1986). *Using the Plan to Achieve Self-support, a SSI work incentive program to fund supported employment: From rationale to case examples.* Manuscript submitted for publication.

Noble, J.H., & Collignon, F.C. (1987). Systems barriers to supported employment for persons with chronic mental illness. *Psychosocial Rehabilitation Journal, 11*(2), 25–44.

Nockleby, D.M., & Deaton, A.V. (1987). Denial versus distress: Coping patterns in post head trauma patients. *International Journal of Clinical Neuropsychology, 9*(4), 145–148.

Rehabilitation Research and Training Center (1988). *Interagency vendorization: Expanded supported employment services.* Richmond, VA: Virginia Commonwealth University.

Rehabilitation Research and Training Center (October, 1988). *Quarterly report: Successful outcomes in supported employment.*

Rusch, F.R. (1986). Developing a long-term follow-up program. In F.R. Rusch (Ed.), *Competitive employment: Issues and strategies* (pp. 225–232). Baltimore: Paul H. Brookes.

Rusch, F.R., Martin, J.E., & White, D.M. (1985). Competitive employment: Teaching mentally retarded employees to maintain their work behavior. *Education and Training of the Mentally Retarded, 20,* 182–189.

Schultz, R.P. (1986). Establishing a parent-professional partnership to facilitate competitive employment. In F.R. Rusch (Ed.), *Competitive employment: Issues and strategies* (pp. 289–302). Baltimore: Paul H. Brookes.

Shafer, M.S. (1986). Utilizing co-workers as change agents. In F.R. Rusch (Ed.), *Competitive employment: Issues and strategies* (pp. 215–224). Baltimore: Paul H. Brookes.

Shafer, M.S., Kregel, J., Banks, P.D., & Hill, M.L. (1988). An analysis of employer evaluations of workers with mental retardation. *Research in Developmental Disabilities, 9,* 377–391.

Stokes, T., & Baer, D. (1977). An implicit technology of generalization. *Journal of Applied Behavior Analysis, 10,* 349–367.

Tyerman, A., & Humphrey, M. (1984). Changes in self-concept following severe head injury. *International Journal of Rehabilitation Research, 7*(1), 11–23.

Wacker, D., & Berg, W. (1983). Effects of picture prompts on the acquisition of complex vocational tasks by mentally retarded adolescents. *Journal of Applied Behavior Analysis, 16,* 417–433.

Wacker, D.P., & Berg, W.K. (1986). Generalizing and maintaining work behavior. In F.R. Rusch (Ed.), *Competitive employment: Issues and strategies* (pp. 129–140). Baltimore: Paul H. Brookes.

Wehman, P. (1981). *Competitive employment: New horizons for severely disabled individuals.* Baltimore: Paul H. Brookes.

Wehman, P., Shafer, M., Kregel, J., & Twardzik, G. (1989). Supported employment implementation II: Service delivery characteristics associated with program development and costs. In P. Wehman, J. Kregel, & M. Shafer (Eds.), *Emerging trends in the national supported employment initiative: A preliminary analysis of 27 states* (pp. 75–96). Richmond, VA: Virginia Commonwealth University.

White, D.M. (1986). Social validation. In F.R. Rusch (Ed.), *Competitive employment: Issues and strategies* (pp. 199–213). Baltimore: Paul H. Brookes.

Zarsky, J.J., Hall, D.E., DePompei, R. (1987). Closed head injury patients: A family therapy approach to the rehabilitation process. *American Journal of Family Therapy, 15*(1), 62–68.

Chapter 10

Quantifying Consumer Outcomes

R. Timm Vogelsberg

Issues related to the community reintegration of individuals who have experienced a traumatic head injury are complex. Recent areas for attention include the development of supported employment programs for this population (Kreutzer & Morton, 1988; Wehman et al., 1988) and the effect of supported employment services on the individuals' quality of life (Schalock, 1988). Existing literature on the quality of life (Borthwick-Duffey, 1989; Bunge, 1975; Campbell, 1976; Campbell, Converse, & Rogers, 1976; Flanagan, 1978; Goode, 1989; Matson & Rusch, 1988) and suggested research approaches to community integration (Heal, 1985; Heal & Chadsey-Rusch, 1985; White, 1988) are establishing an improved understanding of the support needs of the individual.

Successful reintegration of multiple populations who experience significant disabilities (Rusch, 1988; Vogelsberg & Richard, 1988; Wehman & Moon, 1988) and evaluation of their physical integration and social interaction (Bacon & Crimmins, 1989; Chadsey-Rusch, 1986) are awakening the service community to the competence these individuals can demonstrate if given adequate community supports.

Implied within this focus on community reintegration is the establishment of sophisticated service coordination and community activities for the individual (Mayer, Keating, & Rapp, 1986). The hypothesis appearing in the rehabilitation literature is that an increase in activity patterns of daily living (inpatient and outpatient) has a positive effect upon rehabilitation outcomes for the individual (Mayer & Keating, 1988; Mayer, Keating, & Rapp, 1986). These approaches are evident within the establishment of supported employment as a major component of community reentry for the individual.

There are many foundations to the establishment of supported employment throughout the nation. Perhaps the most important concepts for the rehabilitation professions include community reintegration, environmental orientation, accountability, and a true multiple agency–profession approach. Residential and educational services have initiated the progression towards community reintegration and the present decade has witnessed the beginnings of the present focus on community employment.

COMMUNITY REINTEGRATION

Contemporary service development focuses on services that return the individual to the mainstream of society. Previous opinions that individuals benefit from isolated and segregated services have fallen into disrepute as the success of integrated services has been demonstrated (Heal, Haney, & Novak, 1988; Horner, Meyer, & Fredericks, 1986). Empirical studies concerning institutional settings (Bruininks, Meyers, Sigford, & Lakin, 1981) and facility-based vocational settings (Greenleigh Associates, 1975; Whitehead, 1979) have proven that individuals with the most severe disabilities seldom grow, prosper, or move within specialized but isolated environments.

ECOLOGICAL-ENVIRONMENTAL ORIENTATION

Traditional service development focuses on the individual and variables used to predict recovery and identify preparatory activities for the eventual reintegration of the individual. Contemporary service development continues to focus on the individual but provides an equal emphasis on the community that the individual is expected to occupy. A better understanding of the community effect (both positive and negative) is emerging by placing the individual in the desired environment and identifying the supports necessary to maintain the person there. The previous readiness (preparation for community) orientation has been greatly reduced or totally removed.

ACCOUNTABILITY-OUTCOME FOCUS

With new approaches to service delivery, the concept of an accountable service system continues to be a priority. Supported employment was established on empirical evidence of effective outcomes for individuals and the demonstration that existing traditional service models seldom maximized community independence. This same outcome focus must be maintained as individuals who require new types of support gain access to supported employment. Basic research questions, such as prediction and evaluation, must be separated from immediate applied (employment) outcomes for the individual. Research that focuses on the actual implementation of community reintegration will provide valuable information.

PREDICTION VS. IMPLEMENTATION

A constant issue among rehabilitationists is the relationship between the level of severity of the disability and prediction. Multiple areas of research have focused on the ability to predict the future capability of the individual based on injury, amount of time in coma, post-traumatic amnesia, and other indicators. While these measures may prove valuable in the future, they currently do not predict the support needs of the individual in relation to the community environment.

A continual desire within the service community is to predict future levels of community functioning based on demographic and descriptive information on work history and more recent trauma. Although the benefits of this approach are obvious, it continues to be a difficult orientation that categorizes the individual, the injury, and the future without attention to the support capabilities of the environment or idiosyncratic differences of the individual.

MULTIPLE AGENCY-PROFESSION APPROACH

Within the multiple disciplines available in medicine, rehabilitation, psychology, therapy, and education, a continual need exists to communicate and coordinate efforts that focus on outcome for the individual. Professional separation, approaches, ideology, focus, and competition for funding and for individuals limit the amount of sharing that is possible, desirable, or manageable and detract from the best outcome for the individual.

Multiply agency and professional support requires increased communication and coordination to be successful (Vogelsberg, Williams, & Ashe, 1981), but consumer measurement is frequently related only to that level (or section) of rehabilitation. A total outcomes orientation to measurement across services, agencies, and professions is necessary for adequate service delivery to occur. Independent evaluations and measures of progress are valuable, but they must be combined within a total outcome focus to really benefit the individual.

These team activities that focus on the future outcome for the individual are time consuming and indicate a loss of autonomy (or control) by each agency or profession. They continue to be a challenge, but a necessary challenge for success. The transfer (transition) from one service to another (hospital to community and inpatient to outpatient) requires tremendous efforts to guarantee adequate communication is provided to implement the most successful service.

APPROACHES TO MEASUREMENT

When approaching measurement of consumer outcomes across medical rehabilitation, physical and occupational therapy, psychology, social work, and related disciplines, first identify the intent of the analysis. Multiple interim reasons for measurement lead to the developing focus on the actual outcomes to the individual: Perceived improvement (or lack thereof) to the quality of an individual's life.

Data collection and evaluation can be driven by a requirement for funding, a need to measure status or progress of service variables, implementation of research, a court order (mandated), or a need to evaluate experimental treatments. Service projects seldom have extensive data that prioritize the improvement of the service. The common driving force for the collection and analysis of data is the need of the service provider (funding, compliance, research, etc.), rather than the recipient of that service.

The concept of social validity (White, 1988; Kazdin, 1978) identified the necessity to consider the service outcomes in relation to the individual, the environment, and quality of life indicators. "Successful" services that could not verify an improvement to the life of the individual were questioned. The challenge facing supported employment was to guarantee that an immediate, measurable outcome occurs to document the actual benefit to that individual (from society's, the service's, and the individual's perspective).

Measurement approaches concentrate on one small component within a field of inquiry. In the academic world, this sometimes means that minute components within a systemic issue are carefully analyzed, researched, and studied for lengthy periods of time. This intricate study of one component of the larger universe is valuable but must become a contributing factor to positive consumer outcomes to be recognized for immediate use. An applied perspective recognizes the importance of each segment within the total but places priority upon the actual outcome. For the individual who has experienced a traumatic head injury, the applied question focuses on successful community reintegration to employment, residence, and family life.

The influence of the environment (support, lack of support, level of intensity, stimulation, etc.) on successful community reintegration has not been accurately determined within standardized approaches to evaluation. The individual must be given the opportunity to interact within the proposed environment and to understand the environmental supports that exist to maintain the individual there.

The importance of the ongoing relationship between the individual and the environment (residential, vocational, etc.) must be understood to initiate successful community reintegration. In fact, it can make the difference between successful and unsuccessful community reintegration.

If the service benefit to the individual becomes the focal point, then multiple disciplines can become essential components to reach this outcome. From this community integrated outcome focus, a consistent measurement system can be initiated that will allow professionals to identify previous, existing, and future approaches that can have an immediate benefit to the individual.

SUPPORTED EMPLOYMENT DATA SYSTEMS

Data systems that have been developed for supported employment implementation in Virginia, Vermont, Washington, Illinois, Pennsylvania, and other states have become the foundation for future development and expansion (Vogelsberg, 1987; Wehman, 1987). These supported employment programs provide on-the-job employment training services to individuals with severe disabilities and use a data system to gather information on individual outcomes (demographic, support, training, follow-up, employment, and financial) and on the program (job development and program costs and savings).

These consumer outcome measurement systems were established to assist in the documentation of service efficiency and they have provided information for advocacy, formative evaluation, technical assistance, program revision, future funding, and applied research (Vogelsberg, 1987). This applied empirical orientation to direct service has improved the quality of service and assisted in the expansion or replication of that service (it is the reason that there is the present expansion of supported employment).

As funding patterns vacillate, specific data are often required on types of service. The documentation of the hours spent providing various services (therapy, case management, job development, evaluation, on-the-job training, and follow-up) can be used to develop a concise service accounting.

If direct service can be accountable by accurate and reliable data, then legislators, administrators, advocates, and concerned citizens have a vehicle for improvement and expansion. Although there are multiple successful employment programs for individuals with severe disabilities, strong documentation of success was rare before the 1970s. Such documentation continues to be necessary for expansion or replication of that service and for acceptance by individuals and agencies that remain skeptical. This documentation of the effectiveness of new service approaches accounts for the present expansion of community integrated services.

Components of Supported Employment Data Systems

The approach to outcome measurement has many varied components. Typical summative evaluation provides measurements of outcomes once a year (or once for each grant funding period) and provides valuable information for future funding, but cannot be used for immediate benefits to the individual. Longitudinal annual data are not adequate to establish immediate revisions or improve outcomes for the individual. These once a year snapshots get buried in yearly reports that only academic or upper level administrators can access.

The developing focus on outcome measurement must include establishment of a dynamic, growing data base for use beyond the traditional funding or snapshot approach. Information on an individual can be recorded once and then training, support, follow-up, employment, and financial measures updated on a monthly (or quarterly) basis.

Data for supported employment programs have been divided into two major categories—individual data and project data. In Pennsylvania, data are entered monthly on a microcomputer system that allows individual projects to generate internal reports and submit data. The variables listed in Appendix 10-A are collected in three different ways. Some data (demographics) are entered only once and seldom revised, other data (employment information) are entered only when a major change has occurred, and still other data (support, training, and follow-up data) are entered monthly to monitor changes in support services to the individual and to assist in program management.

Individual Data

There are four data areas to describe individuals in supported employment programs: Demographic; financial; support, training, and follow-up; and employment. The most important data for ongoing project management and maintenance within the community are data that document support, training, and follow-up hours required by the individual each month. These are characterized by the level of support (intensive or follow-up) and the type of support. They are recorded as total hours required for each month of service. Exhibit 10-1 lists support activities of supported employment implementation in Pennsylvania. More complete descriptions are available from Wehman (1987) and Vogelsberg (1987).

Support hour data can indicate an increase or decrease in level of support necessary to establish and maintain employment. They are correlated with demographic, financial, and employment information over time to help

Exhibit 10-1 Types of Support Activities Measured for Each Individual Placed into Employment

Intensive Support during the Placement Process (8–24 weeks)

Evaluation	Of Support Needs for Employment
Job Development	Time To Develop This Position
Program Design-Implementation	Developing Programs
Service Coordination	Case Management
Direct Training	Training in Vocational Tasks
Indirect Training	Training in Nonvocational Tasks
Observation	Consumer Performance
Employer Assistance	Employer-Coworker Support
Transportation	To Provide Support

Follow-Up Support (Continual To Maintain Employment)

Direct Contact	On or Off the Job
Related Activities	On or Off the Job, Including Service Coordination, Program Design, Other Areas after Intensive Phase
Number of Contacts	Monthly Contacts Made

projects improve their ability to identify areas for future technical assistance (through examining reasons for job loss or identifying support needs not being met) and actual positive or negative outcomes to the individual. They may eventually provide outcome-driven predictors of service need.

Program Data

Two types of data to describe an entire program are job development data and program cost figures. These areas describe the job development efforts and costs of the program. They are typically used at the systemic (funding and management) levels.

The job development data allow a program to monitor the total number of hours spent identifying positions and define the types of employment sites contacted. The average number of contacts and recontacts to the same business for job development can also be determined. Program and consumer cost data are important to analyze costs of each form of service delivery. Existing resource limitations make it imperative that service delivery focus on consumer outcomes and cost efficiency of the service being delivered. Cost data provide programs with useful directions for the future.

Pennsylvania Data Reporting Format

Consistent data systems that are reviewed and updated monthly assure ongoing communication and quality of replication across 17 programs in

Pennsylvania. These monthly data are reported during staff and Advisory Board meetings, compared with previous monthly data and data from similar programs, and then widely disseminated.

This monthly submittal of data to a central location and the development of a quarterly reporting format, guarantees reliability of the existing data. Summaries are reported on a quarterly schedule. Annual reports (Vogelsberg, Richard, & Nicoll, 1989) provide the ability to do summative evaluations in addition to the ongoing formative evaluations. This objective information has proven to be a valuable addition to program meetings and a guarantee of consistency and quality control.

Appendix 10-B contains a data-based quarterly reporting format developed and implemented in Pennsylvania. Perhaps the most challenging aspect to these data is the fact the projects that produced the data differed widely in approach to community reintegration. The Competitive Supported Employment of Pennsylvania (CSE PA) Project data are generated from a series of projects that provide competitive supported employment to individuals who have many forms of severely disabling conditions (mental retardation, mental illness, severe physical disabilities, and traumatic head injury). The Moss Rehabilitation Hospital Project data are from a project that provides community reintegration and supported employment only to individuals who have experienced a traumatic head injury. The outcomes for both projects are similar, which challenges the assumption that services must be separate by disability.

SUMMARY

As new community reintegration services develop for individuals who have experienced a traumatic head injury, multiple professions will expect verification of the effectiveness of these approaches. The two major areas that will be questioned at the administrative levels are cost effectiveness and positive quality of life changes. Specifically the questions will focus on the expense of new approaches in relation to existing service costs and a more thorough understanding of the service effects on the life of the individual.

Administrations use data at a systemic level for long-term decision making and these data are frequently summative and have little relationship to immediate service implementation issues. Data can also be used for advocacy, formative evaluation of program development, identification of technical assistance and training needs, and financial reimbursement (based on the service received). Until efforts at quantifying outcomes to individuals with severe disabilities result in reliable data that can be utilized by all levels within the service community (administration, direct management, and direct service), the science of quantifying outcomes for consumers with disabilities will continue to be incomplete.

REFERENCES

Bacon, A., & Crimmins, D.B. (1989). Enhancing functional social capabilities: New developments in instructional technology. In W.E. Kiernan & R.L. Schalock (Eds.), *Economics, industry, and disability: A look ahead*. Baltimore, MD: Paul H. Brookes.

Borthwick-Duffey, S.A. (1989). Quality of life: The residential environment. In W.E. Kiernan & R.L. Schalock (Eds.), *Economics, industry, and disability: A look ahead*. Baltimore, MD: Paul H. Brookes.

Bruininks, R.H., Meyers, C.E., Sigford, B.B., & Lakin, K.C. (Eds.). (1981). *Deinstitutionalization and community adjustment of mentally retarded people*. Washington, DC: American Association on Mental Deficiency.

Bunge, M. (1975). What is a quality of life indicator? *Social Indicator Research*, *3*, 65–79.

Campbell, A. (1976). Subjective measures of well-being. *American Psychologist*, *31*, 117–124.

Campbell, A., Converse, P.E., & Rogers, W.L. (1976). *The quality of American life: Perceptions, evaluations, and satisfactions*. New York: Russell Sage.

Chadsey-Rusch, J. (1986). Identifying and teaching valued social behaviors. In F.R. Rusch (Ed.), *Competitive employment issues and strategies*. Baltimore, MD: Paul H. Brookes.

Flanagan, J.C. (1978). *Adolescent community integration*. Paper presented at the National Invitational Conference on Traumatic Brain Injury Research, Tysons Corner, VA.

Goode, D.A. (1989). Quality of life and quality of work life. In W.E. Kiernan & R.L. Schalock (Eds.), *Economics, industry, and disability: A look ahead*. Baltimore, MD: Paul H. Brookes.

Greenleigh Associates (1975). *The role of the sheltered workshop in the rehabilitation of the severely handicapped*. New York: Report to the Department of Health, Education, and Welfare, Rehabilitation Services Administration.

Heal, L.W. (1985). Methodology for community integration research. In R.H. Bruininks, C.E. Meyers, B.B. Sigford, & K.C. Lakin (Eds.), *Deinstitutionalization and community adjustment of mentally retarded people* (pp. 199–224). Washington, DC: American Association on Mental Deficiency.

Heal, L.W., & Chadsey-Rusch, J. (1985). The lifestyle satisfaction scale (LSS): Assessing individuals' satisfaction with residence, community setting, and associated services. *Applied Research in Mental Retardation*, *6*, 475–490.

Heal, L.W., Haney, J.I., & Novak Amado, A.R. (Eds.) (1988). *Integration of developmentally disabled individuals into the community, (2nd ed.)*. Baltimore, MD: Paul H. Brookes.

Horner, R.H., Meyer, L.H., & Fredericks. H.D. (1986). *Education of learners with severe handicaps: Exemplary service strategies*. Baltimore, MD: Paul H. Brookes.

Kazdin, A.E. (1978). Assessing the clinical or applied importance of behavior change through social validation. *Behavior Modification*, *1*, 427–451.

Kreutzer, J.S., & Morton, M.V. (1988). Traumatic brain injury: Supported employment and compensatory strategies for enhancing vocational outcomes. In P. Wehman & M.S. Moon (Eds.), *Vocational rehabilitation and supported employment*. Baltimore, MD: Paul H. Brookes.

Matson, J.L., & Rusch, F.R. (1988). Quality of life: Does competitive employment make a difference? In F.R. Rusch (Ed.), *Competitive employment issues and strategies*. Baltimore, MD: Paul H. Brookes.

Mayer, N.H., & Keating, D. (1988). *Concepts in day programming: What is day programming?* Unpublished manuscript, Moss Rehabilitation, Philadelphia, PA.

Mayer, N.H., Keating, D.J., & Rapp, D. (1986). Skills, routines, and activity patterns of daily living: A functional nested approach. In Uzzell & Gross (Eds.), *Clinical neuropsychology of intervention*. New York: Martinus Publishing.

Rusch, F.R. (1988). *Competitive employment issues and strategies*. Baltimore, MD: Paul H. Brookes.

Schalock, R.L. (1988). Critical performance evaluation indicators in supported employment. In P. Wehman & M.S. Moon (Eds.), *Vocational rehabilitation and supported employment*. Baltimore, MD: Paul H. Brookes.

Vogelsberg, R.T., Williams, W.W., & Ashe, W. (1981). Improving vocational services through interagency cooperation. In C.L. Hansen (Ed.), *Severely handicapped persons in the community*, Seattle, WA: University of Washington Program Development Assistance System.

Vogelsberg, R.T. (1987). *Supported employment data system: SEDS (17th revision)*. Philadelphia, PA: Temple University Center for Research in Human Development and Education.

Vogelsberg, R.T., & Richard, L. (1988). Supported employment for persons with mental retardation: Programmatic issues for implementation. In P. Wehman & S. Moon (Eds.), *Vocational rehabilitation and supported employment*. Baltimore, MD: Paul H. Brookes.

Vogelsberg, R.T., Richard, L., & Nicoll, J. (1989). *Pennsylvania Competitive Supported Employment: Second annual report (1986–1988)*. Philadelphia, PA: Temple University Center for Research in Human Development and Education.

Wehman, P. (1987). *Data management system operations manual*. Richmond, VA: Virginia Commonwealth University Rehabilitation Research and Training Center.

Wehman, P., Kreutzer, J.S., Stonnington, H.H., Wood, W., Sherron, P., Diambra, J., Fry, R., & Groah, C. (1988). Supported employment for persons with traumatic brain injury: A preliminary report. *The Journal of Head Trauma Rehabilitation*, *3*(4), 82–94.

Wehman, P., & Moon, M.S. (1988). *Vocational rehabilitation and supported employment*. Baltimore, MD: Paul H. Brookes.

White, D. (1988). Social validation. In F.R. Rusch (Ed.), *Competitive employment issues and strategies*. Baltimore, MD: Paul H. Brookes.

Whitehead, C.W. (1979). *Sheltered workshop study: A nationwide report on sheltered workshops and their employment of handicapped individuals*. Washington, DC: U. S. Department of Labor.

Appendix 10-A

List of Variables for Supported Employment Data Systems

At this stage in the development of supported employment programs, we know that the careful monitoring of individual performance can greatly assist in training, evaluation, advocacy, and future funding efforts. The following variables have been identified as important for monthly monitoring by previous supported employment programs in Washington, Illinois, Virginia, Oregon, Pennsylvania, and Vermont.

Data about Individuals

I. Demographic Information

1. Name
2. Social Security Number and Other ID Number
3. Placement Number
4. Consumer Number
5. Birth Date
6. Sex
7. Race/Ethnicity
8. Case Manager Name and Telephone Number
9. Provider Name (s)
10. Provider Type (s)
11. Provider Office Number
12. Provider Service Coordinator and Telephone Number
13. Referral Source
14. Referral Number
15. Referral Date

16. Primary Disability
17. Secondary Disability
18. Functional Level
19. Ambulation
20. Intellectual Functioning
21. Full Scale IQ
22. Supported Employment Code (type)
23. Description
    a. Date of Accident
    b. Length of Coma
    c. Post-Traumatic Amnesia
    d. DSM III-R
    e. Medication
    f. Other
24. Living Arrangement
25. Previous Vocational Training
26. Previous Program Training
27. Community Paid Work History (if any)
28. Facility Paid Work History (if any)
29. Pre-Employment Benefits
    a. SSI
    b. SSDI
    c. Other (type)

II. Financial Information

1. Type of Employer Assistance
    a. TJTC
    b. NARC-OJT
    c. Other (list)
2. Benefits
    a. Sick Days/Month
    b. Insurance (types)
    c. Vacation (type)
    d. Other
3. Pay Per Hour
4. Gross Income
5. Taxes Paid
6. Post Employment Benefits
    a. SSI
    b. SSDI
    c. Other (type)
7. Previous Program Costs
    a. Accurate

b. Estimate
8. Previous Transportation Costs
   a. Accurate
   b. Estimate

III. Support, Training, and Follow-Up Information

1. Hours of Project Time Spent Performing
   a. **Intensive Support**
      (1) Evaluation
      (2) Job Development
      (3) Service Coordination
      (4) Program Design and Implementation
      (5) Direct Training
      (6) Indirect Training
      (7) Observation
      (8) Employer/Coworker Assistance
      (9) Transportation
   b. **Follow-Up Support**
      (1) Direct Consumer Contact
      (2) Consumer-Related Activities
      (3) Number of Consumer Contacts in Follow-Up
2. Present OVR Status and Services
3. Type of Supported Employment
4. Transportation Utilized
5. Comments on Present Support, Training, and Follow-Up

IV. Employment Information

1. Employer Name
2. Total Number of Employees
3. Job Title
4. Days Worked Per Week
5. Hours Worked Per Week
6. Amount of Supervision by Employer
7. Date Job Began
8. Date Job Ended
9. Hours Worked Per Month
10. Days Absent
11. Days Tardy
12. Present Job Status
13. Change in Job Status
14. Reason for Change in Job Status
15. Primary Reason for Termination

16. Secondary Reason for Termination
17. Comments on Termination

Data about the Project As a Whole

V. Job Development

1. New Contacts
2. Businesses Contacting Project
3. Repeat Contacts
   a. Consumer Present
   b. No Consumer Present
4. Service Occupation Contacts
5. Other Occupation Contacts
6. Jobs Developed
   a. New Jobs Developed
   b. New Jobs Filled
7. Presentations
8. Total Hours of Job Development

VI. Program and Consumer Cost Figures

1. Program Costs
   a. Total Staff Salaries
   b. Total Fringe Benefits
   c. Total Operating and Indirect Costs for Program
2. Consumer Cost Figures
   a. Salaries Earned
   b. Taxes Paid
   c. Previous Program Costs Saved
      (1) Actual
      (2) Estimated
   d. Transportation Costs Saved
      (1) Actual
      (2) Estimated
   e. SSI/SSDI/Other Costs Saved

Appendix 10–B

Quarterly Data Report Format

Table 10-B1 Demographic Information on Persons with Traumatic Brain Injury

PROJECT: COUNTY / DATA	# PLACEMENT/ # PEOPLE/ # STILL WORKING	# WOMEN # MEN	MEDIAN/AVERAGE AGE	LIVING ARRANGEMENT	SUPPORTED EMPLOYMENT CODE
1. CSE PA 7/86 - 12/88	At 60 days: 85% 25/23/10 40%	3/22	29/29	18 Nat. Fam. 5 Own A/H 2 CLA 0 Other	5 PD 20 Other
2. Moss Rehabilitation 10/87 - 12/88	At 60 days: 66% 17/14/7 50%	1/16	30/29	14 Nat. Fam. 3 Own A/H 0 CLA 0 Other	0 PD 17 Other
TOTAL	At 60 days: 76% 42/37/17 45%	4/38	30/29	32 Nat. Fam. 8 Own A/H 2 CLA 0 Other	5 PD 37 Other

Note: A/H, Apartment/home; CLA, Community living arrangement; CSE PA, Competitive supported employment of Pennsylvania; PD, Physical disabilities

Table 10-B2 Financial Information on Persons with Traumatic Brain Injury

DATA / PROJECT: COUNTY	EMPLOYER ASSISTANCE	PAY PER HOUR		AVERAGE GROSS SALARY/MONTH	AVERAGE TAXES PAID/MONTH
		RANGE	AVERAGE		
1. CSE PA 7/86 - 12/88	TJTC: 20	3.35 - 6.48	4.06	445.15	91.55
2. Moss Rehabilitation 10/87 - 12/88	TJTC: 1	2.30 - 14.30	4.95	543.45	132.29
AVERAGE	TJTC: 12.3	2.30 - 14.30	4.42	484.93	108.04

Note: CSE PA, Competitive supported employment of Pennsylvania; TJTC, Targeted jobs tax credit

Table 10-B3 Training Information on Persons with Traumatic Brain Injury

DATA / PROJECT: COUNTY	AVERAGE HOURS/PLACEMENT								
				TRAINING					
	Evaluation	Service Coordination	Job Development	Direct	Indirect	Observations	Follow-up	CoWorker Assistance	TOTAL
1. CSE PA 7/86 - 12/88	5.7	38.5	13.3	12.3	14.2	73.4	16.9	7.2	292.2
2. Moss Rehabilitation 10/87 - 12/88	6.7	2.9	8.6	22.7	11.6	50.4	11.5	10.6	125
AVERAGE/ PLACEMENT	6.1	24.1	11.4	82.4	13.1	64.1	14.7	8.6	224.5

Note: CSE PA, Competitive supported employment of Pennsylvania

Table 10-B4 Employment Information on Persons with Traumatic Brain Injury

DATA / PROJECT: COUNTY	AVERAGES				
	DAYS/WEEK	HOURS/WEEK	HOURS/MONTH	ABSENCES	TARDINESS
1. CSE PA 7/86 - 12/88	5	31.3	108.2	1.5	.5
2. Moss Rehabilitation 10/87 - 12/88	4.7	32	109	1.2	.6
AVERAGE/ PLACEMENT	4.9	31.6	108.5	1.4	.5

Note: CSE PA, Competitive supported employment of Pennsylvania

Chapter 11

Generalization Strategies

William W. Woolcock

According to Stokes and Osnes (1988), generalization involves the development of widespread behavioral change across "diverse stimulus conditions, responses, and time without comprehensive programming" (pp. 6–7). They also state that determining whether a behavior or set of behaviors generalizes requires that instructors note "when or where apparent generalization occurs" and ask the "critical functional question 'why?' " (pp. 6–7). Central to this definition is the notion that programming for generalization leads to more efficient instruction (Horner, Sprague, & Wilcox, 1982). Instruction on a restricted selection of stimulus or response examples results in a person's enhanced ability to perform "similar yet different" behaviors in the presence of a larger set of "similar yet different" examples.

Instruction that results in prescribed generalization provides learners with: (1) the adaptability to perform correctly across a variety of environments and tasks and (2) the autonomy to perform the appropriate tasks without the need for additional instruction (Gifford, Rusch, Martin, & White, 1984). From a vocational perspective, these qualities may be essential for a worker to perform variations of trained job tasks and independently respond to novel or new variations. These worker qualities are also necessary in building a repertoire of marketable job skills, the development of which facilitates

- a higher level of worker competence upon job entry (thus, a shorter period of job training)
- the ability of the worker to independently perform task variations within the work site

- the ability of the worker to adapt to new tasks, materials, and environments when changing jobs

This chapter describes instructional procedures that have led to the development of generalized job skills by using

- settings and materials other than those in the community work settings in which the skills are ultimately performed (simulation instruction)
- designated community work settings and materials in training for generalization across work settings and materials (in vivo instruction)
- combined simulation and in vivo instruction, particularly within a representative training sample of the larger set of stimuli and responses that will be encountered in generalized job task performance, e.g., general case instruction (Horner, Sprague, & Wilcox, 1982)

Although the procedures described in this chapter were conducted with participants who experienced severe to moderate levels of mental retardation, the procedures may be replicated using materials and settings appropriate for individuals who experience less-pronounced levels of cognitive impairment. Indeed, procedures designed to teach generalized performance of entry-level tasks (floor mopping, table busing, etc.) may be equally effective in teaching generalized performance of advanced skills such as cash register operation and computer use.

TOWARD AN APPLIED TECHNOLOGY OF GENERALIZATION

Recent literature concerning generalization has emphasized active programming for generalization rather than assuming that generalization occurs as a natural function of stimulus control (Hull, 1943) or discrimination learning (Skinner, 1953). In a synthesis of relevant literature Stokes and Baer (1977) identified nine common strategies to produce generalization:

1. Train and hope
2. Sequential modification
3. Introduce to natural maintaining contingencies
4. Train sufficient exemplars
5. Train loosely
6. Use indiscriminable contingencies
7. Program common stimuli
8. Mediate generalization
9. Train to generalize (pp. 351–362)

Stokes and Baer (1977) further delineated seven specific tactics to facilitate generalization:

1. Look for a response that enters a natural community; in particular, teach subjects to cue their natural communities to reinforce their desirable behaviors.
2. Keep training more exemplars; in particular, diversify them.
3. Loosen experimental control over the stimuli and responses involved in training; in particular, train different examples concurrently and vary instructions, discriminative stimuli, social reinforcers, and backup reinforcers.
4. Make unclear the limits of training contingencies; in particular, conceal the point at which contingencies stop operating, possibly by delayed reinforcement.
5. Use stimuli that are likely to be found in generalization settings as well as in training settings; in particular, use peers as tutors.
6. Reinforce accurate self-reports of desirable behavior; apply self-recording and self-reinforcement techniques whenever possible.
7. When generalizations occur, reinforce at least some of them at least sometimes, as if to generalize were an operant response class. (p. 364)

Stokes and Baer (1977) stated that these general strategies and specific tactics not only provide a set of what-to-do possibilities, but emphasize the limitations of generalization technology. Additionally, the occurrence of nonprogrammed generalization and nongeneralization of programmed behaviors underlines the "need to develop a technology of generalization, so that programming will be a fundamental component of any procedures when durability and generalization of behavior changes are desirable" (p. 364).

Of the nine general strategies, "train sufficient exemplars" and "program common stimuli" (Stokes & Baer, 1977) are most relevant to instruction on generalized job skills. These strategies require that instruction use a sufficient number of diverse training examples that share common stimulus and response characteristics with examples found in generalization examples. Therefore, programming for generalized job skills often requires (1) defining the range of stimulus/response variation found in the generalization examples and (2) selecting a number of instructional examples that fully sample this range of variation.

GENERAL CASE INSTRUCTION

General case instruction provides a mechanism through which effective data-based instruction may efficiently produce generalized task performance. It is a method for selecting and teaching a minimum number of teaching examples, which sample the range of stimulus/response variation present in a larger targeted class, or instructional universe, of untrained examples (Horner, Sprague, & Wilcox, 1982). "The general case has been taught when, after instruction on some tasks in a particular class, any task in that class can be performed correctly" (Becker & Englemann, 1978, p. 325). This involves defining the "instructional universe" of "all stimulus situations in which the student will be expected to produce this outcome and all behavior the learner should perform to achieve the outcome" (Horner, Sprague, & Wilcox, 1982, p. 47). Horner, Sprague, and Wilcox's (1982) process for developing a general case instruction strategy involves

- defining the instructional universe
- defining the range of relevant stimulus and response variation within that universe
- selecting examples from the instructional universe for use in teaching and probe testing
- sequencing teaching examples
- teaching the examples
- testing with untrained probe examples to determine whether the student can perform ______ examples without training (p.74)

Define the Instructional Universe

In this step, tasks first are analyzed as to the amount of behavior required or task components typically required to perform the task(s). These task components are referred to as *generic responses* because variations of each will be performed in a similar yet different manner across instructional and generalization examples. Then, the variation in generic responses and stimuli is defined for all of the possible task examples the learner will encounter. Table 11-1 defines an instructional universe for fast-food restaurant lobby cleaning. Each task and generic response is delineated with variations noted for each of four different restaurants (Woolcock, 1989).

Define the Range of Relevant Stimulus and Response Variation

Following the definition of the instructional universe, the range of relevant stimulus and response variation for each task and generic response needs to be defined. For example (Woolcock, Lyon, & Woolcock, 1987), this range could consist of differences in the amount of responding necessary—washing wheelchairs as opposed to washing patient beds in a hospital setting—or differences in response topography—mopping with a large "S" stroke versus mopping with a small "S" stroke.

Select Examples from the Instructional Universe for Use in Teaching and Probe

The instructor should select teaching examples that sample the determined range of task and generic response variation. The object of selection is to identify the minimum number of logistically feasible teaching examples necessary to produce generalization across the defined instructional

Table 11-1 Task Variation Matrix
Instructional Universe: Fast-Food Restaurant Lobby Cleaning (University Ave.

Tasks	Generic Responses	Arby's	Burger King	McDonald's	Wendy's
Clean Tables, Chairs	1. Clean Tables 2. Clean Chairs 3. When Appropriate 4. Clear Trash 5. Arrange Tables	Use sponge from two Compartment Pail Customer takes tray N/A	Damp towel with detergent solution Customer takes tray N/A	Spray bottle with McD, damp towel Customer takes tray N/A	Damp towel wash, dry towel dry Customer leaves on table When leaves
Clean Condiment Stand, Restock, Arrange Condiments, Straws, Napkins etc.	6. Clean Main Stand 7. Restock Condiments, Straws, Napkins,etc. 8. Arrange Condiments, Ashtray on Tables	Use Sponge Get from storage, line up on main stand Sauces, S & P, Ashtray	Damp towel Packets, Straws Wipe napkin holder; arrange with ashtray	McD, damp towel Napkins, Straws Arrange ashtray, salt and pepper, back, middle of table	Damp towel, hot soapy water Fill bins, straws. napkins, ketchup Arrange ashtray, salt and pepper, back, middle of table
Return Trays, Empty Trash Containers	9. To Cleaning Area 10. To Dumpster	To back of store Not on sidewalk	To back of store Not on sidewalk	To cleaning area Not on sidewalk	To cleaning area Not on sidewalk
Clean Floor	11. Pick Up Trash 12. Sweep Area 13. Carpet Sweep 14. Spot Mop-Wet Mop	Around tables when customers not present. In case of spills	Around tables when customers not present In case of spills	Around tables when customers not present In case of spills	Around tables with carpet sweeper Spills- blot with paper towel
Customer Relations	15. Hello 16. Excuse Me 17. Thank You 18. Refer Questions To Manager	Customer arrives Cleaning around customers If customer moves to allow cleaning, when customer leaves If customer has a question concerning service or food, take customer to manager			

Source: From *Generalization Curriculum Instruction: Inschool Instruction on Validated Work Skills* by W.W. Woolcock, 1989, unpublished study, University of Arkansas at Little Rock.

universe (Horner, Sprague, & Wilcox, 1982). In making a sample selection (such as mop small room-move furniture and mop large room-move furniture) the instructor makes a value judgment about which example will work best for teaching the important generic response (mop floor in a floor mopping program). If possible, examples that present significant exceptions to the defined variations (move furniture-don't move heavy furniture in a floor mopping program) should also be selected.

In the Task Variation Matrix provided in Table 11-1, the Clean Tables, Chairs task has four discrete variations across four restaurants. In this case, an instructional sequence was designed in which each participant received instruction on each variation during each instructional session. When discrete variations occur across several or all examples it may be desirable to arrange instructional procedures to incorporate all important variations, if feasible. In this manner, although job training may be taking place at McDonald's, instruction may include one or more trials using Wendy's, Arby's, and Burger King's methods and materials.

In selecting untrained probe examples instructors should look for examples in the instructional universe that learners are likely to encounter as a function of their present job placement or examples that will be encountered in another work setting using similar yet different job skills (e.g., different fast-food restaurants). Further, it is important to use logistically feasible examples that may be readily accessed during untrained probe sessions and possibly during follow-up instruction at the job site.

Finally, select a feasible number of representative untrained probe examples on which the learner may be tested during a designated time without fatigue or failure to complete the examples. Although it may be desirable to test learners on all of the possible examples they may encounter for a particular task or set of tasks, testing all possible examples is often impossible due to time constraints (testing unfamiliar tasks may take more time than criterion performance of those tasks). Testing all possible examples may also be unnecessary because some variations may be closely related to others.

Sequence Teaching Examples

In designing instructional programs, decide the number of teaching examples to use in each instructional session and number of teaching trials to be conducted with each example. If possible, instructors should include all selected teaching examples in each instructional session. Exposing the learner to all task variations during each session allows the learner to generalize across variations within the same session. The use of multiple instructional trials on each teaching example also facilitates generalized learning, although a massed trial strategy (in which the learner is exposed to a massive number of trials) may decelerate learning (Holvoet, Guess, Mulligan, &

Brown, 1980). Two or more trials on each example provide the learner with repeated practice and perhaps the opportunity to correct errors committed during previous trials (while the information is still fresh).

Instructors also may alternate trials on different examples so each example is repeated after instruction on other examples (Mulligan, Lacy, & Guess, 1982). This distributed trial strategy permits repeated practice and error correction while permitting the learner to sample all task variation within each trial sequence. Instructors should be cautioned, however, that repeating the same sequence of examples over time and trials may lead to a situation in which the learner is stimulus bound to the sequence and fails to generalize to novel sequences during untrained probes. Therefore, it may be beneficial to randomly sequence distributed trials unless instruction is conducted on serial order tasks (e.g., cleaning hotel rooms, where the development of a routine order of teaching and probe examples is desired).

Teach the Examples

The development of a data collection system permits measurement of the learner's discrete trial performance and accommodates instructional decisions concerning learner progress. Exhibit 11-1 is a data sheet used to teach fast-food restaurant lobby cleaning skills to high school students with moderate to severe mental retardation (Woolcock, 1989). The task variations on the data sheet provide a representative sampling of the major variations encountered in the instructional universe for fast-food restaurant lobby cleaning (Table 11-1).

Teaching procedures incorporated a "least-intrusive-prompts strategy" (Snell, 1983, p. 123) using a hierarchy of instructional prompts cuing students to initiate generic responses and correct errors in performance. Instructional procedures for persons who experience less severe cognitive disabilities may include a frequency/event data collection system that may measure independent performance "+" and verbally/gesturally prompted performance "−".

Test with Untrained Probe Examples

Testing with untrained probe examples may serve three functions in general-case instruction: (1) determine whether a general case has been learned; (2) identify common errors in generalization; and (3) combine with instructional data as a criterion measure for terminating instruction using the instructional examples. Untrained probe sessions serve to validate the efforts of instruction by verifying that the instruction results in generalized performance of the untrained probe examples. Untrained probe sessions also provide the instructor with information about the learner's failure to generalize to identified variations of generic responses within the probe examples. This information is vital to instructional decisions concerning:

Exhibit 11-1 Sample Data Sheet for Instructional Example for Fast-Food Restaurant Lobby Cleaning

GCI Project
Data Sheet

Site/ Restaurant: J.A. Fair High School Cafeteria

Student: ______________________________

Tasks	Dates											
Clean Table/Seats												
1. Clear if appropriate												
2. Clear trash from tables												
3. Damp sponge												
4. Damp sponge												
5. Spray bottle, damp towel												
6. Damp cloth, dry cloth												
Clean Floor												
7. Pick up trash at tables												
8. Sweep around tables												
9. Spot mop spills												
Trays/Trash												
10. Return trays												
11. Empty trash												
Customer Relations												
12. Hello												
13. Excuse me												
14. Thank you												
15. Refer to teacher, or cafeteria personnel												
Number Independent												
Number of Tasks												
% Independent												
Instructor Initials												
Data Collector Initials												

Key: 3 = Independent
2 = Verbal Prompt, Gesture, Model
1 = Physical Prompt
0 = Incorrect, Incomplete (Probe Only)

Source: From *Generalization Curriculum Instruction: Inschool Instruction on Validated Work Skills* by W.W. Woolcock, 1989, unpublished study, University of Arkansas at Little Rock.

- whether the instructional procedures are resulting in improved learner responses in the absence of prompts and correction procedures used during instruction
- whether the instructional examples adequately sample the range of variation encountered on the probe examples and whether the instructional examples require modification
- whether the learner will require additional instruction on identified components of the probe examples following general case instruction.

The preferred scheduling of probe sessions is at regular intervals during the general case instruction phase (Horner, Sprague, & Wilcox, 1982). This concurrent scheduling with instructional sessions uses probe data to assess the cumulative generalized effects of instruction and pinpoint common errors. Concurrent probe sessions also assist the learner in making the "crucial connections" (Giangreco, 1983, p. 48) between performance on the instructional examples and performance of the generalization probe examples, particularly during simulation instruction.

Horner, McDonnell, and Bellamy (1984) stated that future research is needed to investigate "the overall relationship between generalized performance and the criterion used to terminate training" (p. 21). In a study of janitorial and housekeeping skills instruction using general case instruction, Woolcock, Lyon, and Woolcock (1987) combined a criterion of 90 percent correct independent performance on general case instructional examples with a criterion of 70 percent on probe examples in arriving at criteria for terminating general case instruction and initiating instruction on all of the examples to correct errors in generalization. At issue in this study was the determination of criteria for terminating general case instruction upon a learner's inability to generalize. In such cases, a second decision rule needs to be implemented whereby an inadequate level of generalized performance on a predetermined number of untrained probe sessions results in an instruction change on the generalization examples. This permits error correction on the generalization examples and a continuation of job training, particularly when general case instruction is in a simulation setting.

During probe sessions, the instructor presents the learner with the tasks and steps back to observe and measure the learner's performance of each example. The instructor does not cue the learner during the performance of each probe example, but records learner correct/incorrect performance. Should the learner's failure to perform a particular generic response result in an inability to complete the task or task sequence, the probe on the particular example is discontinued and the remainder of the generic responses for that example are scored incorrect.

EXAMPLES OF GENERAL CASE INSTRUCTION IN VOCATIONAL SETTINGS

Horner and McDonald (1982) compared the generalized effects of teaching one example versus the effects of teaching three general case examples in a study of four high school students with severe to moderate mental retardation. The students were taught to cut and crimp two wire leads on each electronic capacitor within an instructional universe of 20 different capacitors (cut leads to 1 cm. with a half-circle bend on each lead; cutting tool does both operations at the same time). Students initially received one-to-one instruction on one capacitor through the presentation of 30 trials (same type capacitor) per instructional session. When each subject had attained criterion on the capacitor, he or she was provided with untrained probes of the 20 different capacitors. The instruction-probe sequence then was repeated for each student with one-to-one general case instruction provided on three of the capacitors using 10 trials each capacitor/each session. After training criterion was attained on the three capacitors, each student was again provided with untrained probes of the 20 different capacitors. Figure 11-1 provides a diagram of the capacitors used during the instruction and untrained probe sessions.

Results indicated that, after instruction on the single capacitor, none of the students could correctly cut and crimp more than 5 of the 20 untrained capacitors. However, after learning to cut and crimp the three general case capacitors, each student could correctly cut and crimp 15 to 20 of the untrained capacitors during each of the final probe sessions.

In a study by Woolcock and Lengel (1987), three adults with visual impairments and moderate mental retardation were taught to sort the instructional universe of 100 national 2-digit zip code prefixes (the first two zip code numbers), identifying the zip code prefixes on 3-inch by 5-inch note cards on which actual addresses were typed. Participants received instruction on sorting nine zip code prefixes (three initial, three medial, and three final) in one-to-one instructional sessions using five cards for each assigned zip code prefix variation. The addressed note cards were sorted on a 66-inch by 44-inch sheet of 3/8-inch plywood on which vertical columns and horizontal rows of 4-inch by 6-inch sorting rectangles were marked in the following manner:

- Twenty 3-inch by 5-inch note cards were glued to the top and left side of the sorting board and used as cue cards.
- Ten first-digit cue cards, divided into five sections, were marked with the first digits (0-9), 1-inch high in the first section of each card and placed serially across the top of each vertical column.
- Ten second-digit cue cards were marked with second digits in the second section and placed serially down the left side of each horizontal column. Exhibit 11-2 diagrams the sorting board. Instructional zip code prefixes were assigned to each participant (Vernon, Mike, and Gail), whose names were not included on the actual sorting board.

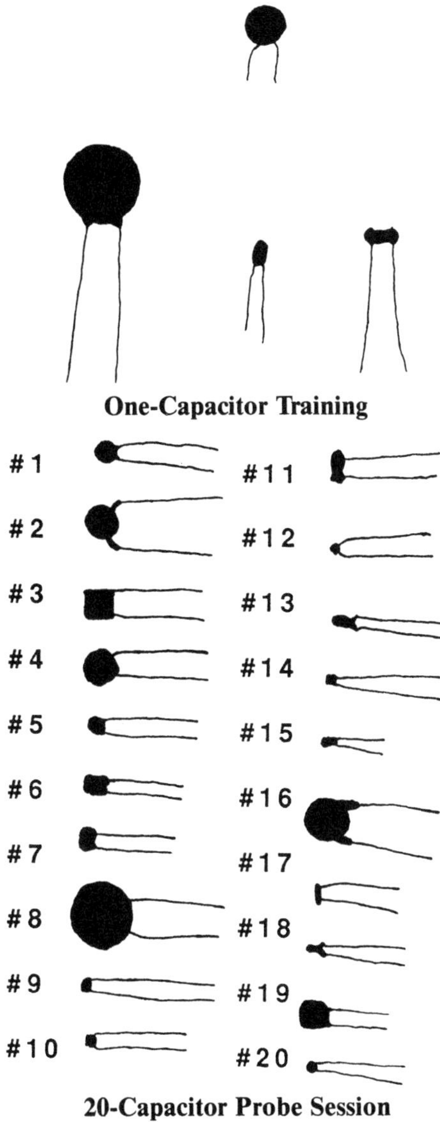

Figure 11-1 Diagram of Single, General Case, and Untrained Probe Capacitors. *Source:* From "Comparison of Single Instance and General Case Instruction in Teaching a Generalized Vocational Skill" by R.H. Horner and R.S. McDonald, 1982, *The Journal of the Association for Persons with Severe Handicaps, 7*(3), pp. 7–20. Copyright 1982 by the Association for Persons with Severe Handicaps. Reprinted by permission.

Exhibit 11-2 Diagram of the Sorting Board

	0	1	2	3	4	5	6	7	8	9
0										
1		Vernon			Vernon			Vernon		
2			Gail			Gail			Gail	
3				Mike			Mike			Mike
4		Vernon			Vernon			Vernon		
5			Gail			Gail			Gail	
6				Mike			Mike			Mike
7		Vernon			Vernon			Vernon		
8			Gail			Gail			Gail	
9				Mike			Mike			Mike

Note: The first digits on the cue cards are at the top, and the second digits on the cue cards are on the left side. Instructional prefixes are delineated by the subjects' names, which were not included on the actual sorting board.

Source: From "Use of General Case Instruction with Visually Impaired, Multiply Handicapped Adults in the Sorting of National Zip Codes" by W.W. Woolcock and M.B. Lengel, 1987, *Journal of Visual Impairment & Blindness, 81*(3), pp. 110-114. Copyright 1987 by American Foundation for the Blind, 15 West 16th Street, New York, NY 10011. Reprinted by permission.

Participants were required to sort cards by matching the first zip code digit with the correct number at the top of the appropriate vertical column and go down that column to match the second digit with the appropriate number at the left side of the horizontal row. Weekly untrained probes of all 100 variations (00 through 99) were conducted using 500 addressed cards (five for each prefix), which each participant was to sort within 1 hour.

Results indicated that two of the participants, Mike and Gail, demonstrated improved performance on 1-hour probes during the general case instruction phase. Although they failed to completely sort all 500 cards during that time, 80 to 95 percent of the cards placed during their last probe session were placed correctly. Thus, a combination of criterion performance on the general case examples and improved performance on the probe examples permitted the instructors to terminate general case instruction. The performance of Mike and Gail on subsequent 2.25-hour untrained maintenance probes indicated that each participant could successfully sort 80 to 100 percent of the probe cards. Two months later, Gail and Mike worked on national mailing contracts. Each was assigned to sort the 2-inch by 3-inch labels for the 217 labels (Contract 1) and 66 labels (Contract 2) using the sorting board. Both subjects demonstrated continued generalized performance on these mailings ranging from 83 percent to 96 percent accuracy (see Figure 11-2, Multiple Baseline Across Subjects Design).

These studies demonstrate the effectiveness and efficiency of general case instruction in producing work skill performance across "diverse stimulus conditions, responses, and time without comprehensive programming" (Stokes & Osnes, 1988, p. 6). Indeed, instruction on all the examples in either study would have been exhausting. However, these studies provide demonstrations of general case instruction in controlled environments (classroom and work activities center) using tasks that incorporated a single response (cut/crimp) or a short sequence of responses (discrimination by first and second digits). At issue is the utility of using general case instruction on more complex competitive job task sequences in simulation environments and actual community work environments.

GENERAL CASE INSTRUCTION ON COMPETITIVE EMPLOYMENT SKILLS

In supported employment, or competitive job-skill training, workers are often presented with job tasks that require similar yet different responses for a number of different examples. Floor mopping, dish washing, window washing, dusting, damp wiping, vacuuming, lawn mowing, and innumerable other tasks require that workers appropriately respond to learned or novel task variations. Even computer operation requires general case learn-

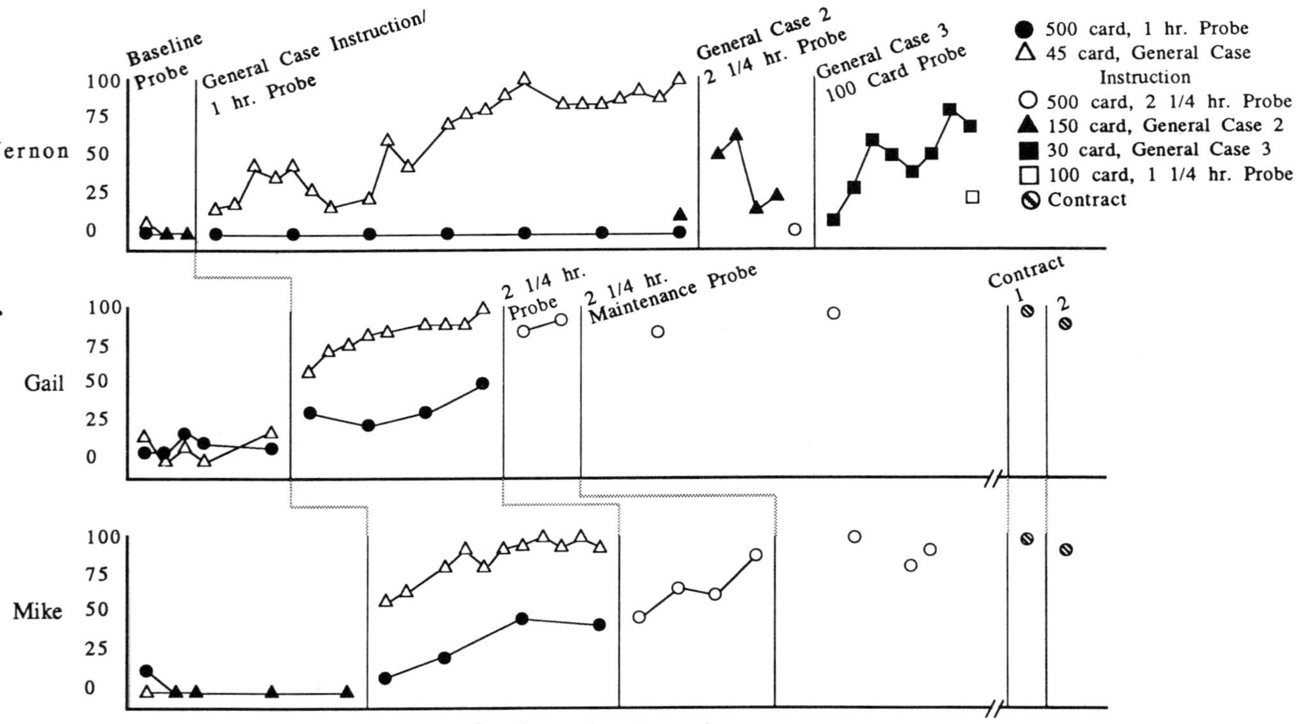

Figure 11-2 Multiple Baseline across Subjects Design. Percentage of Accuracy in Sorting by the First Two Digits (Prefix) of National Zip Codes. *Source:* From "Use of General Case Instruction with Visually Impaired, Multiply Handicapped Adults in the Sorting of National Zip Codes" by W.W. Woolcock and M.B. Lengel, 1987, *Journal of Visual Impairment & Blindness, 81*(3), pp. 110–114. Copyright 1987 by American Foundation for the Blind, 15 West 16th Street, New York, NY 10011. Reprinted by permission.

ing to interact with variations in word processing programs, spreadsheets, data bases, graphics programs, and so on. Thus, the challenge is to deliver instruction that reliably and efficiently results in work skills "that endure over time, are performed under the full range of appropriate stimulus conditions and are not performed under inappropriate stimulus conditions" (Horner, Bellamy, & Colvin, 1983, p. 4).

The following sections will examine the influence of setting on general case instruction, specifically:

- whether a general case response can be taught in an environment other than a targeted work environment (simulation instruction)
- the relative effectiveness of simulation instruction versus instruction in the natural environment (in vivo instruction)
- a strategy for combining simulation and in vivo instruction.

This information may present curricular implications for job training programs inside and outside of a rehabilitation center. Combining general case instruction with on-the-job instruction or probes in a job-skills training program may allow learners to begin full-time on-the-job training with an increased level of relevant job skills resulting from previous and/or concurrent instruction that focused on the range of task variation they will face on job entry.

SIMULATION INSTRUCTION

"Simulation is a training format in which the stimuli used during instruction are different from, yet similar to, the stimuli available in the target performance environment" (McDonald, Horner, & Williams, 1984, p. 123). Simulation is "designed to approximate the natural environmental context but does not involve the conditions under which the behavior ultimately is to be performed" (Nietupski, Hamre-Nietupski, Clancy, & Veerhusen, 1986, p. 12). Simulation instruction may therefore be viewed as a maximally representative "concurrently provided adjunct" (Nietupski et al., 1986, p. 14) to community training, providing for initial skill development and repeated practice of community skills in a simulated setting.

Even though simulation instruction may reduce an individual's involvement in community environments and may not result in generalized skill acquisition, it may be useful in situations in which instruction in the natural environment may be dangerous or require inordinate expenditures of staff time, travel mileage, or financial costs. Instructional efficiency may be increased in cases where natural trials are infrequent or relevant stimuli cannot be controlled systematically in the natural environment (Horner, McDonnell, Williams, & Vogelsberg, 1983; Horner, McDonnell, & Bellamy,

1984). Additionally, simulation instruction provides opportunities to use group instruction on skills usually performed individually in the natural environment (Page, Iwata, & Neef, 1976).

Although instruction and untrained probe sessions were conducted in community environments (three university cafeterias), Horner, Eberhard, and Sheehan (1986) simulated cafeteria conditions when teaching and probing the instructional universe of table bussing skills with four high school students with moderate to severe mental retardation. The students were taught which tables to bus and which not to bus (negative teaching examples) in instructional sessions in which six general case training tables were set up with various combinations of strategically placed people (university graduate students), possessions, food, dishes, and garbage (see Table 11-2). When each participant attained criterion on the training examples, they were provided with untrained probes (in a different cafeteria) on variations of tables that presented "to-be-bussed" or "not-to-be-bussed" decisions. In each untrained probe session, 15 tables were set up with various combinations of people (university graduate students), possessions, food, dishes, and garbage (Table 11-2). These untrained probes following general case instruction indicated that each participant could correctly bus (or not bus) from 60 to 100 percent of the probe tables.

Woolcock, Lyon, & Woolcock (1987) used a simulation environment to teach general case examples for a damp wiping (housekeeping) task sequence and a floor mopping (janitorial) task sequence to four participants with moderate to severe mental retardation. Simulation instruction was conducted in the basement of a church that housed a work activities center the participants attended. During simulation instruction sessions, each participant was provided with group instruction (two groups of two participants) on two trials for each of two examples for both the janitorial task sequence and housekeeping task sequence.

Participants then were provided with weekly untrained probe sessions for both task sequences during which they were to damp wipe and floor mop six actual response examples located in patient rooms (housekeeping) and first floor rooms and halls (janitorial) at a community convalescent hospital. Table 11-3 lists the simulation response examples and actual response examples used in teaching and conducting untrained probes of both task sequences. The weekly probes indicated generalized performance of the task sequences and served as a criterion measure for the termination of simulation instruction and weekly probes. Each student then participated in four consecutive follow-up probe sessions to assess maintenance of generalized task sequence performance. After that, they received instruction on all six actual response examples at the hospital (actual job instruction) to correct errors in generalization and increase fluency of task sequence performance. For two of the participants, criterion performance of 100 percent accuracy on each example during actual job instruction led to an instructor withdrawal phase in which the instructor's presence was systematically faded and the participants performed the task sequences independently (they were offered jobs at the hospital).

For three participants on both task sequences, and the fourth participant on the housekeeping task sequence, untrained probe performance improved over multiple weekly probe sessions and corresponded, at a lower rate, to improvements during general case simulation instruction. The criterion of 70 percent accuracy in weekly probe sessions proved to be a functional means of determining when to end general case simulation instruction, particularly when combined with a criterion of 90 percent performance on the simulation response examples. The weekly probes also helped participants make the crucial connection between the instructional and probe examples and interact with an integrated work environment before ending general case simulation instruction. As a result of this simulation instruction/weekly probe sequencing, participants entered 5 day per week actual job instruction with the ability to perform 70 percent or more of the generic responses required in the task sequences.

SIMULATION AND IN VIVO INSTRUCTION

In comparing the relative effectiveness and efficiency of simulation versus natural instruction, Domaracki (1988) taught four young adults with severe to moderate mental retardation to perform the general case of tasks required of floor housemen and lobby attendants at a large metropolitan hotel. Participants received simulation instruction in a special education center and natural instruction in the hotel lobby and individual floors. Periodic untrained probe sessions were provided in the hotel to assess

1. generalized performance resulting from simulation instruction
2. untrained performance of the job tasks during the natural instruction phase
3. whether participants had achieved a criterion of 70 percent independent performance on the probe measures

A large university classroom/office building and a human service agency lobby area also were used during untrained generalization probes of novel settings.

Data indicated that instruction in the natural setting resulted in faster acquisition of both task sequences and more cost efficiency than did simulation instruction. However, generalization probes conducted in the novel settings during all phases of the study revealed that, although generalization did improve over time and probe sessions, levels of generalization did not correspond with acquisition data. Of particular interest in this study was the introduction of a rule that if a participant performed at or below

Table 11-2 Training Examples and Probe Items for Table Bussing

Training Examples

Training Examples	*Presence of People and Possessions*	*People Eating or Not Eating*	*Dishes: Empty/Part/ New Food*	*Garbage: Present or Not Present*	*Location of Garbage and Dishes*	*Correct Response*
1	0 People + Poss.	N/A	Partial	Present	Table Chairs	Don't Bus
2	0 People	N/A	Partial	Present	Table Floor Chair	Bus
3	2 People	Eating	New Food	Present	Table Chair Floor	Don't Bus
4	0 People	N/A	Empty	Present	Table Floor	Bus
5	1 Person	Not Eating	Empty	Present	Chair Floor	Bus
6	2 People	Not Eating	Empty	Present	Table	Bus

Probe Items for Table Bussing

Probe Table Number	*Probe Setting*	*Presence of People and Possessions*	*People Eating or Not Eating*	*Dishes: Empty/Part/ New Food*	*Garbage: Present or Not Present*	*Location of Garbage and Dishes*	*Correct Response*
1	A	0 People	N/A	Dishes Empty	Present	Table Chair Floor	Bus
2	A	0 People	N/A	New Food	Not Present	N/A	Don't Bus

3	A	1 Person	Not Eating	Dishes Empty	Present	Table	Bus
4	A	3 People	Eating	Partial	Present	Table	Don't Bus
5	A	1 Person	Not Eating	New Food	Not Present	N/A	Don't Bus
6	A	0 People	N/A	Dishes Empty	Present	Chair	Bus
7	A	0 People	N/A	Partial	Present	Floor Table	Bus
8	B	0 People + Poss.	N/A	New Food	Present	Table Floor	Don't Bus
9	B	0 People	N/A	Empty	Present	Chairs Table	Bus
10	B	2 People	Not Eating	Empty	Present	Table Floor	Bus
11	B	1 Person	Eating	Partial	Not Present	Table	Don't Bus
12	B	3 People	Not Eating	Empty	Not Present	Table	Bus
13	B	0 People	N/A	Partial	Present	Table Chairs	Bus
14	B	0 People	N/A	Empty	Present	Table Floor	Bus
15	B	0 People	N/A	Partial	Present	Table Floors Chairs	Bus

Source: From "Teaching Generalized Table Bussing: The Importance of Negative Teaching Examples" by R. H. Horner, J. M. Eberhard, and M. R. Sheehan, 1986, *Behavior Modification, 10*(4), pp. 451-471. Copyright 1986 by Sage Publications, Inc. Reprinted by permission.

Table 11-3 Simulation and Actual Response Examples Used in General Case Instruction and Untrained Probes on the Damp Wiping (Housekeeping) and Floor Mopping (Janitorial) Task Sequences

Simulation Response Examples	*Actual Response Examples*
Response Examples	
Housekeeping Task Sequence	
2 Wheelchairs	1 Wheelchair
2 Sinks and Lavatories	1 Sink and Lavatory
	1 Counter, Shelves, Cabinet
	1 Patient Bed
	1 Chair, Stand, Tray Table
	1 Drinking Fountain
Janitorial Task Sequence	
Simulation Response Examples	*Actual Response Examples*
2 Small roms—Move Furniture	1 Small Room—Move Furniture
2 Large Rooms—Move Furniture	1 Large Room—Move Furniture
	1 Midsize Room—Move Furniture
	1 Midsize Room—Don't Move Furniture
	1 Small Room—Don't Move Furniture
	1 Large Area—No Furniture (Hallway)

Source: From "General Case Simulation Instruction and the Establishment and Maintenance of Work Performance" by W.W. Woolcock, S. Lyon, and K.P. Woolcock, 1987, *Research in Developmental Disabilities, 8*(3), pp. 427–447. Copyright 1987 by Pergamon Press Inc. Reprinted by permission.

the same level of independent performance on two consecutive untrained probes during the simulation instruction phase, simulation instruction was terminated and natural instruction introduced to remediate errors in generalization to the hotel setting.

COMBINED GENERAL CASE SIMULATION INSTRUCTION AND IN VIVO INSTRUCTION

By combining general case instruction provided in a high school cafeteria with twice weekly instruction in a local fast-food restaurant, Woolcock (1989) taught a general case of fast-food restaurant lobby cleaning skills to four high school students with severe to moderate mental retardation. Based on an analysis of the task variations present in four local fast-food restaurants (Table 11-1), each participant received daily inschool instruction that included the representative four variations for cleaning tables (Exhibit 11-1, Tasks 3 through 6). Each participant also received instruction twice a week in one of four assigned restaurants.

A decision rule required termination of combined instruction when participants achieved 90 percent independent task completion in both instructional settings (with the exception of participant Brenda, see Figure 11-3). Each participant then received consecutive untrained probes in all four fast-food restaurants and subsequently received instruction only in their assigned restaurants. Results indicated that each participant improved in independent task completion in both instructional settings during the combined instruction phase. During subsequent untrained probes in all restaurants, participants performed at higher levels of independent task completion in novel restaurants than during probes at their assigned restaurants.

This combined instructional strategy permitted the participants to learn representative task variations for the four restaurants (in the high school cafeteria) while receiving instruction in an integrated community vocational environment twice a week. This combination led to high levels of generalized task performance during the restaurant probe phase. Participants also improved in independent task completion upon entry into daily instruction at their assigned restaurants during the community instruction phase.

SUMMARY

These studies document the effectiveness of using general case instruction in simulation and community vocational settings. Whether general case instruction is most effective in producing generalized performance when examples are taught in a simulation environment or an in vivo setting appears to depend on the degree to which general case instruction examples represent the range of variation present in the generalization examples and the functioning level of individual learners (Bates & Cuvo, 1985; Domaracki, 1988). Another important variable may be the relationship of untrained probe sessions or in vivo instruction sessions to general case instruction sessions. With the exception of the study by Horner, Eberhard, and Sheehan (1986), it is apparent that concurrent untrained probe and in vivo instruction sessions perform key functions in

- assessing the ongoing effects of general case instruction on performance of generalization examples
- allowing learners to participate in integrated vocational environments
- permitting the use of combined criteria from both instruction and untrained probe conditions
- allowing learners to make the crucial connections between instructional expectations and the stimulus/response expectations present in targeted vocational environments

Future research in general case instruction may extend general case technology to an array of different job tasks and environments, and may explore the use of general case instruction with learners who experience

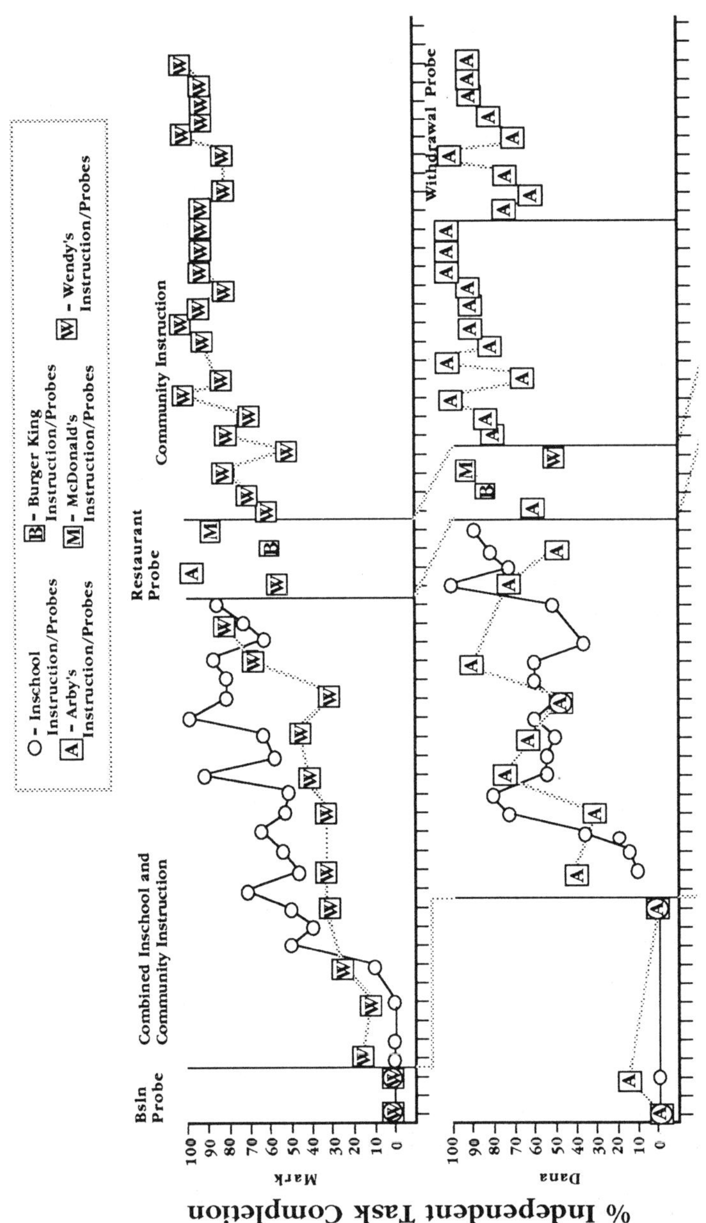
○ - Inschool Instruction/Probes
A - Arby's Instruction/Probes
B - Burger King Instruction/Probes
M - McDonald's Instruction/Probes
W - Wendy's Instruction/Probes
Bsln Probe
Combined Inschool and Community Instruction
Restaurant Probe
Community Instruction
Withdrawal Probe
% Independent Task Completion
Mark
Dana
100
90
80
70
60
50
40
30
20
10
0

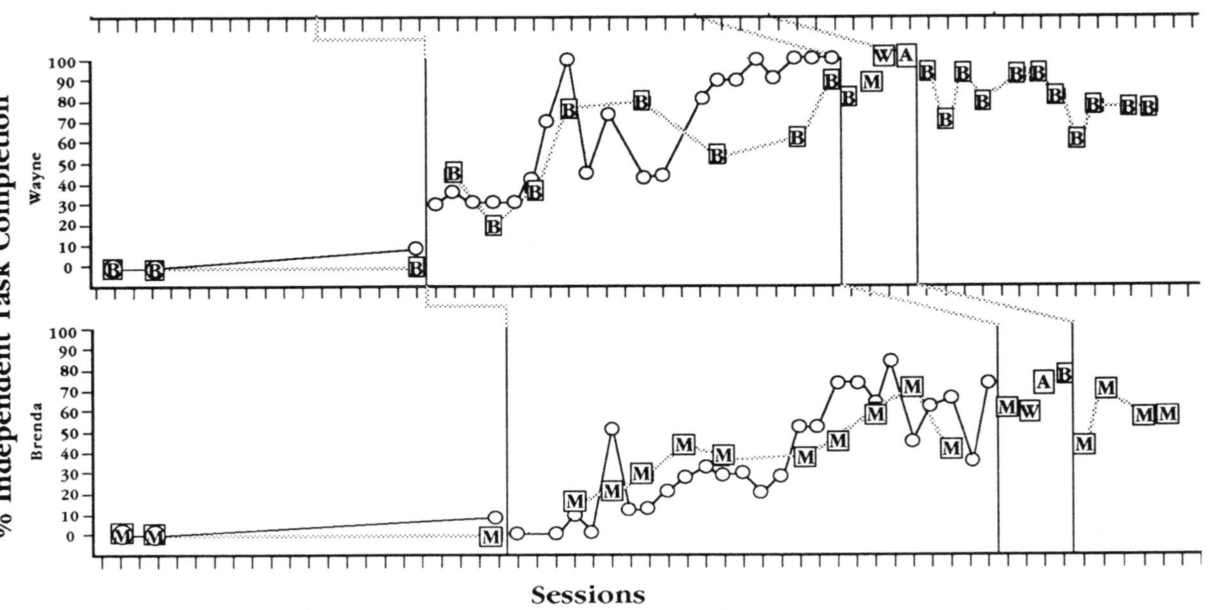

Figure 11-3 Multiple Baseline across Subjects/Settings Experimental Design. Percent Independent Task Completion, Fast-Food Restaurant Lobby Cleaning—High School Cafeteria and Community Fast-Food Restaurants. *Source:* From *Generalized Curriculum Instruction: Inschool Instruction on Validated Work Skills* by W.W. Woolcock, 1989, unpublished study, University of Arkansas at Little Rock.

different disabilities. General case instruction may also be incorporated into competitive employment placement and training programs in instances where the learning of an array of similar yet different job tasks is required. However, given the apparent relationship between general case instruction and untrained probes or in vivo instruction, practitioners are cautioned that conducting training and untrained probe assessment solely within the confines of a job training center or simulation environment may not result in generalized performance of the learned tasks in targeted community environments and may also hinder the learner's access to competitive employment. Therefore, the following recommendations for conducting general case instruction in competitive employment programs are provided:

- delineate the range of task variation and select a minimum number of general case instruction examples that most adequately sample this range in analyzing an instructional universe for particular job tasks
- provide general case instruction in community environments unless the range of task variation cannot be sampled or sufficiently varied without the use of simulation instruction
- provide multiple distributed trials on all of the general case instruction examples during each instructional session
- provide concurrent community instruction on one or more of the general case instruction examples during a general case simulation instruction phase; use data from learner performance during community instruction as a component of the criteria for terminating general case simulation instruction
- provide concurrent untrained probes of all designated generalization examples during a general case instruction phase; use data from untrained probes to assess ongoing generalization and determine criteria for terminating general case instruction
- use untrained probe performance to determine failure to generalize and, in such instances, change to instruction on the generalization examples
- follow-up general case instruction with instruction on all of the generalization examples to ensure fluent performance of all examples and establish a basis for instructor withdrawal from the job training site

General case instruction strategies must, therefore, target specific competitive job skills and environments as opposed to "global approaches, common in some training programs, which teach the general skills deemed necessary without regard for the individual characteristics of specific community environments" (Woolcock, Lyon, & Woolcock, 1987, p. 446).

Ongoing analysis of performance on generalization examples cannot be overemphasized as a means to verify general case instruction procedures and content. This concern is of particular importance when simulation instruction may hinder access to community work settings rather than assist in integrating persons with handicaps into competitive employment.

REFERENCES

Bates, P., & Cuvo, A.J. (1985). *Simulated and naturalistic instruction of community functioning skills with mentally retarded learners: The search for best practice*. Unpublished Manuscript, Southern Illinois University: Carbondale.

Becker, W.C., & Engelmann, S. (1978). Systems for basic instruction: Theory and practice. In A.C. Catania and T.A. Brigham (Eds.), *Handbook of applied behavior analysis: Social and instructional processes* (pp. 325–377), New York: Irvington.

Domaracki, J.W. (1988). *General case simulation instruction and naturalistic instruction: A descriptive and comparative analysis*. Unpublished doctoral dissertation, University of Pittsburgh: Pittsburgh, PA.

Giangreco, M.F. (1983). Teaching basic photography skills to a severely handicapped young adult using simulated materials. *The Journal of the Association for the Severely Handicapped*, *8*(1), 43–49.

Gifford, J., Rusch, F., Martin, J., & White, D. (1984). Autonomy and adaptability: A proposed technology for maintaining work behavior. In N. Ellis & N. Bray (Eds.), *International review of research on mental retardation* (Vol. 12, pp. 285–314). New York: Academic Press.

Holvoet, J., Guess, D., Mulligan, M., & Brown, F. (1980). The individualized curriculum sequencing model (II): A teaching strategy for severely handicapped students. *The Journal of the Association for the Severely Handicapped*, *5*(4), 325–336.

Horner, R.H., Bellamy, G.T., & Colvin, G.T. (1983). *Responding in the presence of non-trained stimuli: Implications of generalization error patterns*. Unpublished Manuscript, University of Oregon: Eugene, OR.

Horner, R. H., Eberhard, J.M., & Sheehan, M.R. (1986). Teaching generalized table bussing: The importance of negative teaching examples. *Behavior Modification*, *10*(4), 457–471.

Horner, R.H., & McDonald, R.S. (1982). Comparison of single instance and general case instruction in teaching a generalized vocational skill. *The Journal of the Association for the Severely Handicapped*, *7*(3), 7–20.

Horner, R.H., McDonnell, J.J., & Bellamy, G.T. (1984). *Teaching generalized skills: General case instruction in simulation and community settings*. Unpublished manuscript, University of Oregon: Eugene, OR.

Horner, R.H., McDonnell, J., Williams, J., & Vogelsberg T. (1983, November). *Simulation training: Strategies for conducting in-class training that results in adaptive performance in the community*. Paper presented at the Tenth Annual Conference of the Association for the Severely Handicapped, San Francisco.

Horner, R.H., Sprague, J., Wilcox, B. (1982). General case programming for community activities. In B. Wilcox & G.T. Bellamy (Eds.), *Design of high school programs for severely handicapped students*, (pp. 61–98). Baltimore: Paul H. Brookes.

Hull, C.L. (1943). *Principles of behavior*. New York: Appleton-Century-Crofts.

McDonnell, J.J., Horner, R.H., & Williams, J.A. (1984). Comparison of three strategies for teaching generalized grocery purchasing to high school students with severe handicaps. *The Journal of the Association for Persons with Severe Handicaps*, *9*(2), 123–133.

Mulligan, M., Lacy, L., & Guess, D. (1982). Effects of massed, distributed, and spaced trial sequencing on severely handicapped students' performance. *The Journal of the Association for the Severely Handicapped*, *7*(2), 48–61.

Nietupski, J., Hamre-Nietupski, S., Clancy, P., & Veerhusen, K. (1986). Guidelines for making simulation an effective adjunct to in vivo community instruction. *The Journal of the Association for Persons with Severe Handicaps*, *11*(1), 12–18.

Page, T.J., Iwata, B.A., & Neef, N.A. (1976). Teaching pedestrian skills to retarded persons: Generalization from the classroom to the natural environment. *Journal of Applied Behavior Analysis*, *9*(4), 433–444.

Skinner, B.F. (1953). *Science and human behavior*. New York: Macmillan.

Snell, M.E. (1983). Implementing the IEP: Intervention strategies. In M.E. Snell (Ed.), *Systematic instruction of the moderately and severely handicapped, 2nd Edition* (pp. 113–145), Columbus, OH: Merrill.

Stokes, T.F., & Baer, D.M. (1977). An implicit technology of generalization. *Journal of Applied Behavior Analysis*, *10*, 349–367.

Stokes, T.F., & Osnes, P.G. (1988). The developing applied technology of generalization and maintenance. In R.H. Horner, G. Dunlap, and R.L. Koegel (Eds.), *Generalization and maintenance: Life-style changes in applied settings* (pp. 5–19), Baltimore: Paul H. Brookes.

Woolcock, W.W. (1989). Generalization curriculum instruction: Inschool instruction on validated work skills. *Unpublished study*, University of Arkansas at Little Rock: Little Rock, AR.

Woolcock, W.W., & Lengel, M.B. (1987). Use of general case instruction with visually impaired, multiply handicapped adults in the sorting of national zip codes. *Journal of Visual Impairment and Blindness*, *81*(3), 110–114.

Woolcock, W.W., Lyon, S., & Woolcock, K.P. (1987). General case simulation instruction and the establishment and maintenance of work performance. *Research in Developmental Disabilities*, *8*(3), 427–447.

Chapter 12

Turning Myths into Reality: Job Coaching

Mary C. Stapleton and Patricia L. Bennett

There have been many theories and models proposed for successfully returning traumatically brain injured persons to work. This chapter will focus on job coaching brain injured persons and how the concept used in many work reentry programs does not always result in success. This is largely due to the fact that little is known about which variables distinguish between those who will and will not return to work.

The clinical experience gained from the use of the job coaching model at the Maryland Rehabilitation Center will assist head trauma professionals in clarifying in their own minds which assumptions are true and which are myths.

Job coaching is intensive and highly individualized job-site intervention and client advocacy directed toward successful placement in a competitive workplace. It does not imply continuing lifetime support and, in the context of this chapter, does not refer to the classic supported employment model described earlier in this book.

Job coaches attempt to deal with the array of complex reentry challenges that face persons with brain injury. These can include the individual's reduced physical coordination and slowness of motor functions; difficulties in attention, concentration, and memory, which limit speed of information processing; psychiatric problems such as depression and explosive behavior; and impaired interpersonal skills, including problems with receiving information and working harmoniously with coworkers and supervisors.

Job coaching teaches traumatic brain injured persons an actual job to be performed on the work site. The concept involves attempting to obviate the need for transfer of learning from therapy or classroom. The concept of domain-specific learning is applied on a job site with the individual having little need to transfer skills from a formal training area to a job site. However, even given this model there are difficulties in applying the job coaching concept to the traumatically brain injured.

A survey on job coaching (Parenté & Stapleton, 1988; Stapleton, Parenté, & Bennett, 1989) assessed the difficulties job coaches encounter in assisting clients on the job. These coaches had worked on a one-to-one basis with eight traumatic brain injured clients, for time periods ranging from 2 weeks to 3 months, at jobs including warehouse work, landscaping, and clerical receptionist work. The results indicated that job coaching did not solve the individual problems returning to work, but did minimize them. The major client problems encountered by the job coaches were inflexibility of thought, poor judgment, reduced memory, slow acquisition of job skills, and anxiety.

Because of the unique and varied pattern of a brain injured individual's deficits, job coaching models that work with groups of clients on a job site may not meet the needs of a brain injured person, whose problems tend to be more different than the same. More than any other disability group, traumatically brain injured persons appear to have a need for an individualized program and a job coach with a thorough understanding of the individual's own style of learning on the job site. Critical differences in learning, environment, and spared cognitive systems must be taken into account and merged with each person's cognitive style.

THE PATHWAYS VOCATIONAL REENTRY MODEL

The Pathways model was developed in part by a federally funded grant project supported by the U.S. Office of Special Education and Rehabilitation Services. The underlying assumptions of the model are that effective services for successful return to employment of traumatic brain injured persons must be comprehensive, individualized, and use a case management system and integrated multidisciplinary approach. The Pathways model includes readiness activities, a modified place-train model, and a constellation of services that could be fitted to design a mosaic appropriate to each individual.

Assessment services include clinical interviews with the client and family or significant other, neuropsychological testing, and a learning style assessment.

Therapeutic services in the model include the option for intensive assessment or individual treatment in occupational therapy, physical therapy, or speech and language therapy. The project focuses interventions primarily on group modalities for addressing memory and psychosocial needs, and clients participate in a memory group and a psychosocial group. Although the focus of this chapter is the job coaching component of the model, our preliminary findings suggest that participation in a group, which provides peer support as well as an environment to work through adjustment to disability issues, may be equally as important for affecting vocational outcome.

Pathways vocational services include vocational evaluations oriented to work sampling and simulated job tasks and environments; vocational skills training in a self-paced, competency-based model for clients who need to refresh technical skills or redirect their careers to related job skills; and a full range of rehabilitation engineering services to identify options for the client or to consult on the job site.

Supportive services of this model include a specialized predriving assessment, driver's education for improved mobility, leisure activities, and therapeutic recreation. All of these assist with reintegration into the community as well as cognitive, social, and physical goals. A family support group assists the families and significant others in supporting the client's progress and in adjusting themselves to the changed family system.

Job coaching, placement, and follow-along services are provided by a staff of two job coaches who

- screen clients for motivation, mobility and financial disincentive issues, salary requirements, and vocational interests
- do job development and job analysis to match each client to a specific job
- provide travel training, if necessary, to get the client to the job site
- develop the job-site training by applying compensatory strategies developed by other specialists on the interdisciplinary team in conjunction with the client
- intervene at the job site to include behavior management, job-site modification, or personal and work adjustment
- act as the client advocate to educate the peers and supervisor

All job coaching placements are individualized and one on one because enclaves and mobile work crews were not appropriate for this population.

An Overview of the Model

A major principle underlying the supported employment model is provision of services at the job site where the person is employed. A staff professional who provides such support is often called a job coach (Wehman, Kreutzer, et al., 1988).

The Pathways job coaching approach is similar yet different from supported employment. Like supported employment, clients are partners in the service and do not need to be "job ready" to be placed. Both models include ongoing assessment and performance monitoring as well as follow-along and job retention assistance. Key activities of the job coach include job matching, job analysis, travel training, job-site training, advocacy, and assistance with non-work-related issues, such as benefits and housing. Both Pathways and supported employment provide competitive wages in real work, integrated settings.

There are, however, important differences in the Pathways and supported employment models. Pathways is job coaching, not supported employment. The service is time limited not a lifetime support system. The focus is full-time rather than part-time employment. All placements are individual rather than enclaves and work crews. As a result of the wide diversity and level of preinjury employment of traumatic brain injured clients, the Pathways program does not guarantee the employer that a job coach will do the job if the client cannot. For example, a job coach could never master the complexities of Blue Cross/Blue Shield claims processing that one of our clients had learned in years of previous employment. Instead of doing the job for the client, the focus was on facilitating the client's application or new strategies and helping the manager and coworkers learn how to reintegrate a former employee.

The approach is interdisciplinary and may include consultations for work site issues from as many as five professionals during the job coaching intervention. Another key characteristic of the Pathways model is the introduction to and practice of compensatory strategies in simulated environments before placement at the work site—a modified place-train model.

Job Coach Intake Interview

The prospective job coaching client's first contact with the coach includes an intake interview (see Exhibit 12-1) to assess the degree of realistic understanding of work and what it entails. The coach and client discuss issues of vocational choice, assessment of work skills, and parameters of availability for employment.

Willingness to relocate is a critical issue which we have learned may have a significant impact upon outcome. Often, a prospective client will answer with an enthusiastic, "yes" to the question, "Are you willing to relocate to become employed?" If an individual lives in an area of high unemployment or a rural part of the state, he or she sees this as a necessity. However, this is not always an easy or realistic task. The person may lack the survival skills to function in a new community; the probability of beginning at entry level at minimum wage may make relocation financially impossible.

We have found two questions to be a good barometer of client self-insight: (1) What importance (besides money) does being employed have for you? and (2) What task can you do as well now as before your injury?

Exhibit 12-1 Sample Job Coach Intake Interview

Job Coach Intake Interview

Date of Screening: ________________ SSN: ________________________

Name: ________________________ Date of Birth: ________________

Interviewers: ____

1. What kind of employment are you interested in? ________________
   Premorbid work history? ________________________________
   What skills do you have to help you do this job? ________________
   ____
   Are you willing to relocate to become employed? ________________
2. When are you available to work? ________________________
   How many hours per week? ________________________
3. If you were an employer, what characteristics would you be looking for in an employee? ________________________________
4. What importance (besides money) does being employed have for you? ________
5. What task can you do as well now as before your injury? ________________
6. What tasks do you have more trouble with now than before your injury? ________
7. What motivation do you have for becoming employed? ________________
8. What does working with a job coach mean to you? ________________
   ____
9. How would you feel with the job coach always being present with you on the job?
   ____
10. Suppose you have now been on the job for 2 months and are getting frustrated with the presence of your job coach. How would you handle this situation? ______
    ____
11. How would you define commitment? Give some examples of your experience with commitment. ________________________________
    ____
12. How do you spend your spare time? ________________________
    ____
13. Who gets you up in the morning? Who is responsible for getting you to work on time? ________________________________
14. What are your strong points? ________________________
    ____
15. If you have been employed, what did you like and dislike about each job you had? ________________________________
    ____
16. What would you like to be doing in 5 years? What kind of job would you like to have in 5 years? ________________________
    ____

The expected response might include some positive and negative descriptions. However, all too frequently, traumatic brain injured persons see no change in their pattern of functioning or may believe they can be better than before the trauma.

The Pathways intake process also includes a family interview (Exhibit 12-2) with a social worker who poses these same questions to someone who

Exhibit 12-2 Sample Family Pre-Admission Interview

Family Pre-Admission Interview

Name ______________________________ Date of
Last First Middle Interview ____________

Address ______________________________ Home Phone ____________
Street

______________________________ ____________
City State Zip Code

Date of Birth ____________ Sex ________ Marital Status ____________

Date of Injury ____________ Social Security # ____________

Education

Highest level of education completed ________ GED? ________ College? ________

Did client receive special help in school (special ed., tutoring, etc.) prior to injury? ___
Explain ______________________________

____

Other training ______________________________

Family Information and History

Please list family members and/or significant others, including parents, step-parents, spouse, siblings, children, and other dependents, and supply information requested. (If deceased, place (*) beside individual's name.)

Name	Age	Relationship	Marital Status	Education	Occupation

Person to contact in case of emergency ______________________________

____

Family Questionnaire

Explain any lawsuit pending as a result of the accident.

____

____

1. How does client get along with other members of the family?

____

____

2. How would you describe client's personality before the injury?

____

____

3. What changes in personality or character have you noticed since the injury?

____

____

4. Is client realistic about the future? ______________________________
5. Is client aware of his/her deficits? ______________________________

____

6. Is client generally oriented to date, time, place, etc.? (e.g., tell time; use a schedule)

____

____

Exhibit 12-2 continued

History of Injury and Rehabilitation

Length of Coma ______________ Length of Post-Traumatic Amnesia ______________

Diagnosis ____

____

Type of Accident ____

____

Type of Treatment Currently Receiving	Frequency	Location	By Whom
Medical			
Orthopedist			
Occupational Therapy			
Physical Therapy			
Speech Therapy			
Psychological			
Neuropsychological			
Vocational			
Recreational			

What Medication Is Currently Used To Control Seizures?

____

Who prescribed and monitors them? ____________________________________

How often are medication levels checked? ______________________________

Date of last medication checkup: _____________________________________

Check areas of difficulty experienced by client as a result of the injury: None (N); Little difficulty (L); Great difficulty (G).

______ Concentration

______ Complex Problem Solving

Memory:

______ Long Term

______ Short Term

______ Sensory Loss

______ Self-Initiating

______ Motivation

______ Reading or Writing

______ Flexibility

______ Tires Easily

______ Control of Emotions

______ Visual Perception

______ Receptive Language

______ Expressive Language

______ Depression

______ Remembering When To Take Medication

continues

Exhibit 12-2 continued

Can candidate reliably engage in two-way communication? ______________________

____

How many hours can client work before becoming tired? ______________________

____

Has client ever been convicted of a crime? If yes, list and explain. ______________

____

Independent Living Criteria

With whom did candidate live prior to injury? ______________________________

____

With whom is candidate living currently? __________________________________

____

Is candidate his/her own legal guardian? __________ If no, then who? __________

____

What were the client's goals and future plans prior to injury?

____

____

Does client exhibit acceptable behavior in public? ___________________________

____

____

Work history:

What is a normal day?

knows the prospective client well, both preinjury and postinjury. It is critical to compare observations from these interviews to assess the level of realistic understanding the prospective client has of his or her own ability levels. Discrepancies between objective and subjective accounts are a strong factor in choice of candidates for coaching. Unrealistic expectations of job choice, salary level, and skills have proven to be a barrier to successful placement.

The intake interview includes discussion of the role of the job coach and the feelings and concerns a traumatic brain injured person may have about this approach. The individual may express concern about being perceived as intellectually impaired by a prospective employer because a coach is needed. Clients have fears of being monitored or watched by someone always looking over their shoulders. These issues need to be discussed and fears alleviated as soon as possible in the plan of services. Obviously, the individual situation must be closely evaluated to assess what will and will not work on a given work site. This is one of the major challenges for a job coach in an individualized model.

Although disorders secondary to frontal lobe damage play a role in initiation, motivation, and tenacity, nevertheless it is important to confront the prospective clients with their motivational responsibility. The client must see the coaching experience as a dynamic partnership between two individuals who are equally committed to achieving a mutual goal—returning the client to work.

Job Coach Contract

The need for a written agreement between coach and client appeared quite early in our experience with traumatic brain injured persons (Exhibit 12-3). Among the reasons for a contract were to

- serve as a memory cue
- provide realistic time limits for completion of the service
- reinforce the commitment made by the client to remain long enough on a job to give it a realistic trial

The contract spells out the duties and responsibilities of client and coach, heightening the experience of a partnership between the two and deemphasizing dependency on the coach. The Pathways model is focused upon eventual independence from coaching. Consequently, independence is emphasized from the beginning of service.

The experience of our coaches led us to create a time limit of 6 months to decide whether the job was a good match for the client's interests and skills. Clients tend to make up their mind too quickly that they do not like a placement because novel situations are difficult adjustments for them. Six months was chosen because this much time is needed to create a learning set, develop a comfort level with coworkers and supervisors, and create and modify (if necessary) strategies on the job.

Job Coaching Criteria

The Pathways model has three specific prioritized criteria for inclusion into the job coaching component of the project:

1. the presence of *spared work skills* and/or the willingness of a former employer to rehire the individual
2. recommendations from a *vocational evaluation* for direct placement and job coaching with specific job areas targeted for development and placement
3. completion of a *vocational training* program

Exhibit 12-3 Sample Job Coach Contract

Job Coach Contract

I, ______________________________, would like to participate in the job coaching project provided by the Pathways project at the Maryland Rehabilitation Center.

I understand that time and effort will be involved in finding employment for me.

The services that my "job coach" will provide will include:

1. An initial interview to determine my interests, my salary requirements, and my job location preference.
2. Location of a job to meet above information.
3. Assistance with interviewing techniques.
4. On-the-job training.
5. Follow-up.

I will be responsible to:

1. Demonstrate motivation to work.
2. Maintain my job by:
   a. accepting supervision
   b. performing appropriate social behavior
   c. demonstrating good relations with coworkers.
3. Consult with my job coach should problems occur.
4. Perform job duties as assigned.
5. Follow rules and regulations on my job.

I agree to give the job a realistic trial that may be as long as 6 months.

I understand that if I must leave my job for whatever reason, I will give at least 7 days notice. If I choose to leave my job before my 6 month trial is over, I know that I will lose my job coaching services.

This contract will result in job interview opportunities (resulting in offers).
If I choose not to take advantage of any of these offers, I agree to give up my job coaching services.

I understand and agree to the provisions of this contract.

______________________	______________________
Job Coach	Client
______________________	______________________
Date	Date

Individuals were chosen from a population of individuals for whom a reasonable expectation of employment had already been determined. Individuals also were chosen in order of priority in keeping with the above criteria.

Spared Work Skills

The first criterion, the willingness of a former employer to rehire the individual, was based on the hypothesis that overlearned skills would provide more transfer of learning than newly learned skills.

For example, one individual preinjury was a systems analyst for Blue Cross/Blue Shield Insurance Company. After 2 years of intensive rehabilitation, however, he could perform only data entry activities. The employer worked in a partnership with the job coach to rehire the individual performing data entry work. The individual was given a job trial at the rehabilitation facility using a simulated sample of work that he would be performing at the actual job site. This model provided maximum transfer of learning for the man to work successfully.

Vocational Evaluation Recommendations

The second criterion, recommendation from a vocational evaluation, was a service of our rehabilitation facility. The evaluation, from 4 to 6 weeks in duration, requires a prospective job coaching client to attempt a variety of simulated hands-on job tasks. The vocational evaluator observes the individual's habits, attitudes, punctuality, attendance, and work speed. Specific job areas, such as stock clerk, are recommended and can then be developed by the job coach. Successful placements occurred when this criterion was used to identify brain injured individuals for job coaching services.

Successful Vocational Skill Acquisition

The third criterion, completion of a vocational training program, involved a prospective client in a formal training program for a job in which he or she had shown potential. This criterion required the most generalization from one learning area to another.

The intent of our methodology, as stated above, was to minimize the need for formal retraining and maximize the use of previously learned skills. The job coaching model used was one-on-one interaction to specifically develop and tailor a job to the interests, needs, deficits, and assets of the brain injured individual. The individual was evaluated and then a job developed for them. This model involves a labor-intensive effort and individualized placement.

Learning Style Assessment

Prior to job coaching, each individual was given a Learning Style Assessment developed at the Maryland Rehabilitation Center (Winner, 1988).

The Learning Style Assessment can be used with any battery of tests. It is not itself a standardized test, but a framework for interpreting results (Wheatley & Rein, in press). It is similar to a qualitative analysis of a battery of tests done by a neuropsychologist, a vocational evaluator, or cognitive therapist.

First, an occupational therapist administers a group of measures, including visual-perceptual tests, memory tasks, and functional activities of daily living. From these varied sources of information, an assessment of learning style is deduced. The Learning Style Assessment focuses on capacities and limitations to determine what interventions and strategies will work best and to relate learning characteristics to potential work tasks and job settings.

Optimal Method of Presentation

Because new information can be presented in a variety of ways, it is important to ascertain the best presentation method for receptivity by each brain injured individual. Each client has specific deficits and assets resulting from his or her own lesion site and preexisting learning abilities. Consequently, the best method of presenting material is not so much a result of one standardized test, but rather a way of interpreting and qualitatively assessing the individual's manner of approach to any one of a variety of problem-solving tasks.

For example, an individual who clearly has a stronger visual than verbal memory would learn best when presented tasks in a visual manner. This information is then given to the job coach to use on the job site in presenting any type of learning task to that individual. For example, an extremely aphasic (expressive/receptive language disorder) individual was given a picture chart of a variety of flowers to use in the landscaping store where he was employed. He was unable to verbally learn flower names, but could recognize them visually and sort incoming packs of flowers into their proper places by using this method, i.e., a color-coded chart. This strategy worked so well for our client that the employer adopted it for his other employees.

Retention Strategy

This process refers to assessing whether the individual can use internal mnemonic strategies or whether retention of information can be mediated best by an external source, such as a written reminder or audiotaped employer instructions. This information is used on a job site by the job coach to provide an individualized external memory device that can record the coach's and/or employer's instructions. The client also may be provided with a data bank watch in which to store relevant information to compensate for a damaged memory system.

Optimal Environment

It is critical for a brain injured person that the best possible environment for both learning and adjustment be provided in the work situation. The environment needs to be assessed as part of a job analysis based on a job-site visit. The coach then can be aware of the details in this environment that may be best suited to the client's individual needs.

For example, a young woman was easily overwhelmed by multiple stimuli and would not do well in a busy office. The optimal working environment for her turned out to be a one-person office, which we initially thought she might have great difficulty handling because of the level of independence required. The Learning Style Assessment provided us with information that this individual's most significant deficits were distractibility and an inability to stay on a task when others were present in the environment. The one-person office worked out well because she could organize the work area and attend to the work task without distraction of other persons and any stimulus for socializing. In this way the optimal environment was identified before placement rather than attempting to remediate this woman's level of distractibility.

This woman's case is further illustrated below to demonstrate the specific job coaching technique used and application of Learning Style Assessment.

Case Illustration

C. was a college student at the time of her accident. She was approximately 2 years post-trauma when she entered the rehabilitation center. She displayed significant memory deficits that interfered with her overall function, but distractibility and difficulty staying on task were the most significant variables. It was hoped that her past office experience and skills could be used in an office setting. Moreover, interpersonal skills were generally quite good, although C. had a tendency to oververbalize when with others.

The plan for placing C. was to use her overlearned skills. Although it was impossible to place her in the previous employer's setting, we attempted to find a placement as similar as possible. The Learning Style Assessment suggested that rehearsal was the best strategy for retention and that visual cues were most effective for presentation. The optimal environment was found to be one that was distraction free.

C. was placed in an office in which her basic job involved giving information by phone to customers wishing to enroll in a driver's education school. A script written by the job coach contained the information to be given to prospective customers. When a call came in, a major decision involved giving different sets of information, which depended on whether the caller was over or under 18 years old. The two sets of information were written on a blackboard in different colors in a very visible area across from C.'s desk.

Staff in the rehabilitation center called approximately five times per day, playing various roles and scored C. on her level of correctness. This individual's memory deficits were also managed by having her generate her own script rather than remembering or reading verbatim. It had been our experience that self-generated, personally relevant information increases the likelihood of retention.

We were aware that the optimal learning environment for C. was as distraction free as possible, as she talked incessantly when in any group situation. The one-person office was a perfect match that lessened the need to totally modify her verbalism.

This case exemplifies using spared work skills as well as the Learning Style Assessment to provide: the optimal method of presentation, the best retention strategy, and the optimal environment.

JOB COACHING MYTHS AND REALITIES

This part of the chapter will explain the realities that the Pathways project has experienced in day-to-day service delivery working with traumatically brain injured survivors. Over the years, we have concluded that some of our basic assumptions might better be seen as myths. If these myths are not turned into realities, the model of a job coaching system for traumatic brain injured persons may lead to massive frustration on the part of staff, employers, and clients involved in a program.

The following assumptions (myths) are not always true or are complicated by a myriad of other factors that must be taken into consideration before job placement can be a successful outcome. Each myth will be followed by a statement of reality, then by a relevant case illustration.

Myth 1—Traumatic brain injured persons with marketable job skills are able to function in a work environment.

Reality 1—The traumatic brain injured individual who has difficulty with psychosocial functioning may sabotage positive vocational outcome by difficulties in getting along with coworkers and supervisors and displaying inappropriate behavior on the job.

Case Illustration—D.D. was a 26-year-old man who was 4 years post-trauma when referred to our program for rehabilitation. He had sustained his trauma secondary to an assault, during which he received a skull fracture and subdural hematoma (localized blood clot) in the left frontal region. He also had a diagnosis of depression.

D.D. had received extensive psychosocial rehabilitation in a prevocational program specifically oriented to head trauma survivors. A vocational evaluation yielded recommendations for employment in factory work, food service, or as a construction trades helper. It was felt that D.D. could benefit from job coaching, as he had marketable job skills and had demonstrated them in the structured environment of a vocational evaluation.

Moreover, D.D. had a work history in unskilled labor and, therefore, met the second criterion for inclusion into the job coaching service.

D.D. had an eleventh grade education but also had a self-reported drug and alcohol abuse problem of long duration.

D.D. was assigned to a job coach with whom he initially worked quite well and a placement was found in a position as a factory worker at a plastics company, which manufactured Halloween masks and party goods.

D.D. was very suspicious of coworkers on the job; he demanded frequent smoking breaks and could not tolerate that his supervisor was able to have longer breaks than he. He became very agitated about the perceived inequalities and was unable to work through these problems with his job coach. This depression, which also seemed to have paranoid overtones, sabotaged this placement attempt. D.D.'s suspiciousness intensified and he believed that his coworkers were infected with the AIDS virus. He refused to touch objects or packages with which they had been working. After 2 days of employment, D.D. became agitated and walked off the job and refused to return.

These behaviors and problems were not exhibited in the structured vocational evaluation program, nor did they emerge in the structured environment of a psychosocial program in which D.D. had participated. He had received strong recommendations from the vocational evaluation; the Learning Style Assessment revealed that he easily could follow verbal directions and appeared ready to work with others in a small company. However, the real environment of a job site proved to elicit unanticipated behaviors and reactions.

Subsequently, D.D. experienced paranoid ideation off the job site and was incarcerated the following weekend for an assault apparently based on misperceptions of intent in a neighborhood dispute. Recommendations for psychiatric intervention were implemented.

The lesson from this placement was that a traumatic brain injured individual who does extremely well in a structured program may have quite a different, and unpredictable, result on the actual job site. The lack of control over the reactions of other people in a real environment, even given the presence of the job coach, was enough to precipitate the underlying psychiatric problem. Frontal lobe dysfunction aggravating D.D.'s lack of ability to inhibit his response to his paranoid feelings also played a significant role in D.D.'s problems.

Myth 2—Traumatic brain injured persons who can hold a job successfully also can live independently because both tasks require similar skills.

Reality 2—Traumatic brain injured individuals may be able to work quite successfully but have extreme difficulty structuring life outside of the work environment. This can adversely affect ability to work if there are no programs for independent living supportive of the work placement.

Case Illustration—D.R. was a 20-year-old woman who was injured in a motor vehicle accident. She sustained a bilateral frontal contusion and multiple fractures of the right arm (D.R. was left-handed).

She was comatose 1 month postinjury and was in a rehabilitation hospital for 8 months. She subsequently received cognitive rehabilitation, physical therapy, occupational therapy, and psychosocial skills training in a structured program.

Before her injury, D.R. had completed high school and 1 year of community college. The medical records on D.R. revealed a group intelligence test score (Otis-Lennon) I.Q. of 117. D.R. had worked after high school as a bartender and cocktail waitress. She had admitted to alcohol and drug abuse for many years.

The neuropsychological evaluation revealed both focal and diffused cerebral dysfunction. Impairment in higher level learning, abstracting, and problem solving; disinhibited, and at times, inappropriate interpersonal interaction; and sexual disinhibition were documented. Moreover, D.R. had a tendency to become verbally aggressive when she was frustrated in an interaction.

At the time of referral, D.R. was attending both Alcoholics Anonymous and Narcotics Anonymous and was residing at the rehabilitation center. D.R. had previous work experience and had good bimanual skills and agreed to work upon a vocational goal of a retail stock clerk. A placement was developed in a discount clothing retail store, where D.R. would be performing stock work. Visual learning was a strong modality for D.R. and an approach to learning inventory tasks was devised by the job coach. Behaviors to be targeted were temper outbursts, voice modulation, and inappropriate language on the job site. These proceeded quite successfully, with the job coach intervening directly with D.R., as well as educating coworkers about D.R.'s disability. The supervisor was pleased with her ability to learn the task.

Although this individual was able to work quite successfully, problems developed when D.R. left the job site in the evening. For example, she became sexually involved with coworkers. D.R.'s problems with both drugs and alcohol re-emerged, as she began to earn her own income and feel more independent. She began to resent structure because she was doing so well on her job and was moving towards more independence. This precipitated actions involving poor judgment in choice of social companions and sexual partners. She eventually drifted back into high-risk behavior involving drugs and alcohol. The placement was terminated for these reasons, not because of lack of work skills or lack of success in the workplace.

D.R.'s family felt that a return to her community in a rural area where she would reside with family members would obviate some of the problems in living in a large city where the likelihood of high-risk behavior would continue to be a concern. The need for supervised living and the intact and supportive family network precluded a relocation even though the employment was successful. Unfortunately, work opportunities were not as available in D.R.'s rural community. Consequently, a successful vocational outcome was complicated by D.R.'s difficulty with judgment, which was a direct result of frontal lobe dysfunction, and her history of disinhibited social behavior seemingly exacerbated by her brain injury.

Clearly, D.R.'s poor judgment put her at great risk if she lived independently in an apartment. This original plan had to be significantly altered due to D.R.'s inability to function independently. Although she did indeed possess the functional skills to live in an apartment, including financial management, activities of daily living (ADL), etc., she involved herself in dangerous situations beyond the "dignity of risk."

Myth 3—In placing the traumatic brain injured individual, memory problems are apt to pose the most significant barrier to employment success.

Reality 3—A person's unrealistic job expectation poses more of a barrier to successful placement than do memory problems, which can be worked with rather successfully by means of the job coach model. Unrealistic expectations tend to result in a myriad of barriers to successful coaching.

Case Illustration—This particular difficulty was revealed across a number of individuals with whom we worked. However, it is most poignantly demonstrated by a man 2 years post-trauma when he began his vocational program. R.H. was a 24-year-old man injured in a motorcycle accident resulting in right hemiplegia, ataxia, and brain stem deficits. He was comatose for 5 months and had sustained significant cognitive deficits. R.H. was a high school dropout who acquired his high school equivalency while in the Marine Corps. He was working as a night manager at a gas station at the time of his injury. The neuropsychological evaluation revealed general I.Q. scores in the average range and evidence of short-term memory problems.

R.H. was involved in every phase of rehabilitation services. He received occupational therapy, physical therapy, cognitive retraining, and psychosocial skills training. An extensive vocational evaluation recommended him for computer programming. However, upon entrance into this training area, R.H.'s short-term memory problems surfaced in his inability to learn the basics of COBOL and difficulty with reading and comprehending textbook material. Consequently, this training endeavor was terminated and R.H. began a program in business education, where the problems repeated.

At this juncture, a referral for Pathways job coaching services was thought to be feasible. R.H. appeared to have marketable skills in data entry and basic entry-level stock work. He expressed a strong interest in job coaching and the service was begun.

Throughout the coaching experience, R.H. maintained that he "really wanted to be a marine biologist or an electrical engineer." These goals had been laid to rest prior to R.H.'s involvement in training programs but reemerged when job development activities began. Still, he agreed to a position as a stock clerk, with eventual opportunities in data entry inventory work. Initially, R.H. was enthusiastic about this placement—he was able to work significant overtime, was earning a good salary, and had heightened self-esteem. However, his original goal of becoming a marine biologist or electrical engineer began to haunt him. He compared his present job as a stock clerk unfavorably with his previously stated goals. He began to complain bitterly that he could have performed these job functions while "I was in high school." He failed to take into account the presence of his traumatic brain injury as a factor that had changed his skill level.

After working successfully for 6 months with a job coach, R.H. was performing stock work quite well with the opportunity to begin data entry in the near future and with the possibility of upward mobility in the organization because management liked his work. However, R.H. began to focus upon unrealistic goals, maintaining that he had actually done well in computer programming, denying memory problems, and maintaining that he could return to college and work toward a degree in engineering. Attempts were made to encourage R.H. to stay with his job and perhaps take a course at a community college to see how he would fare in basic level coursework involving pre-engineering. He declined and R.H. eventually asked his employer to "lay him off" so that he could return to school.

Various interventions were attempted to maintain employment, but R.H. insisted he could earn a degree in engineering. His lack of insight into his own deficits and refusal to compromise about employment versus return to school resulted in termination of services to R.H., who eventually was unhappy with the outcome.

Many brain injured survivors like R.H. are shadowed by an image of their former selves. Some have done extremely well in school and could have been high achievers professionally. Their lack of insight and inability to perceive their deficits results in difficulty in service delivery.

M.P., for example, had been gifted academically, earning a college degree preinjury. During postinjury, he refused to admit any difficulty in acquiring a graduate degree. He received multiple recommendations for employment and training in a variety of areas, including accounting, drafting, and basic clerical jobs. When these options were discussed, he was extremely distressed about these employment options. M.P. became depressed about the reality of the situation and maintained he was going to complete his application to graduate school to pursue an advanced degree.

Memory deficits and organizational problems associated with frontal lobe dysfunctioning clearly precluded the likelihood of success. However, he maintained his unrealistic expectations and would not consider attending school part-time while working in the Pathways program with an employment goal. Consequently, an individual who had a very high likelihood of success in employment with a job coach left the program.

Myth 4—Traumatic brain injured persons will work as equal partners in setting realistic employment goals and can work together with a coach on the job site.

Reality 4—Traumatic brain injured persons with frontal lobe dysfunction may not see the need for any type of assistance from a job coach, probably because they deny the deficit. Their lack of insight into the deficits that the job coach is attempting to remediate often means they cannot collaborate with a coach's rehabilitation plan on the job site.

Because the job coach approach is basically a collaborative one in which the coach and client work in conjunction to accomplish a task, an individual whose job expectations and unrealistic goals are completely at a variance with skills and ability cannot function in this manner.

Case Illustration—Unreality in this regard is a theme that affects a number of individuals with whom we could have predictably had a success, based on job skill ability. The individual listed above, M.P., who was a scholar before his injury, clearly lacked the organizational strategies to perform tasks. His abilities to categorize material and deal in the abstract were quite well developed preinjury, making him unable to see that this indeed was now a deficit. This was not only psychologically overwhelming and a blow to his self-esteem and self-image, it precluded our efforts to assist him with organizational strategies.

M.P. was involved in a memory group to assist him with organizational strategies. He rationalized that he did not need this type of therapy. Consequently, as we neared job coaching, M.P. resisted the need for the service, as well as the job options that were to be explored. M.P. spent a great deal of time verbally rationalizing, seeking to negate the therapist's findings by pursuing psychological consultations to argue in his favor about his level of impairment. Unfortunately, M.P. became obsessed with this task and was unable to energize his efforts toward working with us in any collaborative manner, which was critical to the job coaching model.

Failure experience and reality testing may be necessary to precipitate more realistic goal setting and self-evaluation. It would appear that the experience of attempting to work independently, being fired from positions, or having other difficulties may be a necessary, albeit painful learning experience that is a prerequisite to a traumatic brain injured person being ready to be a partner in a job coaching endeavor.

PRELIMINARY RESULTS FROM THE MARYLAND PATHWAYS MODEL

Preliminary findings suggest that job coaching is an effective method of returning traumatic survivors to work. However, a good job match, the willingness of the employer to work hand in hand with the coach, and a

Table 12-1 Employment Outcome Data

Status	*Number*	*Percent*
Working	10	35%
In Job Training	8	28%
Not Working	9	32%
	N (Project Participants) = 27	

Table 12-2 Demographic Variables

Race	White	70%	Black	27%	Other	3%
Sex	Male	82%	Female	18%		
Education	$\bar{X}$ = 12 years					
Age	$\bar{X}$ = 28.4 years		Range 18–44 years			
Time Post-Trauma	$\bar{X}$ = 18 months					

Note: $\bar{X}$ = Average number.

strong commitment by the client to return to work are factors of a great significance. Table 12-1 portrays our initial results.

Our preliminary results with a group of 28 persons with traumatic brain injury suggest that 35 percent have had a successful employment outcome. An additional 28 percent of this group are currently in job skills training in our facility in a variety of programs and will have a high probability of successful outcome. These eight individuals will be provided services by coaches in the form of job development, marketing, and on-site coaching. The probability for employment is high, and their success would raise the employment rate.

The typical traumatic brain injured client served is a young, white male who was involved in a motor vehicle accident and who has a history of substance abuse. A clinical observation, corroborated by a review of history and neuropsychological test results, suggests a high likelihood of pre-existing learning problems in our population. These factors combined to form a unique client population. Comparable programs for the traumatically brain injured often exclude clients with psychiatric, preexisting learning, or substance abuse problems as part of the admission's criteria. Table 12-2 reveals the demographic composition of the clients we have worked with to date.

FUTURE DIRECTIONS

While the preliminary results of this project and others are very promising, especially for this project population with a high incidence of preexisting substance abuse and learning difficulties, the study highlights how far we have to go to return traumatic brain injured clients to the work place. Several major barriers that still need to be addressed by the rehabilitation community and consumer and advocacy groups are described below.

Independent Living

Independent living is defined as control over one's life based on choice of acceptable options and independence in making decisions and in performing everyday activities (Pfluger, 1979). This focus on consumer choice can complicate independent living rehabilitation for individuals with brain injury. Unlike many other disabling conditions, brain injury typically affects cognitive functioning. This complicates the individual's potential for independent living, although it appears it is a critical issue in successful job placement outcomes.

Choosing between relocating for reasons of job availability and the need for guidance from an existing support system and lifestyle may be incompatible in terms of an overall workable plan. Consequently, the choice may be to remain in the community without the type of job that would be available if the individual was free to relocate. Clearly, this kind of choice is not acceptable but rather a forced choice between less than satisfactory options.

The afterwork hours also pose a dilemma for the traumatically brain injured individual. Independent living assumes the right to take risks and to fail (Pfluger, 1979). However, an issue of great concern to families of brain injured persons and to vocational rehabilitation professionals are fears that risk taking based on severely impaired cognitive function can be very dangerous. Poor choices in nonwork hours complicate and sometimes destroy the entire vocational outcome.

Support Systems

Isolation is a major issue for the traumatic brain injured client in the community. Social isolation and lack of effective personal and social support systems are major factors in interrupting or preventing a successful return to work. The survivor often finds that marriages disintegrate, family members become burned out or dysfunctional, and friends move on to other relationships. The constricted social support system of the average disabled person is the immediate family; for a person with traumatic brain injury, that system has often meant simply the mother. The challenge of finding and nurturing new systems is often beyond the cognitive and interpersonal skills of these survivors. Rehabilitation will have to find methods to salvage old support systems or new and creative ways to assist the client to meet this need.

Accessible Affordable Housing

Without an accessible, affordable home, it is impossible to obtain or maintain employment. In addition to being accessible and affordable, there is a need for housing options that provide various levels of services and supervision whether it is dispensing medication, monitoring diet and nutrition, or some assistance with ADL. Services programs can benefit from the pioneering work of many of the independent living centers and the providers of the developmental disabilities systems in creating levels of community-based housing options for traumatic brain injured persons.

Transportation

Transportation is essential to employment and can sometimes be the deciding factor. Many clients cannot or should not drive or may drive but cannot afford a car and insurance. Many areas do not have reliable, timely, or accessible public transportation. Traumatic brain injured persons and rehabilitation advocates will need to join hands with other disabled persons to solve this continuing barrier to workplace entry.

Disincentives

Social security benefits, workers' compensation benefits, insurance settlements, and government-sponsored health care present major disincentives to return to employment just as they do with other disability groups. This issue can present some new dimensions with the traumatic brain injured client who does not perceive his or her deficits and who may have had a well-compensated, high-status position before injury.

One of our clients had been an executive with a large wine company before he was injured. Although he was quite functionally capable of employment, he could no longer generate an executive level income and could not earn the level of income he received from his benefits. He continued to associate income level with self-worth and rejected any opportunities that would not improve his income standard. The shadow of his former self and his benefit level continued to reinforce his reluctance to accept his new limitations. This mutual reinforcement of a distorted reality orientation creates an environment for negative outcomes far beyond employment and presents immense challenges to families and rehabilitation.

Psychosocial

While housing, transportation, and disincentive barriers are shared with other disability groups, residual psychosocial issues are more closely associated with the traumatic brain injured client. Residual behavior and personality changes, such as depression or dysfunctional interpersonal skills, often can be the determining factor in an unsuccessful return to work. These can manifest as denial of new self-image or disability, which needs to be explored and addressed further.

Substance abuse and lack of treatment programs and resources for clients with this diagnosis combine as another psychosocial barrier. The traditional detoxification and inpatient treatment programs do not seem to work with this population. This is an area requiring further study and the development of new treatment strategies.

A support group to deal with psychosocial issues, according to preliminary findings from the Pathways project, is of equal significance to job coaching in determining which individuals are successful. Unfortunately, persons who are employed full-time may have difficulty attending such support groups. More need to be developed in the community or in the rehabilitation facility so they are readily available to individuals who are moving into the vocational reentry phase of their recovery.

In our experience, the psychosocial barriers are the most formidable and immutable.

LONG-TERM FOLLOW-ALONG

Our original model assumed that job coaching would have a beginning and ending point. While this has been true for a significant group, it appears that there must be other options as well for long-term follow-along. Individuals tend to change jobs five to seven times in their working life and over time even the same job will change. While some clients appear to require continuing ongoing support such as that provided by supported employment, it appears there is also a need for models that can provide intermittent assistance for clients who have made a successful return to employment. Our experience suggests that psychosocial follow-along needs are as great as are employment-related needs.

In addition to time-limited job coaching and supported employment, other models for long-term follow-along are needed within both public and private sector rehabilitation.

SUMMARY

Our experiences and data indicate that it is possible using current methods and technologies to resolve the vocational issues to successfully return traumatic brain injured clients to employment and to integrate them full time into the competitive marketplace. We are also able to do this at a higher success rate than before. A method with great promise in vocational rehabilitation is the job coaching approach that is such an integral part of the supported employment model.

Many independent living issues remain as barriers for these persons who seek to be fully integrated into society. These critical issues must receive national advocacy and creative problem solving to ensure the continued success of those who are currently in the marketplace and to remove barriers that prevent other traumatic brain injured persons from achieving their employment potential.

REFERENCES

Parenté, R., & Stapleton, M.C. (1988, March). *Job coaching TBI individuals: Lessons learned*. Paper presented at the Fourth National Traumatic Brain Injury Symposium. Maryland Institute for Emergency Medical Services Systems.

Pfluger, S. (1979). *Independent living*. Washington, DC: Institute of Research Utilization.

Stapleton, M.C. (1986, September). Maryland Rehabilitation Center closed head injury study; A retrospective survey. *Cognitive Rehabilitation*, *4*(5), 34–40.

Stapleton, M.C., Parenté, R., Bennett, P. (1989, July–August). Job coaching traumatically brain injured individuals: Lessons learned. *Cognitive Rehabilitation*, *7*(4).

Wehman, P., Kreutzer, J., Wood, W., Morton, M.V., & Sherron, P. (1988, June). Supported work model for persons with traumatic brain injury: Toward job placement and retention. *Rehabilitation Counseling Bulletin*, *31*, 296–310.

Wheatley, C.J., & Rein, J. (in press). The challenge of head trauma returning the brain injured to work. *Work program guidelines*. Rockville, MD: American Occupational Therapy Association.

Winner, D.M. (1988). *Protocol for learning style assessment*. Unpublished manuscript. Baltimore, MD: Maryland Rehabilitation Center.

Chapter 13

Returning to Work: Illustrations of Competence

Paul Wehman

Vocational outcome studies do not tell a positive story as far as success in returning to work for persons following severe head injuries. Kay, Ezrachi, and Cavallo (1986) summarized 46 outcome studies, including one by Peck, Fulton, Cohen, Warren, and Antonello (1984) investigating vocational outcome in a group of 60 severely head injured patients from the Richmond, Virginia, metropolitan area. Patients were a mean of 3.5 years postinjury, all were initially admitted in a comatose state, and 82 percent were between 16 and 40 years of age. Only 13 percent of the sample had returned to preinjury vocational levels, whereas 35 percent were employed in less-demanding or sheltered workshop settings and 52 percent were unemployed. Factors most strongly related to vocational adjustment included physical status, thinking efficiency, concentration ability, and motor coordination. Problems with remote memory, depression, and seizures were reported by 88 percent, 78 percent, and 15 percent, respectively. Furthermore, 56 percent reported that they relied on their spouse or other family member as a primary source of income. Disability compensation was received by 27 percent of the sample. The authors concluded that diminished status is common, even years after injury, and suggested a need for supplementary rehabilitation programs to reduce symptomology related to reduced vocational status.

Similarly, Jellinek, Torkelson, and Harvey (1982) completed an investigation of functional, emotional, and occupational status involving 23 brain injured patients in the Madison, Wisconsin, area. Mean age and time post-injury were 27 and 4 years, respectively. Of the sample, 82 percent were unmarried, 55 percent were women, and 68 percent were independent in mobility and self-care. The investigators found that 41 percent of the sample were involved in education or work activity. Unfortunately, no data were provided regarding level of employment, average number of hours worked per week, or type of educational activity.

The earliest investigations of postinjury vocational status were done in Great Britain and Scotland. Even though these countries differ socioeconomically from the United States, the investigations provide insight into the long-term consequences of head injury. When Weddell, Oddy, and Jenkins (1980) studied 31 male and 13 female patients approximately 2 years postinjury, all patients had experienced more than 1 week of posttraumatic amnesia, were aged 16 to 39, and lived in the London area. Mean duration of coma was 4.2 weeks. Only five patients had returned to their former employment, all after absences of more than 6 months. Of these, two were skilled manual laborers, one was a teacher, and two were employed in unskilled jobs. Eleven patients returned to full-time work at a reduced capacity between 6 and 18 months postinjury. Notably, nearly one half of the sample, 20 patients, were reportedly unable to work at all and parents often sacrificed their own employment to care for the disabled person at home. Unemployment was linked to memory dysfunction and personality changes (e.g., increased irritability, childishness, and disinhibition) and to poor neurophysical status.

Brooks, McKinlay, Symington, Beattie, and Campsie (1987) recently completed an investigation of employment status within 7 years postinjury. Of 98 patients with a preinjury unemployment rate of 14 percent, the unemployment rate was 73 percent at 4 years postinjury and 70 percent at 5 years postinjury. Brooks et al. indicated that there was not a significant change in work status for the sample between 2 and 5 years postinjury. They found the significant contributors to unemployment were personality problems, behavioral disorders, and cognitive impairments, including deficits in attention, memory, and communication.

These studies all yield similar conclusions. First, the severity and type of head injury are clearly determinants of postinjury employment potential. Patients with more severe injuries (e.g., long coma duration and more severe physical, emotional, and cognitive problems) have a smaller likelihood of returning to work. Second, less than one third of patients with severe head injuries are likely to be competitively employed postinjury. The likelihood of returning to work at preinjury levels is considerably smaller, and there are long delays for those who do return to work. Finally, the family members often sacrifice their own employment to care for the unemployed head injured person at home.

STUDYING SUPPORTED EMPLOYMENT OUTCOMES

To examine the effects of an individual placement model of supported employment on the wages and hourly work outcomes of five traumatic brain injury survivors who have consistently been unable to gain competitive employment and/or hold employment, a small-scale supported employment program was initiated and monitored. Competitive employment is defined as earning at least the federal minimum and working in integrated work environments within business or industry.

Subjects

The five subjects were selected in early 1988 from referrals made by parents, private and public rehabilitation counselors, physicians, local hospitals, and insurance providers. The age range of the subjects was from 20 to 37 years. They were selected for the study based on the following criteria: (1) a Glasgow Coma Score < 10 on initial admission, (2) a record of post-traumatic amnesia exceeding 24 hours, and (3) a minimum age of 17. Table 13-1 lists demographic characteristics and major vocational problems of the five subjects. Table 13-2 shows their neuropsychological and cognitive characteristics based on a full neuropsychological battery given by a Ph.D. level neuropsychologist. This table indicates that the participatory subjects were below the average of 50 percentile on most relevant items of cognitive functioning.

This was a group of persons with long-term chronic unemployment or periodic work in sheltered workshops. Some exhibited serious alcohol or substance abuse problems and acting out behaviors and were viewed as being at risk for employment by vocational rehabilitation counselors, family members, and physicians. All subjects were injured due to motor vehicle accidents and, as the mean length of coma (118.6 days) indicates, were very severely injured.

Individual job placement into supported competitive employment was based on a variety of factors, such as client interest, job compatibility, job availability, availability of transportation services, and family support. There was less emphasis on the entry skill level of the person because the supported employment approach is designed to overcome whatever client deficits are present. No criteria for excluding persons from the program exist based on the severity of the brain injury.

Setting

The program is based in central Virginia at a large university medical center. All placements are in competitive employment with coworkers who are predominantly nonhandicapped.

Table 13-1 Client Demographic Profiles

Client Number	*Gender*	*Age at Injury*	*Cause of Injury*	*Length of Coma (days)*	*Current Age*	*Preinjury Educational Level*	*Residential Status*	*Major Presenting Vocational Problem Areas*
1	M	23	Auto Accident	233	31	Some high school	Parents' home	Ambulation Fine motor coordination
2	M	20	Auto accident	153	33	College student	Supervised apartment	Short term memory, thinking, motor/coordination
3	M	27	Motorcycle accident	59	29	High school graduate	Parents' home	Vision, coordination, communication
4	M	9	Auto accident	138	20	Elementary student	Parents' home	Work speed, compliance with instructions
5	M	16	Auto accident	10	37	High school student	Independent	Seizures, attention span, memory
Means =		19		118.6	30			

Table 13-2 Neuropsychological Test Scores of Subjects

Test	*1* *Client Total*	*2* *Mean Score*	*Standard Deviation*
GOAT = T (modified: max = 70)	4	69.00	2.00
Token Test	3	57.33	23.12
Control Oral Word Association	4	33.50	16.11
Information (WAIS-R)	4	.39	.23
Spelling (WRAT-R)	4	.50	.43
Passage Reading (GORT-R)	3	.37	.43
Reading Comprehension (GORT-SF)	4	.37	.42
Digit Span Forward (WAIS)	4	5.25	.50
Immediate Verbal Memory	4	6.00	2.31
10' Delayed Memory	4	6.50	2.08
60' Delayed Memory	4	6.50	2.08
Verbal Learning (total T1-T5)	4	41.25	6.99
Verbal Learning Recognition	3	13.37	2.89
Left/Right Body Parts	4	19.00	1.41
Right Hand Pegboard (seconds)	4	117.25	46.87
Left Hand Pegboard (seconds)	3	142.33	86.18
Rey Osterrieth Copy	3	33.33	3.79
Rey Osterrieth Memory	3	17.00	1.73
Visual Reproduction	3	11.00	2.00
Time Recognition	4	8.00	0.00
Block Design	4	.41	.36
Symbol Digit Modalities/Written	4	29.50	12.48
Symbol Digit Modalities/Oral	3	44.00	10.44
Category Test	4	43.50	11.62
Judgment of Safety	4	12.25	1.26
Logical Deductive Reasoning	4	4.75	.50
Similarities (WAIS-R)	4	.57	.49
Arithmetic Reasoning (WAIS-R)	4	.32	.29
Arithmetic Calculation (WRAT-R)	4	.05	.02

[1]Not all clients could be tested or would agree to be tested.
[2]Where possible, scores were converted to percentile ranks. Means < 1 indicate mean percentile; means > 1 indicate means of raw scores.

Independent Variable

The independent variable is the supported employment individual placement model, which is a treatment package that includes job placement, job-site training and advocacy, assessment, and job retention strategies. Table 13-3 describes the methods involved in the supported employment intervention.

Dependent Variables

Two dependent variables were measured: wages earned per week and hours worked per week. These were the key outcome measures for assessing

Table 13-3 Checklist of Activities in Supported Work Approach to Competitive Employment

Program Component I	Job Development and Job Placement	• Conducts structured efforts to find job for client and match client strengths to job needs • Plans transportation arrangements and/or travel training • Is actively involved with parents on identifying appropriate job for client • Communicates with Social Security Administration
Program Component II	Job-site Training and Advocacy	• Trained staff provides behavior skill training aimed at improving client work performance • Trained staff provides necessary social skills training at job site • Staff works with employers/coworkers in helping client • Staff helps client and coworkers adjust to each other
Program Component III	Ongoing Assessment	• Provides for regular written feedback from employer on client progress • Utilizes behavioral data related to client work speed, proficiency, need for staff assistance, etc. • Implements periodic client and/or parent satisfaction questionnaires
Program Component IV	Follow-up and Retention	• Implements planned effort at reducing staff intervention from job site • Provides follow-up to employer in form of phone calls and/or visits to job sites as needed • Communicates with employer regarding staff accessibility as needed • Helps client relocate or find new job if necessary

Source: From "A Supported Work Approach to Competitive Employment of Persons with Moderate and Severe Handicaps" by P. Wehman and J. Kregel, 1985, *The Journal of the Association for Persons with Severe Handicaps, 10*(1), pp. 3-11. Copyright 1985 by Association for Persons with Severe Handicaps. Reprinted by permission.

the efficacy of the intervention. The data were collected by four professional service staff persons who work as industry-based employment specialists. Each has either a bachelor's or master's degree in special education, psychology, rehabilitation, or social work, and/or at least 2 years experience working with persons who have severe disabilities. The employment specialist computes the two variables by

- wages earned per week—multiplying wages earned per hour by the number of hours worked per week
- hours earned per week—verifying the total with the client and then with employer each Friday

During the *intervention* phase by employment specialists, data were collected using the Data Management System developed at the Rehabilitation Research and Training Center at Virginia Commonwealth University (Hill, 1988).

Staff Intervention Time

The employment specialist also tracked total staff intervention time beginning with job development activities and ending with ongoing follow-up and on-site consumer advocacy. These data were collected to evaluate costs associated with placement of these clients.

Total intervention time included all hours staff spent in job development, consumer assessment, job-site analysis, direct job-site training activities (hands-on training and direct observation of subject performance), and indirect job-site training activities (e.g., travel/transport time, writing behavioral programs, and on-site consumer advocacy). Employment specialists turned in their time records each Friday to the programmer/analyst of the Data Management System.

Reliability

The accuracy of the wages accumulated and hours worked were computed by having two or more job coaches collect these data independently and then corroborate the accuracy of this information with the employer. There was a 100 percent reliability level for each time this was done, which was monthly.

The accuracy of the staff intervention data was checked every other week by a senior research staff person against the data submitted by the employment specialists. There was also a 100 percent level of reliability for this measure.

Experimental Design

A multiple baseline design across subjects was used in this study (Hersen & Barlow, 1976). In this design, the wages earned and hours worked by the five subjects were identified and measured over time. The baselines then were used to compare the effects of supported competitive employment training for each individual as well as across individuals. As the supported competitive employment model is applied to succeeding subjects, the baseline for each subsequent subject increases in length.

Baseline

During the baseline phase, each subject's earning power and hours were assessed before supported competitive employment services were initiated. The baseline phase extended from January 1987 to January 1988 for all five subjects. Baseline levels of wages earned and hours worked per week were assessed retroactively through extensive interviews with each subject, parent/guardian, vocational rehabilitation counselor, and, when possible, employer.

Intervention Procedures

The supported competitive employment model emphasizes vocational intervention directly at the job site after the person is hired. This approach requires the use of skilled human services professionals who can provide specialized placement and training support. As noted in Table 13-3, the major components in this model include: job placement, job-site training, ongoing assessment, and permanent follow-along through the subject's life of employment (Wehman & Kregel, 1985). This model differs from traditional job placement practices by placing individuals who are not "job ready" and by having an on-site employment specialist or job coach provide training and advocacy support. The employment specialist begins with intensive one-to-one support and fades this support as the individual gains independence at the job site. A training curriculum that describes specific elements of the model in more depth can be found in Moon, Goodall, Barcus, and Brooke (1985).

This model is modified for traumatic brain injured clients by emphasizing more development of cognitive compensatory strategies at the job site and, when appropriate, physical modifications of the work environment. Because short-term memory and planning are a major deficit of most traumatic brain injured clients, the employment specialist had to resolve these problems at the job site. Also, employment specialists spent a great amount of time in away-from-work counseling activities and community resource coordination (e.g., substance abuse counseling and residential assistance).

Results

The data in Figures 13-1 and 13-2 and Table 13-4 indicate that each of the five persons were able to be placed into competitive employment. Figure

Table 13-4 Consumer Outcomes

Client	*Type of Placement*	*Type of Company*	*Weeks Employed*	*Wages Accumulated*	*Staff Intervention to Stabilization*[1]	*Hours: Total*
1.	Maintenance Worker	Children's Retail Outlet	47	$7,092.00	299:20	321:30
2.	Activities Assistant	Child Service Center	37	$2,220.00	183:05	252:55
3.	Price Ticket Changer	Children's Retail Outlet	32	$4,675.95	125:30	154:15
4.	Stock Clerk	Drug Retail Outlet	12	$1,206.00	138:49	138:49
	Sales Associate	Children's Retail Outlet	16	$1,530.00	287:00	287:00[2]
5.	Assistant Cook	Nursing Home	23	$4,293.00	417:25	451:05

[1]As defined by the Virginia Department of Rehabilitative Services, stabilization occurs when staff intervention time required for job maintenance remains at or below 20 percent of the consumer's work time for a period of 30 consecutive days.

[2]Stabilization did not occur for either of these placements.

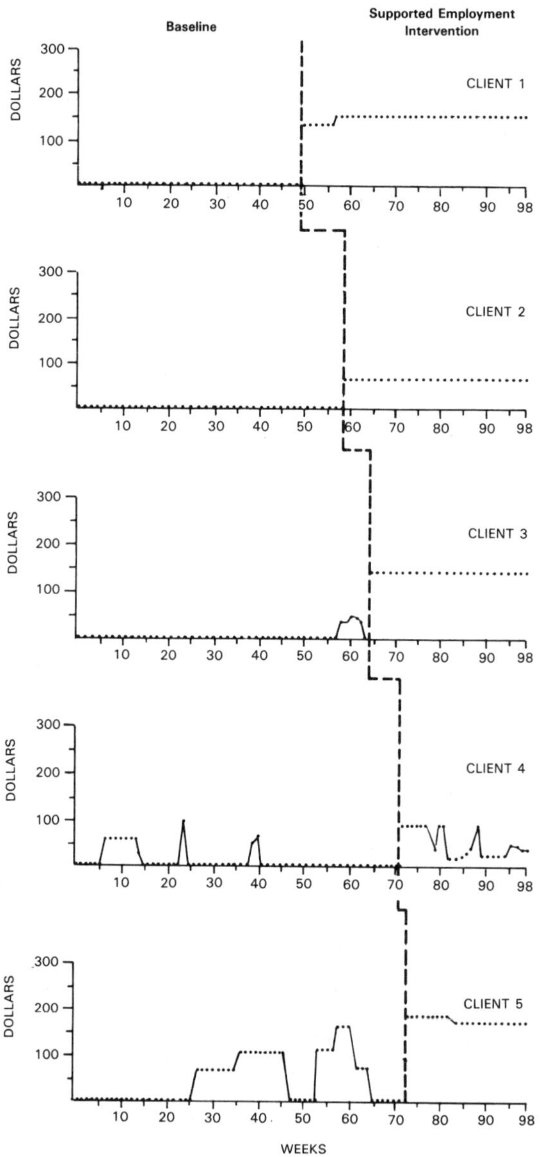

Figure 13-1 Earnings per Week

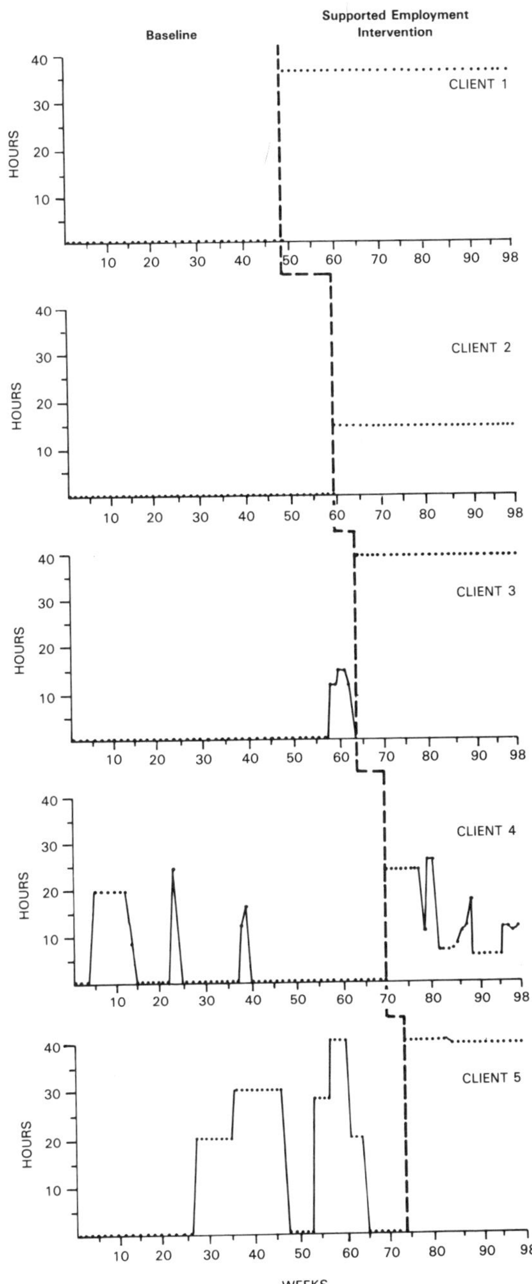

Figure 13-2 Work Hours per Week

13-1 shows the lengthy period of unemployment or unstable employment experienced by each individual. Upon the intervention of a supported employment specialist, meaningful competitive work was located and on-site training and support were provided. The range of wages was from $4.25 to $5.00 per hour, above the existing federal minimum wage of $3.35 per hour. The range of hours worked weekly varied from 15 to 40, as displayed in Figure 13-2. Client #2 was receiving social security disability income; he and his mother were concerned about jeopardizing these payments so he chose to work only 15 hours per week although more hours could have been made available.

Table 13-4 also indicates the employment specialist intervention hours, which ranged from 154 to 451, with a mean of 321. At a rate of $25 per hour, which is an average vendor rate in Virginia for rehabilitation service providers, the costs per placement averaged $8,015. The mean hours to stabilization (that is, until staff time on the case has been reduced to 20 percent or less) were 256 for 4 cases; client #4 never attained stabilization. He was laid off from his first job in a drugstore and was quickly replaced in a children's retail store.

SUMMARY

The data presented in this study indicate that a supported employment intervention program was functionally related to job placement into competitive employment for persons who have been unable to gain or maintain jobs since their injury. The first three clients had been unable to find competitive work either by themselves or with the help of family members or professional counselors due to the perceived disability impairments they exhibited. Clients #1 and #3 had worked periodically in sheltered workshops; clients #4 and #5 repeatedly proved unable to hold any employment for more than a few weeks or months at a time. In fact, Client #5 reportedly had 18 jobs over the preceding 6 years.

The purpose of this study was not to isolate and evaluate different components of the individual placement model of supported employment. It was to show that this model has some efficacy with a small population of persons who have sustained severe head injuries and who had been comatose for a long period of time (average = 118 days). There have been no applied behavior analysis demonstrations of the relationship between supported employment and return to work outcomes for persons who have experienced traumatic brain injuries in the published research literature that we could locate. This pilot study represents a small beginning in this direction.

It is noteworthy that none of these persons earned enough money to live totally independent lives. Some help from family and/or other sources will be necessary until they can establish a sufficiently positive work history to move up into better paying positions. However, the cognitive and psychiatric impairments presented by these persons raise the questions of how much upward mobility will ever be possible and to what degree ongoing staff support can be withdrawn. Although the answers are unknown, it may be that steady competitive work is actually a positive facilitator of neuropsychological improvement given that traumatic brain damage is not a static phenomenon and long-term physiological improvement can occur in the brain.

While the intervention activities identified for each case were individualized to the job site and person's needs and although the work environments and jobs were each different for the five persons, clearly similar problems had to be worked on in every case. For example, getting to work on time, transportation arrangements, inappropriate verbal behavior at the job, planning and sequencing work activities, remembering work tasks, and inappropriate sexual behavior at the job site were common problems that needed to be managed by the employment specialists in conjunction with the business supervisors. The challenges to the employment specialist in placing, training, and retaining a person with these complex problems are substantial indeed. A highly experienced or trained counselor who is well compensated is essential.

The cost of placing these persons and training them through supported employment was high, certainly relative to costs for persons with mild and moderate mental retardation in similar supported employment programs (Rusch, 1986). The range of staff intervention hours was 154 to 451, with a mean number of 321 hours. Hence, the average cost was over $8,000 per case.

The financial cost of not helping these victims return to work, however, is far higher. These cases are known as "catastrophic" cases in the insurance industry, because usually the victims are young males who have their entire life of work ahead of them. Therefore, the cost reserves that must be set up to compensate these victims run into the millions of dollars for just one case. Tens of millions of dollars are also spent by the Social Security Administration on Social Security Disability Income cases. It is not difficult to see how a 25-year-old person who worked as a carpenter preinjury with $20,000 a year earnings, would, with projected inflation increases, easily be able to command a minimum settlement of $750,000 to $1,000,000. Obviously, with settlements this large, a placement cost of even $10,000 is quite small if and when a client's earned wages can be used to offset the liability exposure incurred by the insurance firm.

This study has been an evaluative demonstration of how supported employment can enable postacute traumatic brain injured victims to become competitively employed. It represents a step in the right direction to focus upon critical employment outcomes, such as wages earned, hours worked, and staff intervention hours expended. Future research activities must look at the positive role, if there is one, of preplacement activities such as cognitive retraining, improvements of cognitive ability over time as a function of job placement, the most efficient mechanisms for making a job match, and appropriate ways of staff intervention at the job site for inappropriate acting out behaviors.

REFERENCES

Brooks, N., McKinlay, W., Symington, C., Beattie, A., & Campsie, L. (1987). Return to work within the first seven years of severe head injury. *Brain Injury, 1*, 5–19.

Hersen, M., & Barlow, D.H. (1976). *Single case experimental designs: Strategies for studying behavior change*. New York: Pergamon Press.

Hill, M. (1988). Supported competitive employment: An interagency perspective. In P. Wehman & M.S. Moon (Eds.), *Vocational rehabilitation and supported employment* (pp. 31–54). Baltimore: Paul H. Brookes.

Jellinek, H., Torkelson, R., & Harvey, R. (1982). Functional abilities and distress levels in brain injured patients at long-term follow-up. *Archives of Physical Medicine and Rehabilitation, 63*, 160–162.

Kay, T., Ezrachi, O., & Cavallo, M. (1986). Annotated bibliography of research on vocational outcome following head injury. New York: New York University Head Trauma Center.

Moon, M.S., Goodall, P., Barcus, J.M., & Brooke, V. (1985). *Job coach training manual.* Richmond, VA: Rehabilitation Research and Training Center on Supported Employment.

Peck, E., Fulton, C., Cohen, C., Warren, R., & Antonello, K. (1984). Neuropsychological, physical, and psychological factors affecting long term outcomes following severe head injury. Paper presented at the annual meeting of the International Neuropsychological Society, Houston, Texas.

Rusch, F.R. (1986). *Competitive employment: Issues and strategies*. Baltimore: Paul H. Brookes.

Weddell, R., Oddy, M., & Jenkins, D. (1980). Social adjustments after rehabilitation: A two year follow-up of patients with severe head injury. *Psychological Medicine, 10*, 257–263.

Wehman, P., & Kregel, J. (1985). A supported work approach to competitive employment of individuals with moderate and severe handicaps. *Journal of the Association for Persons with Severe Handicaps, 10*, 3–9.

Wehman, P., Kreutzer, J., Sale, P., West, M., Morton, M.V., & Diambra, J. (1989). Cognitive impairment and remediations: Implications following traumatic brain injury. *The Journal of Head Trauma Rehabilitation, 4*(3): 76–85.

Chapter 14

Community Factors and Successful Work Reentry

Al Condeluci

The move toward supported employment is one step to improve work reentry outcome for persons with traumatic brain injury. But the devastating reentry prognosis for this population may demand we also shift the very foundations of their rehabilitation programs. If present methods in vocational rehabilitation for people with head injuries are falling short, what might be done to inspire a greater success in job finding and retaining?

This chapter suggests a shift from a medical-based foundation to a community-based one. It does not minimize the importance of appropriate medical personnel and treatments to vocational rehabilitation for persons with head injury but suggests a thorough consideration of community factors as equally important. Survivors, their families, and their home situations and lifestyles all need to be linked together in a gestalt if we are to better our outcomes.

THE PHILOSOPHY SWITCH

Most rehabilitation efforts for persons with head injuries are framed from a medical model (NHIF Directory, 1987). This is particularly appropriate when the goal in the early stages of the rehabilitation process is to save or stabilize the individual. As the person proceeds in rehabilitation, however, the goals and challenges begin to shift. By the time the individual is ready for rehabilitation discharge, the major goal is community reentry.

In human services today, the challenge of community integration is taking on a focus area of its own (Taylor, Racino, Knoll, & Lutfiyya, 1987). Researchers and practitioners are recognizing that traditional and medical models need to give way to newer foundations (Zola, 1986). It is becoming commonly accepted in the disability movement that community success and support systems around people with disabilities must take on a broader, empowerment focus (DeJong, 1983).

A client's overall community integration goals are

- *A viable place to live*—All people need a place to live, where they feel private, safe, and in control.
- *Meaningful day activities*—All people seek and can benefit from daily activities and rhythms that are meaningful to not only them but society at large.
- *Viable, supportive relationships*—No person can really exist without relationships that are intimate and meaningful.
- *Opportunities to rejuvenate*—People must have opportunities to replenish them well and choices that allow them to relax and recharge.

The common theme that underscores these four goals from a broader, community focus is the concept of valorization (Wolfensberger, 1971). This means to bring value to the person and is especially important in the social role. The major convictions that baseline the valorization concept are (Condeluci, 1988)

- consumer choice and participation
- age appropriateness
- right to choose
- the nonrestrictive environment

In traditional approaches to vocational rehabilitation, the consumer has little input into the process. When occupations or job settings are selected, they are often decided on and obtained autonomously by the vocational rehabilitation professional. In many cases, final choices are sheltered, congregated, or protected settings or no options are available. This is all too common for people with head injuries. In a large study in California (Jacobs, 1987), the researchers concluded that, once active rehabilitation ended, a significant number of survivors with head injuries watch television. This conclusion is particularly biting. Yet the vision and goal of a community philosophy is to avoid isolation or congregation of persons with disabilities. When people are congregated in sheltered workshops or other segregated settings or isolated, negative dynamics occur (Biklen & Knoll, 1987), including

- labeling and stereotyping
- lack of privacy and control

Table 14-1 A Comparison of Human Service Models

Issue	*Medical Models*	*Empowerment Models*
What Is Problem?	The Brain	Lack of Support
Where Is Problem?	The Person	The System
What Is Solution?	Classify-Congregate-Fix	Create Supports
Who Is in Charge?	The Expert	The Consumer
What Is Outcome?	Fix and Accept	Interdependence

Source: From "Independent Living: From Social Movement to Analytical Paradigm" by G. DeJong, 1979, *Archives of Physical Medicine and Rehabilitation, 60*, pp. 435–436. Copyright 1979 by American Congress of Rehabilitation Medicine.

- linking with other devalued people
- lessening of standards
- promotion of dependency

These dynamics create powerful and often devaluing images of persons with disabilities. They cast a deep stigma in the public's eye that is difficult to erase (Goffman, 1963). This stigma and negative image follow persons with a disability as they reenter communities. Further, given the deep-rooted dimensions of the medical model, there is a propensity for individuals with a disability to perceive themselves within the confines of the stereotype. Not only does society see them this way, but they begin to believe that they are sick and incapable (Illich, 1976).

To better understand the medical model is to contrast it with a community-based empowerment model (DeJong, 1979) (see Table 14-1).

As these models demonstrate, the focus of attention shifts from a microscopic perspective of the individual as the problem, the one to be fixed in the medical model, to a more systematic approach in the empowerment model. In the empowerment approach, the focus is to understand, sensitize, and/or change the environment to which the person with a disability relates.

This type of analysis should offer a real challenge to head injury service systems today. If the medical model leads us into a deficit approach, then it would follow that our programs need deficits and dependency to operate. That is, the commodity can become the ability to fix a person's deficits. This commodity creates a strong dependency on the expert to make the problem better. It implies that experts must make the key decisions. It also continues to keep the survivor in a dependency routine.

On the other hand, the empowerment model challenges this assumption. It starts to reframe the basic question of the problem and suggests a focus on the environment. It assumes that the individual with the disability can and should take a lead role. Finally, it suggests that the target of change is not the person with a disability, but the system and the community. The commodity in the empowerment model is a more open, receptive community.

To operate the empowerment model, however, mandates that we know, understand, and relate to communities. This is where current head injury rehabilitation efforts fall short. Most rehabilitation efforts today attempt to change the person—even those programs that specialize in community reentry (Condeluci, Fawber, & Gretz-Lasky, 1986). When we can no longer dramatically change persons and they still manifest challenging behaviors, then the traditional solution is to create segregated, assisted living or work communities. What has resulted in head injury rehabilitation is the growing development of retreats, ranches, farms, group homes, workshops, and other separate activity milieus.

Before we relegate these more challenging individuals to congregated environments, we can and must do more within our existing environments. We need to test, adjust, and create alternative actions in an effort to promote vocational success. To institutionalize one person because we did not try an alternative community action is not only a tragedy, but a travesty in rehabilitation.

UNDERSTANDING COMMUNITY FACTORS

All of us have dimensions beyond our work persona. We are family members, neighbors, community members, and citizens. Our lives are a blend of these faces and are certainly tied together. To understand how our community perspective impacts and affects our vocational perspective, we must explore the concept of community.

O'Brien (1986) defines community as experiences that lead to mutually supportive relationships vital to living well. It arises when valued personal relationships with connections to others lead to purposeful action and celebration. Often we think of the community as the setting we live in. Yet the concept of community relates to any environment where people come to some common ground. To this extent, the work environment is as vital a community as our neighborhood.

In a broader sense, community relates to vital human interaction. It is when people come together for a common purpose. Community recognizes a need for privacy but equally allows for a fluid flow of integration and interchange (Nisbet, 1953). Given this dimension of communality, it is easy to pervert the nature of community by suggesting that people of common identity *should* all live together. This approach has been followed when groups of people, such as people with mental retardation labels, have been segregated to common environments. Some experts in head injury rehabilitation have argued that such common settings for people with head injuries

Table 14-2 Distinctions between Assisted Settings and Community

IN ASSISTED SETTING . . .	*IN THE COMMUNITY . . .*
people are known by what's wrong, their condition or label	people are known as individuals
people are incomplete, need to be changed or fixed	people are as they are with opportunity to dream
relationships are unequal-workers do for the client	relationships are reciprocal
people are broken into parts, separated into groups	people are accepted as whole and viewed as part of the whole society
problems are solved by consulting authorities, policy, procedure	people seek answers from their own experience and the wisdom of others
there is no room to acknowledge mistakes and uncertainty	people can make honest efforts and acknowledge honest mistakes and fears
all problems have a rational solution	there is room for confusion, mystery, and recognition that some things are beyond human control

Source: From *The Gift of Hospitality* by M. O'Connell, 1988, Evanston, IL: Center for Urban Affairs and Policy Research, Northwestern University.

might be the best long-term solution. This perspective needs to be understood as a perversion of the community definition. A key factor in community is the freedom to choose. There is a fundamental difference between choosing to be with people of common bond, such as ethnic or socioeconomic similarity, and being relegated to such settings by others who think it is best.

An easy way to understand the real nature of community, be it a neighborhood or work environment, is to contrast it to structured human service settings such as sheltered workshops or group homes. McKnight (1987) suggests the opposites between human service settings and natural communities are:

- Human services operate on control.
  Communities operate on consent.
- Human services are often slow and deliberate.
  Communities respond quickly.
- Human services often require solutions to go through channels.
  Communities inspire creative reactions.

The difference between assisted settings and community is further contrasted by O'Connell (1988) in Table 14-2.

Within the past 20 years, when we consider a philosophical shift it is interesting to note that the human service professions have been subconsciously undermining the role of community in supporting all its citizens. That is, as specialists in retardation, mental illness, geriatrics, and other human service interests have endeavored to support their constituencies in communities, most of their actions have been exclusionary or isolating (McKnight, 1987). Witness the advent of senior centers and high rises where elderly folks are corralled and secluded. Other examples can be group homes, separate education settings and the like. We have special transportation, special workshops and special olympics; all in the name of community integration for people with developmental disabilities. Ten to fifteen years ago, we exported retarded and mentally ill persons to the institution; then we returned them to group homes and sheltered workshops, which are often as isolated as the institutions.

These isolated programs or services give a basic message to the community: "Don't worry about these groups, we experts will take care of them." Further, it perpetuates a stigmatic message that these people are strange, different, vulnerable, or dangerous and that they need to be contained. Special service programs imply that people who are head injured, have mental retardation labels, or have some type of physical disability are very different from the average citizen. This isolation further generates the notions that the problems of these groups will be solved by the experts and communities need not worry.

Newer visions in human services are recognizing the inappropriateness of separate settings. Programs that have created group work or group living options are now looking to the next generation of services—those where individuals with disabilities can be a real part of natural settings (Taylor, Biklen, & Knoll, 1987). These newer visions have created service approaches that are supportive, not supervisory; that are integrated, not segregated; that are non-restrictive, not least restrictive. Supported living and supported employment are examples of this thrust and head injury rehabilitation needs to learn from these lessons.

THE CHALLENGE OF SYMBIOSIS

Any personnel director will tell you that work life and home life are symbiotic. What happens in one world is sure to affect another. Absenteeism, tardiness, and difficulties in performance are often related to problems at home and work performance frequently falls when family problems arise. Classic studies in motivation and work directly link the home life with work performance. Similarly, an upswing in performance, attitude, and work interest is often tied to positive areas in the worker's private life. A person establishing a new relationship, getting a new car, or mending a broken fence can lead to an upsurge in performance and productivity.

Studies have proven likewise that most vocational rehabilitation failures of persons with disabilities are related to difficulties in personal relationships (Gold, 1973; Rusch, 1979; Wehman, 1975). This awareness has led to support models that promote a social bonding between coworkers and the person with a disability (Shelton & Lipton, 1983). These models put as much attention on relationships as on skill acquisition.

This information suggests that our home life and personal skills are critical to vocational success. Yet, in most vocational efforts for persons with disabilities, very little attention is paid to community living arrangements, personal skills, and home/community relationships (Nisbet & Callahan, 1987). Vocational rehabilitation efforts for persons with disabilities, including head injuries, still pay little attention to community and home factors (White, 1986). More than any other disability approach, head injury rehabilitation has taken to specialization and segmentation. Most vocational rehabilitationists are experts in job assessment, development, and placement, but know little about communities. In fact, evidence suggests that the primary target to address vocational failure, for most programs, is to attempt more training for the worker with a disability (Gold & Ryan, 1980). Consequently, an approach blending community and personal dimensions with the vocational rehabilitation is rare. We need to reverse these trends.

In head injury rehabilitation, where cognitive challenges are most acute, it seems to follow that strategies applied to personal skills can and should be connected to the work setting. A study of supported employment in Pittsburgh shows that job retention and acceptance are highest with individuals that are receiving holistic support in all aspects of their lives (McCue, 1988). Further research continues to support the holistic approach (Doperak, 1989; Wehman & Kreutzer, 1984).

There are several ways the vocational rehabilitation professionals can consider community factors in their plan and placement actions.

Many vocational rehabilitationists have advocated conducting a community assessment (Hutchings, Renzaglia, Stahlman, & Cullen, 1986; Wehman, Renzaglia, & Bates, 1985). These inventories, emphasizing community skills and abilities, are helpful in developing a target for vocational training but fall short when looking at the important relationship factors.

A different concept, social validation (White, 1986), suggests a social comparison and subjective evaluation of the vocational and social behaviors of the worker. The goal is to develop a treatment plan that will assist the worker to fit into the work environment.

Exhibit 14-1 is a recommended inventory that acknowledges the work site as a community and ties the home life to the work environment. The inventory lists community factors that are essential in developing a holistic vocational support plan.

Exhibit 14-1 Sample Community/Vocational Integration Information Form

Community/Vocational Integration Information Form

NAME ______________________ DATE ______________________
ADDRESS ______________________ PHONE ______________________
____

KEY SUPPORT PERSON ______________________
RELATIONSHIP ______________________ PHONE ______________________
PERSON FILLING OUT FORM:
NAME ______________________
RELATIONSHIP ______________________ PHONE ______________________

NOTE: This form is designed to give the survivor and support person a holistic view of the potential linkages for planning. All sections should be filled out and entered in the support plan.

SECTION I

The Living Environment

- Where does the person live ______________________
- With whom ______________________
- Who provides support ______________________
- What is the setting like
  Is it a home ______________________
  Is it homelike ______________________
  Is it congregate ______________________

SECTION II

The Morning Pattern

- What is the person's morning routine ______________________
- When does the person get up ______________________
- How ______________________
- What assistance does the person need ______________________
- What assistance is provided ______________________
- Who gives the assistance ______________________
- How does the person seem to feel about it ______________________
- What about breakfast ______________________

SECTION III

To Work

- How is transportation handled ______________________

Exhibit 14-1 continued

- Who provides it ______________________________
- Is it reliable ______________________________
- Is it safe ______________________________

SECTION IV

At Work

- What is the work culture ______________________________
- What about work norms ______________________________
- Who is influential ______________________________
- What about lunch routines ______________________________
- How do people dress ______________________________
- What happens during breaks ______________________________

SECTION V

After Work

- Are there patterns ______________________________
- What do people do ______________________________

SECTION VI

Extra Work Activities

- Where are the work celebrations ______________________________
- How are they carried out ______________________________
- Are there work teams (bowling, softball, aerobics, golf) ______________________________
- Are there work-related clubs (poker, bridge) ______________________________

SECTION VII

Evening Routines

- What are the patterns ______________________________
- Where is laundry done ______________________________
- Where is shopping done ______________________________
- Leisure activities
  At home ______________________________
  TV shows ______________________________
  Hobbies ______________________________

continues

Exhibit 14-1 continued

Outside interests ______________________________

____

SECTION VIII

Weekends

- What are the patterns ______________________________

  ____

- Any travel ______________________________
  How ______________________________
  Where ______________________________
- Church activities ______________________________

  ____

SECTION IX

People Dimensions

- Who are friends ______________________________

  ____

- How active is family ______________________________

  ____

- Paid support ______________________________
  From where ______________________________
- Volunteer support ______________________________
  From where ______________________________
- Does dating occur ______________________________

  ____

Answering the inventory questions provides a holistic profile of the individual. Pieces emerge that can be vital to a support plan. At this point, the vocational rehabilitationist should be open and ready to link or relate key community elements in support of the person who is working or to be placed.

DEVELOPING A CIRCLE OF SUPPORT

One way to implement a holistic approach is to orchestrate a circle of support around the person. This circle consists of a variety of players who talk about or commit to a plan for the person with a head injury. This gathering should not be a staffing in the traditional sense, but a brainstorming session where those around the worker with a disability, be they in their home setting or work setting, can speak to or commit to a part of the support plan. The only goal of this gathering should be to promote and keep the individual with a disability integrated into the work place.

This circle of support concept has worked successfully in residential and life support planning (O'Brien & Lyle, 1987). In these residential situations are neighbors, friends, and associates from the church as well as family and paid support personnel—anyone who might have an interest in or commitment to the person with a disability.

This circle of friends approach can work well with the person with a head injury who is reentering the workforce. In fact, there may be many people who knew the individual before the accident and would gladly be a part of the circle. Certainly, people identified in the aforementioned Community/Vocational Integration Information Form can and should play a key part in the circle of support.

Studies are now suggesting that involvement of ancillary support people, such as personal care attendants or case managers, can play an important role in the vocational rehabilitation effort (Nisbet & Callahan, 1987). Further, concepts from supported employment, such as coworker support, job coaching, and job sharing, all inspire fresh ways to promote a comprehensive support team. Outside individuals, services, or concepts to consider in the vocational rehabilitation effort are described below.

Residential/Community Case Manager

This person is a key support to community living. In many situations, the case manager has a solid history with the survivor. This person can play a key role in balancing work-related issues that spill over to the home setting and can help the survivor gear up or adjust to new work demands.

Personal Care Attendant

These individuals provide direct physical and/or cognitive supports for the resident. As the first person to interrelate with the survivor each morning, the personal care attendant can help set a positive tone. Fears, concerns, and anxieties can be talked about before the survivor sets out for work. The personal care attendant may also be the first person to debrief the survivor upon returning home. These times can be vital in establishing a confident and solid work personality. In many cases, workers with disabilities miss out on work-related social activities that help create a work ecology. With prework and postwork personal care attendant intervention, the worker with a disability can attend these most important gatherings.

The Bridgebuilder

A newer residential support person to be considered in the vocational process is the bridgebuilder (Mount, Beeman, & Ducharmer, 1988). Community support people are realizing that it is relatively easy to help the person with a disability move into communities. The real challenge is to ensure that person is a viable part of the community. The bridgebuilder is more concerned about linking the individual with a disability to typical and natural relationships than to changing or fixing the person to fit in. A community bridgebuilder attempts to find an interest or link for the persons with a disability to their neighborhood. This interest, such as a hobby, serves as a "ticket" to commonality. All people have tickets to integration.

For vocational rehabilitation specialists, the bridgebuilding concept serves two important purposes. First, a community bridgebuilder needs to be tied into the vocational rehabilitation process. As part of the plan and action of vocational placements, they may assist the survivor in linking with coworkers.

The other purpose is for the specialist to fold the bridgebuilder concept into the work setting. That is, the vocational rehabilitation support person or coach uses bridgebuilding strategies in coaching or vocational rehabilitation activities. Along with teaching skills of the job, they can help the worker with a disability establish friendships and relationships on the job.

Coworker Linkups

For many persons with head injuries, the cognitive and psychosocial deficits suggest that regular and steady job supports be available. Yet, ongoing job support is either unavailable, financially inefficient, or unrealistic. Consequently, many persons with head injuries fail in jobs after the support has been faded (Gilchrist & Wilkerson, 1979; Matheson, 1982). One way to maintain supports in a cost effective way is to identify and tie coworkers into the long-term support plan. Often such situations are not paid support, but if it is necessary, a minimal contract can be established. The coworker can fulfill support needs to oversee, cue, or monitor work of the head injured person. Further, the connection with a coworker will help to valorize the worker with a disability. In valorization theory, the more time that the disabled individual spends with a valued person, the greater the spread of a positive social role (Wolfensberger, 1972). Coworkers, although not realistic for all supports, can play a key role in general support, acceptance, and valorization.

The Family

As simple as it may seem, vocational rehabilitation success in head injury rehabilitation is critically tied to family intervention. Unofficially, many vocational rehabilitation specialists will tell you that most plans succeed or fail because of family support or sabotage. In many situations, the family takes the place of the case manager and personal care attendant, setting the tone and reacting to work environment dynamics. As with the personal care attendant, the family can hold the key to attitude, motivation, and, consequently, success. Family energy is powerful and needs to be drawn into a holistic approach.

SUMMARY

This chapter has suggested a foundational shift in the vocational rehabilitation process to a community/vocational and holistic support approach. It will extend support to include community and home support people and can adopt key concepts from community integration theory, such as the bridgebuilder and the circle of friends, to ensure success.

Although these ideas will lead to better vocational outcomes for persons with head injuries, there is another important community factor that must be acknowledged and discussed. This is the challenge of long-term funding for continuing vocational supports. Certainly, the debate around the longevity of support is a crisp one in the vocational rehabilitation community (McConnell & Minton, 1985). Traditional vocational rehabilitation efforts have been time-limited and closely linked to closure. If a person with a disability placed in a job can have paid support fade, then the case gets closed as a positive outcome. In most instances, however, if a case cannot be closed constructively over a reasonable period of time, then the case will be foreclosed. In some instances when an individual's situation is very severe, then the vocational rehabilitation counselor may not even open the case in the first place.

It is well documented that psychosocial ramifications from head injury can last a lifetime. Further, it is documented that support systems can offset these psychosocial ramifications (Jacobs, 1987). This reality begs the question: Should people with severe situations receive paid support for an unlimited time period? Advocates of supported employment will argue that this model calls for lifetime support, if needed (Bellamy, 1988). Others suggest that although people may need lifetime support, we cannot expect the public vocational rehabilitation arena to carry these costs; other sources must be tapped. The literature on vocational failure, especially after placement, makes it clear that longer support options must be adopted.

To find the keys to long-term success, basic federal program reform is required. Over the past few years, two federal portals have been identified for change and reform. The Rehabilitation Services Administration (RSA) of the Department of Education, creates the mandate and regulation for state vocational rehabilitation efforts. In 1978, RSA services were extended to include some independent living activities. This change marked a fundamental adjustment to traditional vocational rehabilitation and remains a key area for further reform. Advocates for long-term supports would do well to build on this breakthrough.

The other portal to changes in long-term community and vocational support is Medicaid reform. For the past 6 years, disability advocates have been working to shift the medical and institutional bias of our present Medicaid system. Gains have been made in the past 3 years with the introduction and growing interest in the Home and Community Quality Assurance Act. This bill, if enacted, will shift our present institutional bias of Medicaid toward community services. Projected services of Medicaid reform are long-term case management, attendant care, and job coaching, all of which would be time unlimited and related to the functional needs of the eligible person. Again, advocates for community supports would do well to aggressively promote Medicaid reform in the U.S. Congress.

Until this reform occurs, however, we are forced to demonstrate and show efficacy of community supports within our present system. This calls for creativity, flexibility, and new ideas. We need to reach out in novel ways and the holistic and community model offers a viable option.

The shift from a medical model to a community model will not come easy. Years of conditioning and tradition have taken their toll. Yet, more must be done and we need to start somewhere.

REFERENCES

Bellamy, G.T. (1988). *Supported employment, a community implementation guide*. Baltimore: Paul H. Brookes.

Biklen, D., & Knoll, J. (1987). The disabled minority. In S. Taylor, D. Biklen, & J. Knoll (Eds.), *Community integration for people with severe disabilities*. New York: Teachers College Press.

Condeluci, A. (1988). *Community residential supports for persons with head injuries*. Washington, DC: United Cerebral Palsy Association.

Condeluci, A., Fawber, H., & Gretz-Lasky, S. (1986). A national survey: The need for long term independent living/vocational rehabilitation services. *NHIF Newsletter, 5*(4), 5,8.

DeJong, G. (1979). Independent living: From social movement to analytical paradigm. *Archives of Physical Medicine and Rehabilitation, 60*, 435–456.

DeJong, G. (1983). Defining and implementing the independent living concept. In N. Crew, & I. Zola (Eds.), *Independent living for physically disabled people* (pp. 4–28). San Francisco: Josey Bass.

Doperak, L. (1989). Mental health consequences of brain injury. A paper presented at Western Psychiatric Institute and Clinic, Pittsburgh, PA.

Gilchrist, E., & Wilkerson, M. (1979). Some factors determining prognosis in young people with severe head injuries. *Archives in Neurology, 36*, 355–359.

Goffman, E. (1963). *Stigma*. New Jersey: Prentice-Hall.

Gold, M.W. (1973). Vocational rehabilitation for the mentally retarded. In N.R. Ellis (Ed.), *International Review of Research in Mental Retardation* (p. 6). New York: Academic Press.

Gold, M.W., & Ryan, K. (1980). Vocational training of mentally retarded. In M.W. Gold (Ed.), *Did I say that? Articles and commentary on the try another way system*. Champaign, IL: Research Press.

Hutchings, M.P., Renzaglia, A., Stahlman, J., & Cullen, M.E. (1986). *Developing a vocational curriculum for students with moderate and severe handicaps.* Charlottesville, VA: University of Virginia.

Illich, I. (1976). *Medical nemesis.* New York: Pantheon.

Jacobs, H. (1987). Adult community integration. A paper presented to the National Invitational Conference on Traumatic Brain Injury. Tysons Corner, VA.

Matheson, J.M. (1982). The vocational outcome of rehabilitation in fifty consecutive patients with severe head injuries. In J.F. Garrett (Ed.), *Australian approaches to rehabilitation in neurotrama and spinal cord injury.* New York: World Rehabilitation Fund.

McConnell, L.R., & Minston, E.B. (1985). *If . . . the future of VR.* Morgantown, WV: West Virginia University Research and Training Center.

McCue, M. (1988). Cognitive, behavioral and vocational rehabilitation of persons with traumatic head injury. A presentation to the Annual Conference on Cognitive Rehabilitation, Williamsburg, VA.

McKnight, J. (1987, Winter). Regenerating communities. *Social Policy,* 54–58.

Mount, B., Beeman, P., & Ducharme, G. (1988). *What are we learning about bridge-building.* Manchester, CT: Communitas, Inc.

NHIF Directory of Services. (1987). Southborough, MA: National Head Injury Foundation.

Nisbet, J., & Callahan, M. (1987). Achieving success in integrated work settings. In S. Taylor, D. Biklen, & J. Knoll (Eds.), *Community integration for people with severe disabilities.* New York: Teachers College Press.

Nisbet, R. (1953). *The quest for community.* New York: Oxford University Press.

O'Brien, J. (1986). *Discovering community.* Atlanta: Responsive Systems Associates.

O'Brien, J., & Lyle, C. (1987). *Framework for accomplishment.* Decatur, GA: Responsive Systems Associates.

O'Connell, M. (1988). *The gift of hospitality.* Evanston, IL: Center for Urban Affairs and Policy Research.

Rusch, F. (1979). Toward the validation of social/vocational survival skills. *Mental Retardation, 17,* 143–145.

Shelton, C., & Lipton, R. (1983). An alternative employment model. *Mental Retardation, 33*(2), 12–16.

Taylor, S., Biklen, D., & Knoll, J. (1987). *Community integration for people with severe disabilities.* New York: Teachers College Press.

Taylor, S., Racino, J., Knoll, J., & Lutfiyya, Z. (1987). Down home: Community integration for people with the most severe disabilities. In S. Taylor, D. Biklen, & J. Knoll (Eds.), *Community integration for people with severe disabilities.* New York: Teachers College Press.

Wehman, P. (1975). Toward a social skill curriculum for developmentally disabled clients in vocational settings. *Rehabilitation Literature, 11,* 342–348.

Wehman, P., & Kreutzer, J. (1989). Supported Employment Workshop. Dallas Rehabilitation Institute, Dallas, TX.

Wehman, P., Renzaglia, A., & Bates, P. (1985). *Functional living skills for moderately and severely handicapped individuals.* Austin, TX: PRO-ED.

White, D. (1986). Social validation. In F. Rusch (Ed.), *Competitive Employment Issues and Strategies.* Baltimore: Paul H. Brookes.

Wolfensberger, W. (1972). *Normalization.* Toronto: National Institute on Mental Retardation.

Zola, I.K. (1986). The medicalization of aging and disability: Problems and prospects. In C. Mahoney, C. Estes, & J. Heumann (Eds.), *Toward a unified agenda.* Berkeley: World Institute on Disability.

Chapter 15

A Family Perspective

Evelyn F. Esposito and Frederick W. Esposito

The year was 1977 and our family seemed finally to be on the road to independence. I remember thinking as I was driving home from my job as an assistant teacher in the Richmond, Virginia, public schools that finally, after raising our five children and being concerned about their education and our financial responsibilities, the time was near when Fred and I could begin to think about other things (e.g., trips and pleasures for ourselves). These were our children: Carla, our oldest, married and doing well; Fred Jr., in his third year at the University of Montana; Cindy, in her second year at James Madison University; Bill, a senior at Douglas Freeman High School and the object of recruitment by six or seven major universities because of his selection as outstanding linebacker in the state of Virginia; and our youngest daughter Dory, a sophomore at Douglas Freeman who was already confident she was not going to college.

That is pretty much the scenario of our life in October 1977. Until October 27, when Bill received a concussion in the final game of the football season. It was a goal line stand and Bill stopped the fullback, preventing a score but receiving a hit on his helmet from the ball carrier. The team doctor told us that it was a concussion and all would be well. However, Bill seemed distressed and came home with two of his teammates, who sensed something was wrong with him. After much persuasion, Bill agreed to go to the hospital with his dad and was admitted, checked, and kept overnight for observation. The next morning, he was released from the hospital and told not to play football for two weeks. Within a few days, Bill began having headaches. I took him back to the doctors for examination; the diagnosis was the same postconcussion syndrome and the doctor prescribed medication to relieve Bill's headaches. Ten days after the initial hit on the football field, Bill collapsed and was rushed to the local hospital near death. Our lives have never been the same.

Bill lay in a coma for 10 days, during which our lives and his life became an open book. Because Bill had received a tremendous amount of publicity before his injury (he was named the blue-chip prospect for the state of Virginia), the entire saga received constant media coverage and we were bombarded by the media, friends, relatives, strangers, and classmates during Bill's stay at the hospital. The support was fantastic, but the unwelcome questions were not: "Will Bill be able to play in the championship game? Will Bill be a vegetable?" and on and on. We had absolutely no answers. The medical team attending Bill gave us all the negatives: Bill will probably never talk, he will become obese, there is always hope his brain will come back but how far and how soon no one could answer.

We felt so inadequate and helpless. What was traumatic brain injury? Where could we send Bill for rehabilitation? Would he finish high school? How far could or would he come back? So many questions, so few answers.

COMING HOME: THE SEARCH FOR SERVICES

Bill came home within 6 weeks of his injury and I remember two things the doctors had said: be sure he doesn't fall out of bed and the two best rehab hospitals for head injuries are in California and New York. We were on our own with our son, who 6 weeks before was a 215 lb., bright, articulate athlete on his way to a college scholarship and a law degree, but was now a nonverbal, gaunt, 150 lb., passive young child. The entire family was in shock. Somehow we had to cope with what had happened to Bill and figure out what we were going to do with him. Thus begins the story of how we became brokers for our son.

The focus of our lives became finding services for our son to bring him back to his full potential. My husband became totally absorbed with reading everything and anything he could find about the brain and he spoke to anyone and everyone about what types of programs were available for Bill. In 1977, very little was offered in the field of rehabilitation from a head injury and what was available was costly and not easily accessed. However, we knew we could not let Bill just vegetate on his own.

The first thing we did was contact the Henrico County services and, after many phone calls, we started Bill with a tutor from the school system so he could begin to work on getting his diploma from high school. The county also supplied us with an occupational therapist who came to the house to work with Bill. We then began to investigate the possibilities of Bill going to the Medical College of Virginia for rehabilitation. The word was out that they had some cognitive remediation. (I remember hearing those words for the first time and trying to figure out what they meant.) We visited the outpatient clinic at the Medical College of Virginia, which agreed to take Bill as an outpatient for occupational therapy three times a week. So, for the next 6 months, I would drive Bill the 12 miles to his therapy and the 12 miles back home. Also during this time, we were recommended to a neuropsychologist who began to do some testing on Bill and also did some family counseling. Suffice it to say that the entire family was in turmoil. . . . Fred, trying to hold down his extremely stressful position with a major company (while seeking and searching for Bill's rehab); myself (I had quit my job to be with Bill) struggling to understand and cope with what had happened to my child; and the other siblings going through their own grief without the support of their parents. But we continued on our journey, trying to rehab Bill.

ONE YEAR LATER

November 1978 (1 year postinjury) found Bill doing fairly well physically but still very low cognitively. Each day becomes less and less of a struggle. The shower and shave take only 25 minutes for Bill, instead of the initial 45 to 60 minutes. The progress is slow and we have always in the back of our minds that the progress can stop anytime. As Bill becomes more and more aware, so problems surface we hadn't even thought about. The "why me" syndrome begins and we spend hours and days and months trying to give him some rhyme or reason to what has happened.

Bill begins weekly counseling with a neuropsychologist. His social life becomes null and void. After the first few months of Bill's return home, his friends and football buddies gathered around him and tried to accept this new person. However, unable to cope with what had happened to Bill Esposito, they begin to find their own avenues and Bill is shut out from their lives. How understandable that is now! We, his own loving parents, brother, and sisters could hardly cope and understand what had happened; how difficult it must have been for his peers. And how do you explain to a person who had been so popular with his fellow classmates and so in demand as a friend, that now he was different and his friends could not understand? So, as well as becoming Bill's rehab brokers, we become his social life brokers. I remember visiting Virginia Union Theological Seminary and asking if a young male student would befriend Bill so he could have some contact with people his age. With both his older brother and sister away at college and his younger sister going through her own devastation, Bill was left with his mother as his only contact with the outside world.

TOWARD CONTINUED REHABILITATION

In November 1979 (2 years postinjury), Bill continues to make strides. His psychologist suggests that Bill get a job to begin reentry into the real world. Douglas Freeman awarded him his diploma in June 1979, 1 year after he was supposed to graduate. Again, we act as brokers by calling on friends who owned a sporting goods store and they agree to let Bill work part time. Without any real knowledge of what Bill could or could not do, we took a chance that having a little part-time job would definitely increase his self-esteem.

During this time, we had attended a conference sponsored by the Medical College of Virginia on traumatic brain injury and were introduced to Dr. Yehuda Ben-Yishay, who had an innovative program on cognitive remediation at New York University Hospital. We felt the program would benefit Bill and we talked Dr. Ben-Yishay into testing Bill to see if he would qualify as a candidate. Every day of every week we were constantly striving to find appropriate programs for Bill and keep him stimulated and progressing. During the next few months while we waited to hear from New York University, we devised several programs to keep Bill on track. The part-time job was working out relatively well, but looking back we realize that Bill was really not ready to work, even though it did occupy some of his time. The days had to be structured for Bill and keeping him busy became my full time job. We next tried to get him to take some courses at a community college. And always through all of this was his lack of social life.

The more aware Bill became of his injury, the angrier he became, so now we began to deal with some of that anger. Without any real guidance, much of what we did for Bill was trial and error—the latter of which was often. To help Bill overcome his anger and lack of self-esteem, his father decided to let him purchase an automobile. Thus began a whole series of problems. Although the car provided Bill with an outlet, he began to go to bars (where most of his peers were and he felt more "normal") and began to drink too much and get into trouble with the law. Emotions ran from high to low in our family, almost like sun up and sun down. To watch Bill get dressed up and look so "normal" was a real high, to realize that he might not have the judgment he needed to handle situations that might arise was a real low. We now became brokers to keep him out of trouble. The drinking became a real problem and we struggled with whether he should keep the car.

Test scores continued to show Bill gaining. His I.Q. went from a score of 60 when he first was tested to 98 in 3 years. However, underlining everything were his lack of motivation and judgment. But we continued in all areas to push Bill to the maximum. During the 2 years that followed Bill's injury, I became full-time coordinator for Bill, trying to keep him mentally alert by enrolling him in one course at the community college, giving him some self-esteem with a job, getting him to work out at the health spa so his body would stay in shape, and trying to fill in the gaps for his social life. Meanwhile, my husband investigated Bill's social security benefits and handled a thousand and one forms for securing hospital benefits. We also entered the Department of Rehabilitative Services to see what they had to offer in the way of rehab for the head injured.

Finally Bill was granted an interview with Dr. Ben-Yishay and we drove to New York for the evaluation. The fact that the program was a day program presented a problem for us, but we had relatives living in Connecticut and felt if Bill was accepted he definitely would go. We also had heard about Woodrow Wilson Rehab program for head injured, which was in the beginning stages and the staff had been going to Dr. Ben-Yishay for training. When we visited Woodrow Wilson, we were told that Bill probably would have to wait 1 year to get into the program. One of the most difficult and frustrating problems with our "brokering" for Bill was that at that time head injury didn't fit into a category for services. For all intents and purposes, our son, who looked perfectly normal, did not qualify for services under any state agency. He was not retarded, not physically handicapped, not emotionally disturbed, not visually handicapped, not hearing impaired, not indigent. Yet he could not enter the mainstream of life. He needed help and we could not find it anywhere.

Finally, in September 1980 Bill received his letter of acceptance into New York University's head-trauma program. The program lasted 5 months, and each day, Monday through Thursday, Bill and I commuted via the train from New Haven, Connecticut to New York so Bill could attend the program. The program was and still is, in my opinion, the best in the nation. The main thrust was on cognitive remediation, but the program tried to deal with all aspects of head injuries (i.e., social and emotional problems that follow a severely head injured person). Bill received almost one-on-one services and, although being separated from my husband and other children was a hardship, we decided it was worthwhile to give Bill the opportunity to have the best. When the program began, there was concern among the staff that it would be hard to provide Bill with follow-up services after we went back to Virginia.

When the program terminated in February, the final evaluation confirmed that Bill still suffered many deficits from his trauma, but with proper assistance could become productive, could handle a highly structured job environment, and could begin his reentry into the real world. How we would handle all the emotional and social needs that any young 20-year-old person would have along with Bill's special problems were questions that no one could answer for us or for Bill. So, we returned home to begin another series of brokering for Bill.

COMMUNITY INTEGRATION AND ADJUSTMENT

Although we were connected with the Department of Rehabilitative Services, the paperwork and case loads were tremendous and time lagged for Bill. He needed activity and self-esteem and a job helped both of these. My husband was able to contact a friend who was overall manager for a warehouse and he gave Bill a job. By this time, Bill's car had been sold so I became his driver to and from his job. We felt we had done a good job of educating the warehouse manager as to Bill's problems. What we did not realize was that all the people coming into contact with Bill would not understand the problems he faced, and as a result he was shifted from department to department in the warehouse. After a year, the whole thing fell apart. Bill was easily influenced and in dire need of friends and as a result was easily led and fell into a pattern of drinking again. By this time, he was on his second neuropsychologist.

Emotionally, Bill was devastated because of his inability to hold down a job and the realization that he was out of the mainstream, had no real friends, and all his hopes and dreams were gone. In the meantime, the entire family began to pull away when they saw the devastating effect all of this was having on their parents. It was difficult enough for them to cope with what had happened to Bill, but witnessing what it was doing to their parents lives was beyond belief. And yet they understood and supported us because they knew we had to help Bill; he was our son and we had to try to piece his life back together. Our daughter, Cindy, was a special education teacher and provided ideas and strategies during Bill's rehabilitation. My husband and I held our marriage together in spite of all that was happening. We were strong for each other and used every ounce of energy we had working to bring our son to his full potential.

After Bill lost his job at the warehouse, he began a whole period of job failures. To the average person, Bill looks totally normal and without any physical impairments. He would never have any trouble getting a job—he would simply apply and he would get this position. From Hardee's to K-Mart to construction work to a manufacturing plant to a printing company and on and on the cycle would go. Apply for the position, work 1 week, 1 month, 2 months, and then lose the job. The reasons were varied—lack of concentration, not fast enough, too many breaks, etc., etc. During this 3- to 4-year period, we applied for social security for Bill and he had been turned down three times. Finally, through the Department of Rehabilitative Services, Bill was placed in the Goodwill program. I felt it was inappropriate for Bill from the beginning, but we were at our wits' end and willing to give it a try. Again we educated the counselors who would be working with Bill and devised a behavior modification program for him while he was in the program. The program was not geared to handle head injured persons, who definitely need a specific highly structured environment in which to learn skills. As a result, not only did the program not help to rehabilitate Bill, he lost ground, became involved with another client, and got into serious trouble with the law. We intervened, got him out of the program, and were back to ground zero again.

At this time, his psychologist suggested Bill enter an alcohol rehabilitation program because he felt that Bill's drinking was interfering with his holding down a job. So, now we were faced with another major problem coupled with the head injury. We felt Bill was drinking to escape from the devastation of his injury and we couldn't deal with all the problems at once, so we signed him into an alcohol program for 30 days. Once again we had to educate the people in charge as to just what a head injured person was like. Ironically, many professionals felt they knew and had worked with other head injured clients, but once they were dealing with Bill it really was a first for them. Although many head injured persons do have physical disabilities, many like Bill do not. Hence, it becomes difficult for anyone working with them to recognize the disability until they have been involved for a few weeks. We call them the walking wounded. Bill has the same face, the same body, but in fact is a totally different person. Our first son Bill has actually died, we now have a new son. We are still adjusting. . . .

Fortunately, Bill made it through the 30 days in the program. The last week of it, we received a phone call from the director informing us that Bill might have to be released due to his disruptive behavior during group counseling sessions, but he did complete the program. We now have to begin looking for a halfway house for Bill to go to as that is standard for most coming out of the alcohol rehab. After making 20 or 30 calls throughout the state, we have the name of a halfway house in Harrisonburg, Virginia. We drive to Harrisonburg, visit with the staff, tell them about Bill, his injury and his problems, and ask if they are willing to accept him in their program. With as much information as I have available to me, I try to educate the staff and answer their questions. Bill is accepted into the program and we feel relieved that he will have a chance to be away from home for a few months. However, 6 weeks into the program, Bill was sent home. The other clients felt he was too demanding of their time and not willing to listen in group sessions. We are back to ground zero again.

REACHING OUT FOR SERVICES AND NEW FRIENDS

Two positive things happened during this time: The Virginia Head Injury Foundation is beginning to make some inroads and impact in the state and Bill has met a group of young Christians who become his new circle of friends. In fact, Bill has a wonderful involvement with a young Christian girl for a year and a half. During their courtship, we see strange things happening for Bill. All the problems we faced with Bill begin to disappear. He is motivated, his self-esteem rises, he doesn't drink, his appearance improves, and he seems happy. Having that one person in his life did more for him than any therapist, family member, or psychologist. For Bill and for us it was the best year and a half since his injury. Also during this time, I began working through the Department of Rehabilitative Services to get a job coach for Bill. He had had too many failures and he needed to have some success. So from February 1983, when Bill came home from the halfway house, until December 1984 we waited patiently, went through all the interviews, and finally met with Paul Wehman from Virginia Commonwealth University. We modified his program for the mentally retarded and adapted the program for a job coach for Bill. The next year or so Bill was working part time as a moderately successful salesman in a sporting goods store. This job, coupled with his girlfriend and a strong belief in God, seemed to be the final saga in a long, long challenge. We felt relieved and confident things were settled.

Without getting too specific, when the girlfriend bowed out on Bill, things began again to deteriorate. He left one Sunday morning for church and never came home. Bill was gone, whereabouts unknown, for 10 days with my car. The trauma and emotions were running high again: Would he be arrested? Would he have an accident? Where was he? All attempts to find him proved unsuccessful. . . . He was old enough to be on his own, so the police wouldn't check for the car unless we reported it stolen and then Bill would be arrested . . . so we waited. . . . Finally, he arrived home safe and sound. It seemed he had picked up a young man hitchhiking to his grandmother's home in North Carolina and Bill just decided to drive him all the way. We decided it was Bill's way of getting away from home. Other than a short trip to Alaska to see his brother Fred, Bill had spent the majority of his time with his Mom and Dad. A young adult male with all the normal wants and desires having to live under the same roof with his parents makes for a very unhealthy situation. The trip to North Carolina proved costly: He had left his job for 10 days without notice and the result was he lost his job. We were back to ground zero again. . . .

We go back to his counselor at the Department of Rehabilitative Services (by this time Bill is on his third counselor) and the decision is made that he should go to the workshop for the retarded. Again, I feel the program is not going to be suitable for Bill, but the Virginia Head Injury Foundation has been doing some training at different workshops, so we send Bill to the program. With lots of support, we tell Bill it is temporary and he can learn to become a printer in the program. I drive Bill back and forth to the center each day. Bill does not do well in the program. He feels angry having to go there, doesn't like the environment, and leaves town for another short vacation, this time to New Jersey. We receive a phone call after the third day of his disappearance from the New Jersey police, who have arrested him. Back to ground zero. We now find ourselves with a 25-year-old man back home with no job, no program, and no activity. How do you fill the days for an active, fully functioning human being with a traumatic brain injury? Nothing seemed to fit for Bill. Through his years of rehabilitation, we have tried everything humanly possible to develop some sort of meaningful lifestyle for Bill, but to no avail.

The years have brought much in the field of head injury and things have begun to change for our loved ones. But going through the last 8 years has been most difficult for all of us and mainly for Bill. He sees himself as almost totally recovered and yet the mountains still seem unsurmountable. We brokered for everything imaginable from services to therapy to friends to jobs to benefits and the list goes on and on. Unwritten are the energies and time spent trying to keep his self-esteem up, filling his social life, explaining his injury, and brokering on his behalf. My husband and I felt totally frustrated for years simply because there never seemed to be a spot for Bill. He just never seemed to fit the criteria for services. So we devised and schemed and tried to work the system to give him the best that anyone could get. Society seems to play mean tricks on the human race. When Bill was an up-and-coming star athlete, the world was at his feet; he could pick and choose the college of his choice, friends abounded; life for him was going to be college, a career in law, marriage, children, and living happily ever after. The reality of all that never happened for Bill and society has not created even one little niche for him. He is different, he doesn't fit the criteria for success, there is no place for him. Where and what happens to Bill is a chapter yet to be written.

However, to end this on a little more positive note, it is my pleasure to announce that, again through more brokering, we have opened the first independent living center for head injured in the state of Virginia. Bill was accepted into the program and lived for 12 months with a roommate. The program was initially started in Newport News and most recently was moved to Richmond. Bill recently left the program and was able to buy a small townhouse close to the H.I.G.H. HOPES (Head Injury Group Housing) so he is still in contact with the other clients living in the apartments. All the clients living in the apartments were assigned job coaches to help them find meaningful employment. After several months, Bill was able to find a job at a retirement home as an assistant cook. The job coach investigated the job site, spoke to the employer, and felt confident Bill would be successful. We had specifically asked that Bill be put in an environment that would keep him away from negative influences because he had been influenced so many times by the people he had worked with and Bill did not use good judgment. One of the devastations of Bill's injury is in the area of judgment. His inability to make wise decisions is due in part to the area of his brain that was injured. Coupled with that is his desire to make friends. Therefore, he can be easily manipulated and tends to follow anyone who offers him a sign of friendship. That poor judgment has led Bill down many wrong avenues. The job was perfect for 4 months. Bill seemed to be enjoying the challenge of cooking and with the help and guidance of his coach and employer the "supported employment" seemed to be the answer.

However, Bill went to his high school reunion in late August and within a few days we discovered he was smoking marijuana and had been arrested. Maybe the reunion reminded him too much of who he was before and what he was now. But for days he talked about his friends who had been at the reunion who were real estate agents, lawyers, accountants—all of them had "good jobs." Was that the reason Bill started to lose interest in his job? He began "playing sick" and asking to go home early. At the same time, the retirement home hired a 19-year-old to do groundskeeping and he and Bill became friends. Although Bill talked about him as having "bad habits" and not having a good family, Bill asked him to move into his townhouse as a roommate. We had discussed this possibility with Bill and advised him not to take him in as a roommate.

As the cracks began to appear, his job coach kept us informed as to what was happening and we held several meetings trying to keep Bill in the job. When Bill did not show up for work one Sunday, his employer called and asked for a conference with Bill, myself, and his job coach. The bottom line was Bill would be suspended from work for one week but could come back to the job providing he gave his all to the job. Bill made the decision to quit . . . even though his employer said Bill was doing the job at 99 percent. We tried desperately to convince Bill that he needed the job to support himself and for his self-esteem (for months prior to his getting this job we had heard nothing but "I need a job"). But Bill, for whatever reason, was determined to quit. Why did he quit? We heard him say things like, "I don't like the job," "I don't like my coworkers," "I don't like my boss." However, 3 months before, Bill only had positive statements: "I love this job," "My boss is so fair," "I'm learning to become a chef." Can you imagine how frustrating it is to know that Bill can work and do a job well but something over which we have no control is interfering with his "holding down the job." We may never know the answer to this question. But I strongly believe that every effort must continue to be made to seek employment for our head injured son and all head injured persons.

SUMMARY

The field of head injury has come a long way in the past 11 years since Bill's injury, especially in the areas of rehabilitation and supported employment. However, it is a devastating and complex injury that will require many more years of research and training. Professionals working with head injury need to be innovative, diligent, and persistent. But most of all they need to be careful. Careful that the client is ready to work, careful that the job environment is appropriate, careful that the client is receiving the support he or she requires, and careful that the client does not fail. . . . Success for many head injured persons comes in very small increments over a very long period of time and professionals must be aware that there will be many failures before one small success. Although Bill has had 17 jobs over the past 11 years, we are still confident that someday (maybe some years) he will be working. He has worked, he has had small increments of success, and in spite of his past record we continue to be hopeful.

For anyone to experience losing their "future" has to be one of life's ultimate devastations. All over the country, young men and women lose their future through the tragedy of traumatic brain injury and must begin again. The future that was so bright for them is now filled with anxiety, insecurities, and loneliness. They face a society that wants perfection, that uses drugs and alcohol to cope, that is definitely on the fast track. We say to our young head injury victims, "you must try to fit into society" but without playing by the rules society has made. Each of us has the responsibility to help head injured persons learn to cope with society the best they can and give them all the support they may need. A difficult task. . . . Perhaps for some there will be no reentry to the mainstream. Perhaps the areas of the brain that control motivation, judgment, and responsibility are too damaged and there will be no place for them in our society. However, every effort must be made to work with our head injured, trying to give them a worthwhile life that provides all the basic needs that each of us desires.

We do not know what the future holds for Bill and many others like him. . . . We do not know what new and innovative research lies on the horizon. . . . We do know that we will continue to strive in what we believe . . . that everyone is entitled to the best we can give.

Chapter 16

An Advocacy Perspective

Elizabeth V. Horn

In 1980, 9 in 10 persons sustaining a severe blow to the head died. Today, just one decade later, that statistic is reversed and 9 in 10 survive. Improved rescue and emergency medical techniques are saving lives at the rate of 70,000 per year in the United States. Permanently disabled, these people need an array of services to remain in the mainstream of society and their families need ongoing support and information.

The field of rehabilitation has grown slowly and only recently have there been programs available beyond hospital discharge. Even today only one survivor in 20 can access lifelong adequate care; the others either go without treatment or end up in programs designed for other disability groups.

Equally staggering are the 800,000 Americans each year who sustain mild brain injuries that either temporarily or permanently disrupt their work and family life. Often undiagnosed, these injuries make up what has become known as the "silent epidemic."

WE ARE ALL AT RISK

Head injury can strike anyone at any time. This disability knows no cultural, racial, or socioeconomic bounds; we are all vulnerable. At greatest risk are 15- to 24-year-old males, children, and the elderly. Vehicular crashes cause 50 percent of the injuries, followed by falls, sports and recreation incidents, and interpersonal assaults.

"There is no cure for brain injury and no evidence that the incidence is diminishing," states Janine Jagger, Ph.D., an epidemiologist at the University of Virginia School of Medicine. "Aggressive prevention, program development and research to determine which efforts are the most productive will be the most effective means for dealing with this epidemic."

NATIONAL HEAD INJURY FOUNDATION: A MOVEMENT IS MAKING HEADWAY

In 1980, the National Head Injury Foundation (NHIF) was begun by families and professionals to respond to this emerging population. At the cutting edge of this new social phenomenon, NHIF has led the way to greater public awareness and action. Membership has grown to 21,000 and includes 35 state associations, 5 affiliates, 375 support groups, a survivor council representing 7,500, a professional council representing 7,000, and a provider council of 140 facilities.

NHIF is the only national organization dedicated to preventing head injuries and improving the quality of life for head injury survivors and their families. Its goals include increasing public awareness of the consequences of head injury, developing support systems, encouraging appropriate rehabilitation for head injury survivors, and disseminating information about head injury and head injury prevention. Marilyn P. Spivack, NHIF founder and president, has said of the Foundation's role:

> Advocacy is the prime vehicle used by NHIF to pursue a quality of life for people disabled by head injury. Advocacy involves mobilizing survivors, families and professionals, educating the media, and negotiating with our nation's law and policy makers to recognize and fund this population. For now, our effort must be grass-roots and it must also be well-conceived and executed in a business like manner.

NHIF has made great strides in these areas. It is the collective hope of its members that impressive life-saving measures will one day be matched by the ability to restore quality to these lives.

What began in 1980 as a kitchen table operation with a dozen people has grown to a nationally recognized organization. NHIF has brought together under one organizational roof all parties involved in head injury. Most obvious are the people who have sustained head injuries and their families and friends who must recover indefinitely along with them. Secondly are the providers of service. Although facility administrators and direct care personnel first come to mind, this group also includes social workers, eligibility officers for public entitlements, regular and special education teachers, vocational rehabilitation counselors and college professors, mental health workers, insurance claims adjusters and private rehabilitation case managers, lawyers, and even landlords.

Because the goal of head injury rehabilitation is community integration, the circle of people who ultimately will interface with head injured people is infinite. It is society itself. We are in an age of disability rights and mainstreaming and it is to this end that our advocacy must be directed.

At the very least, everyone directly involved in head injury should view themselves as an advocate for this population. Membership in NHIF is the first step in one's commitment to advocacy. A large and vocal membership is the most effective way to promote systems change.

It is also essential that head injury advocates merge their agenda with the agenda of other disability groups. There is great commonality of need among all people with disabilities in the areas of housing, employment, personal assistance, transportation, education, case management, and ongoing community supports for both the individual and the family.

Often individual disability groups end up pitted against one another fighting for the same piece of the resource pie. For example, mental illness and mental retardation have had whole agencies built up around their needs while those with traumatic brain injury or physical disabilities have no one agency to access for services. One easily assumes that the needs of the mentally ill and mentally retarded persons have been adequately met by their agency and attention, therefore, should be directed at unserved or underserved populations.

A better strategy would be to ally oneself with groups whose needs are already well recognized and simply clarify to policymakers that existing services need to be augmented in order to meet the needs of additional discrete populations.

Even with augmented resources, a clear line of authority must be established to determine which agencies have programmatic and fiscal responsibility for persons with traumatic brain injury. Because of the diversity of needs over time, the resources of many agencies must be made available to this population.

It is safe to say that no state currently has resources adequate to serve the long-term catastrophic needs of brain injured persons. Strategies to generate new revenues will be necessary. A few states have initiated cause-related fees or fines to establish a catastrophic fund earmarked for use by catastrophically injured persons.

Advocacy can also be expressed by program developers and shapers of public policy. The underlining philosophy must be person centered.

In 1987, the Virginia Chapter of the National Head Injury Foundation adopted a philosophy statement to guide the development of permanency planning for head injured people in Virginia. Although it is focused on community living arrangements, it applies to all programming:

> The Virginia Head Injury Foundation recognizes the ongoing need for alternative community living arrangements which meet

the unique challenges of persons with head injuries. We endorse continuous study of the needs of head injured persons and their families and the application of state-of-the-art information to the planning and principles used in making decisions about housing.

- Persons with head injuries must have their needs and preferences met in a residential environment that is normalized and nonrestricted; having the quality of a home rather than a facility.
- A system of integrated community services must be utilized to address the unique residential, vocational, recreational, and social needs of each head injured person.
- Case management and other appropriate supports must be used in a manner which respects the dignity and right to self-determination of the individual, the involvement of the individual and the family, and the concept of permanency planning.
- All persons with head injuries must be encouraged and facilitated to participate in daily affairs of the community, including (but not limited to) political, religious, cultural, recreational, vocational, and interpersonal affiliations with non-head injured persons.
- All persons with head injuries must live in settings which promote physical, psychological, professional, and financial independence.
- All persons with head injuries must live in environments which nurture their capacities to risk, mature, and self-actualize according to their individual abilities, preferences, and aspirations.

Supported employment and supported living options reflect this philosophy. They are good examples of community based services and should be pursued as part of the effort to provide quality services for people who will live with brain injury.

Educating the Media

As a new special interest group, NHIF must compete for visibility with hundreds of other health and social organizations. The media is the playing ground for this competition.

How effective has the media been in telling the story of this new disability? Does the average person know about traumatic brain injury and, if so, is the information they have correct?

Unfortunately, television has been particularly misleading. We see people emerge from coma and resume their lives or, worse yet, characters who sustain a severe blow to the head or experience a car crash without consequences. These messages teach us that we are invulnerable when the opposite is true. This is an especially cruel message to young men who are given to risk taking.

The print and newscast media have also been remiss. Equally serious or even less prevalent issues tend to get more press than traumatic brain injury.

This points up the need for a clear and consistent public relations effort. Myths about head injury have been created by the media and also must be dismantled by the media. These are the messages the media must convey: Coma, amnesia, and unconsciousness are all functions of a damaged brain; brain damage, though not a static condition, can have permanent consequences, hardly ever leaving the injured person the same; and brain damage does not cause mental illness or mental retardation.

Negotiating with Our Nation's Law and Policy Makers

Without proper treatment, brain injury can and is contributing significantly to broken homes, unemployment, homelessness, crime, and a host of other social dilemmas. "Fully forty percent of all death row inmates have suffered brain injury," states Dr. Carl C. Bell, a physician and professor of clinical psychology at the University of Illinois. Ron Savage, Ed.D., Chairman of the National Head Injury Foundation's Education Task Force, conducted a survey of 1,500 special education students in Vermont and found more than 20 percent had a history of traumatic head injury severe enough to require hospitalization; of those listed as emotionally disturbed, 40 percent had a history of head trauma.

Unknown are the number of head injured persons who reside undiagnosed in mental health facilities or who are unidentified on our streets.

The effects of head injury are insidious and to date our nation's response has been fragmented and reactive.

Through the initiative of NHIF, this is turning around. Members of Congress and heads of federal human service agencies are beginning to acknowledge the problem. Traumatic head injury is beginning to be addressed as a single issue with multiple secondary effects.

Though dollars are slow to be appropriated, NHIF has created a permanent stir among those who set the agenda for this country. Each spring, NHIF members from across the United States assemble on Capitol Hill to recount their stories of life after head injury. Equally poignant are their examples of dollars spent fruitlessly by families and the government on inappropriate systems of care and unnecessarily on public assistance that promotes dependence.

From a fiscal standpoint, our policymakers must understand that it makes no sense to spend billions of dollars investing in trauma care and then renege on that investment with policies that promote maintenance rather than independence and productivity.

Prevention

Any national effort to address the consequences of traumatic head injury would be remiss not to address prevention. The refrain of so many survivors and their families is that they don't wish head injury upon anyone. Is head injury here to stay or can we hope for a day when the damage can be reversed or the incidence substantially reduced?

Head injury is America's number one health problem and yet the dollars devoted to research are greatly skewed. In 1987, the United States was spending $1 billion a year paid by taxpayers on cancer research, which takes 1.7 million years of preretirement life, and $624 million on heart and stroke, which take 2.1 million years of preretirement life. In contrast, traumatic head injury takes 4.1 million years of preretirement life (more than cancer, heart, and stroke combined) and only $4 million are spent annually on its research. A further irony is that head injury is largely preventable and prevention is considered to be the only cure.

The single largest cause of head injury is vehicular crashes, thus prevention efforts must be targeted here first. The efforts must be twofold: To reduce the incidence of crashes and to reduce the likelihood of injury or death when crashes do occur. Mothers Against Drunk Drivers should be commended for their efforts in reducing the incidence by ridding our roads of drunk drivers. But in an imperfect world where crashes will occur, we must implement methods to prevent injury upon impact. Seat belts are one method to curb the rate of head injury due to car crashes; for more effective protection against head injury, cars must also be equipped with airbags. As a result of a 1984 ruling by the Department of Transportation, airbags are being introduced by many automobile manufacturers in satisfaction of a passive restraint requirement. It is up to the consumer to drive the airbag market by requesting this safety device.

Other prevention efforts are aimed at bicycle and motorcycle safety with an emphasis placed on helmet use. Some states have sought prohibitions on all-terrain vehicles, which are among the most dangerous of vehicles. Other forms of preventing traumatic head injury include gun control; awareness and reporting of child abuse, including the shaky baby syndrome; a ban on boxing; and institution of stricter regulations governing contact sports. Lastly, the prevention of secondary injury is equally important. Immediate identification and diagnosis of head injury can go a long way to reduce the multiple effects of brain injury.

SUMMARY

The purpose of this chapter has been to describe how advocacy for persons with traumatic brain injury can affect public policy. Clearly, the past 10 years have shown that thousands of survivors will need comprehensive rehabilitation services. Advocates need to build a case for the cost-effectiveness of comprehensive rehabilitation and lifelong supports for persons who have sustained a traumatic brain injury. Identifying and redirecting dollars spent fruitlessly in service systems designed for other populations would provide resources for the development of these services. At the same time, the head injury community and its advocates must build alliances with other disability populations. A multi-disability coalition with a clear and unified agenda is a much greater force to be reckoned with than a single disability group.

With the declaration of the 1990s as the Decade of the Brain, more research and resources will be focused on brain injury and with it will come a new hope for survivors and their families and the service providers who work with them.

Index

C

D

E

G

H

I

J

N

O

P

T